T0264147

Pulmonary Hypertension

Guest Editors

SRINIVAS MURALI, MD, FACC
RAYMOND L. BENZA, MD, FAHA

HEART FAILURE CLINICS

www.heartfailure.theclinics.com

Consulting Editors
RAGAVENDRA R. BALIGA, MD, MBA
JAMES B. YOUNG, MD

Founding Editor
JAGAT NARULA, MD, PhD

July 2012 • Volume 8 • Number 3

SAUNDERS an imprint of ELSEVIER, Inc.

W.B. SAUNDERS COMPANY
A Division of Elsevier Inc.

1600 John F. Kennedy Boulevard • Suite 1800 • Philadelphia, Pennsylvania 19103-2899

http://www.theclinics.com

HEART FAILURE CLINICS Volume 8, Number 3
July 2012 ISSN 1551-7136, ISBN-13: 978-1-4557-3873-1

Editor: Barbara Cohen-Kligerman
Developmental Editor: Donald Mumford

© **2012 Elsevier Inc. All rights reserved.**

This journal and the individual contributions contained in it are protected under copyright by Elsevier, and the following terms and conditions apply to their use:

Photocopying
Single photocopies of single articles may be made for personal use as allowed by national copyright laws. Permission of the Publisher and payment of a fee is required for all other photocopying, including multiple or systematic copying, copying for advertising or promotional purposes, resale, and all forms of document delivery. Special rates are available for educational institutions that wish to make photocopies for non-profit educational classroom use. For information on how to seek permission visit www.elsevier.com/permissions or call: (+44) 1865 843830 (UK)/(+1) 215 239 3804 (USA).

Derivative Works
Subscribers may reproduce tables of contents or prepare lists of articles including abstracts for internal circulation within their institutions. Permission of the Publisher is required for resale or distribution outside the institution. Permission of the Publisher is required for all other derivative works, including compilations and translations (please consult www.elsevier.com/permissions).

Electronic Storage or Usage
Permission of the Publisher is required to store or use electronically any material contained in this journal, including any article or part of an article (please consult www.elsevier.com/permissions). Except as outlined above, no part of this publication may be reproduced, stored in a retrieval system or transmitted in any form or by any means, electronic, mechanical, photocopying, recording or otherwise, without prior written permission of the Publisher.

Notice
No responsibility is assumed by the Publisher for any injury and/or damage to persons or property as a matter of products liability, negligence or otherwise, or from any use or operation of any methods, products, instructions or ideas contained in the material herein. Because of rapid advances in the medical sciences, in particular, independent verification of diagnoses and drug dosages should be made.

Although all advertising material is expected to conform to ethical (medical) standards, inclusion in this publication does not constitute a guarantee or endorsement of the quality or value of such product or of the claims made of it by its manufacturer.

Heart Failure Clinics (ISSN 1551-7136) is published quarterly by Elsevier Inc., 360 Park Avenue South, New York, NY 10010-1710. Months of publication are January, April, July, and October. Business and editorial offices: 1600 John F. Kennedy Boulevard, Suite 1800, Philadelphia, PA 19103-2899. Periodicals postage paid at New York, NY, and additional mailing offices. Subscription prices are USD 224.00 per year for US individuals, USD 347.00 per year for US institutions, USD 76.00 per year for US students and residents, USD 268.00 per year for Canadian individuals, USD 398.00 per year for Canadian institutions, USD 285.00 per year for international individuals, USD 398.00 per year for international institutions, and USD 96.00 per year for Canadian and foreign students/residents. To receive student and resident rate, orders must be accompanied by name of affiliated institution, date of term, and the *signature* of program/residency coordinator on institution letterhead. Orders will be billed at individual rate until proof of status is received. Foreign air speed delivery is included in all *Clinics* subscription prices. All prices are subject to change without notice. **POSTMASTER:** Send address changes to *Heart Failure Clinics*, Elsevier Health Sciences Division, Subscription Customer Service, 3251 Riverport Lane, Maryland Heights, MO 63043. **Customer Service: 1-800-654-2452 (US and Canada). From outside of the US and Canada, call 314-447-8871. Fax: 314-447-8029. For print support, e-mail: JournalsCustomerService-usa@elsevier.com. For online support, e-mail: JournalsOnlineSupport-usa@elsevier.com.**

Reprints. For copies of 100 or more of articles in this publication, please contact the Commercial Reprints Department, Elsevier Inc., 360 Park Avenue South, New York, NY 10010-1710. Tel.: 212-633-3812; Fax: 212-462-1935; E-mail: reprints@elsevier.com.

Heart Failure Clinics is covered in *MEDLINE/PubMed (Index Medicus).*

Printed and bound by CPI Group (UK) Ltd, Croydon, CR0 4YY
Transferred to Digital Print 2012

Cover artwork courtesy of Umberto M. Jezek.

Contributors

CONSULTING EDITORS

RAGAVENDRA R. BALIGA, MD, MBA
Vice Chief and Assistant Division Director,
Professor of Medicine, Division of
Cardiovascular Medicine, The Ohio State
University Medical Center, Columbus, Ohio

JAMES B. YOUNG, MD
Professor of Medicine and Executive Dean,
Cleveland Clinic Lerner College of Medicine;
George and Linda Kaufman Chair, Chairman,
Endocrinology and Metabolism Institute,
Cleveland Clinic, Cleveland, Ohio

GUEST EDITORS

SRINIVAS MURALI, MD, FACC
Professor of Medicine, Temple University
School of Medicine, Philadelphia; Director,
Division of Cardiovascular Medicine; Medical
Director, Cardiovascular Institute, Allegheny
General Hospital, West Penn Allegheny Health
System, Pittsburgh, Pennsylvania

RAYMOND L. BENZA, MD, FAHA
Cardiovascular Institute, Allegheny General
Hospital, Pittsburgh, Pennsylvania

AUTHORS

RICHA AGARWAL, MD
Cardiology Fellow, Heart Failure Transplant,
New York Presbyterian Hospital; Section of
Cardiology, Columbia University, New York,
New York

CHRISTOPHER F. BARNETT, MD, MPH
Assistant Professor of Medicine, Division of
Cardiology, University of California, San
Francisco, San Francisco General Hospital,
San Francisco, California

SONJA BARTOLOME, MD
Assistant Professor, Division of Pulmonary and
Critical Care Medicine, UT Southwestern
Medical Center, Dallas, Texas

D. HUNTER BEST, BS, PhD
Assistant Professor (Clinical), Department of
Pathology, University of Utah School of
Medicine; Assistant Medical Director, Genetics

Division, Associated Regional and University
Pathologists (ARUP), Salt Lake City, Utah

**ROBERT W.W. BIEDERMAN, MD,
FACC, FAHA**
Associate Professor of Medicine, Temple
University, Philadelphia; Director of
Cardiovascular Magnetic Resonance Imaging
Laboratory, Division of Cardiology, Department
of Medicine, Gerald McGinnis Cardiovascular
Institute, Allegheny General Hospital,
Pittsburgh, Pennsylvania

EDUARDO BOSSONE, MD, PhD
Director, Division of Cardiology, Cava
de'Tirreni-Amalfi Coast Hospital; Department
of Cardiology and Cardiac Surgery, University
Hospital "Scuola Medica Salernitana", Salerno;
Consultant, Department of Cardiology and
Cardiac Surgery, IRCCS Policlinico San
Donato, Milan, Italy

TERESA DE MARCO, MD, FACC
Director, Heart Failure and Pulmonary
Hypertension Program; Medical Director,
Heart Transplantation; Professor of Medicine
and Surgery, Division of Cardiology, University
of California, San Francisco, Medical Center,
San Francisco, California

C. GREGORY ELLIOTT, MD
Professor of Medicine, Department of Internal
Medicine, University of Utah, Salt Lake City;
Chairman, Department of Medicine,
Intermountain Medical Center, Murray, Utah

ASGHAR A. FAKHRI, MD
Echocardiography Laboratory and
Cardiovascular Magnetic Resonance Imaging
Laboratory, Division of Cardiology, Department
of Medicine, Gerald McGinnis Cardiovascular
Institute, Allegheny General Hospital,
Pittsburgh, Pennsylvania

VERONICA FRANCO, MD, MSPH
Department of Cardiovascular Disease,
Section Head, Pulmonary Hypertension
Research, The Ohio State University,
Columbus, Ohio

ROBERT P. FRANTZ, MD
Associate Professor of Medicine, Division
of Cardiovascular Diseases and Internal
Medicine, Mayo Clinic, Rochester, Minnesota

MARDI GOMBERG-MAITLAND, MD, MSc
Associate Professor of Medicine, Director
of Pulmonary Hypertension, Section of
Cardiology, Department of Medicine,
University of Chicago, Chicago, Illinois

VEDANT GUPTA, MD
Resident, Departments of Internal Medicine,
and Medicine, The Cleveland Clinic,
Cleveland, Ohio

PAUL M. HASSOUN, MD
Professor of Medicine and Director, Pulmonary
Hypertension Program, Division of Pulmonary
and Critical Care Medicine, Department of
Medicine, Johns Hopkins University,
Baltimore, Maryland

RACHEL A. HUGHES-DOICHEV, MD, FASE
Assistant Professor of Medicine, Temple
University, Philadelphia; Director of Claude
Joyner Echocardiography Laboratory, Division

of Cardiology, Department of Medicine, Gerald
McGinnis Cardiovascular Institute, Allegheny
General Hospital, Pittsburgh, Pennsylvania

MANREET KANWAR, MD
Department of Cardiology, Gerald McGinnis
Cardiovascular Institute, Allegheny General
Hospital, Pittsburgh, Pennsylvania

RICHARD A. KRASUSKI, MD
Director of Adult Congenital Heart Disease
Services, Department of Cardiovascular
Medicine, Heart and Vascular Institute,
The Cleveland Clinic, Cleveland, Ohio

STEPHEN C. MATHAI, MD, MHS
Assistant Professor of Medicine, Pulmonary
Hypertension Program, Division of Pulmonary
and Critical Care Medicine, Department of
Medicine, Johns Hopkins University,
Baltimore, Maryland

DANA MCGLOTHLIN, MD
Associate Professor of Medicine, Division of
Cardiology; Associate Director, Pulmonary
Hypertension Program; Medical Director,
Mechanical Circulatory Support Program;
Medical Director, CCU, University of California
San Francisco, San Francisco, California

MICHAEL D. MCGOON, MD
Professor of Medicine, Division of
Cardiovascular Diseases and Internal
Medicine, Mayo Clinic, Rochester, Minnesota

ROBERT J. MORACA, MD
Assistant Professor of Surgery, Department of
Thoracic and Cardiovascular Surgery, Gerald
McGinnis Cardiovascular Institute, Allegheny
General Hospital, Pittsburgh, Pennsylvania

SRINIVAS MURALI, MD, FACC
Professor of Medicine, Temple University
School of Medicine, Philadelphia; Director,
Division of Cardiovascular Medicine; Medical
Director, Cardiovascular Institute, Allegheny
General Hospital, West Penn Allegheny Health
System, Pittsburgh, Pennsylvania

ROBERT NAEIJE, MD, PhD
Professor of Physiology and Medicine, Director
of the Department of Physiology, Faculty
of Medicine; Consultant at the Department
of Cardiology, Erasme Academic Hospital,
Université Libre de Bruxelles, Brussels,
Belgium

MYUNG H. PARK, MD
Associate Professor of Medicine and Director, Pulmonary Vascular Disease Program, Cardiology Care Unit, University of Maryland School of Medicine, Baltimore, Maryland

GAUTAM V. RAMANI, MD
Assistant Professor of Medicine, University of Maryland School of Medicine; Director of Echocardiography, Baltimore VA Medical Center, Baltimore, Maryland

ROSECHELLE M. RUGGIERO, MD, MSCS
Assistant Professor, Division of Pulmonary and Critical Care Medicine, UT Southwestern Medical Center, Dallas, Texas

BENJAMIN P. SMITH, MD
Division of Pulmonary and Critical Care Medicine, University of Utah, Salt Lake City, Utah

ADRIANO R. TONELLI, MD
Staff, Department of Pulmonary and Critical Care, Respiratory Institute, Cleveland Clinic, Cleveland, Ohio

FERNANDO TORRES, MD
Associate Professor, Division of Pulmonary and Critical Care Medicine, UT Southwestern Medical Center; Head of the Lung Transplant and Pulmonary Hypertension Program, UT Southwestern, Dallas, Texas

Contents

Pulmonary hypertension (PH) can develop in association with many different diseases and risk factors, and its presence is nearly always associated with reduced survival. The prognosis and management of PH is largely dependent upon its underlying etiology and severity of disease. The combination of clinical and hemodynamic classifications of PH provides a framework for the diagnostic evaluation of PH to establish a final clinical diagnosis that guides therapy. As our understanding of the different pathologic mechanisms that underlie the syndrome of PH evolves, so too will the classification and treatment of PH.

Pulmonary arterial hypertension (PAH) is an uncommon disease in the general population, but a disease with significant morbidity and mortality. The prevalence of heritable PAH (HPAH) remains unknown. The reason for incomplete penetrance of HPAH is not well understood. A patient's clinical response to disease-specific therapy is complex, involving the severity of the patient's disease, other comorbidities, appropriateness of the prescribed therapy, and patient compliance. Warfarin is often used as an adjuvant therapy in patients with PAH.

Dilemmas persist in the screening, assessment, and follow-up of patients with pulmonary hypertension, relating to issues of whom and how to screen, how to resolve ambiguities in the clinical classification of patients with multiple potential substrates of pulmonary vascular disease, how to interpret test results, how to integrate multiple clinical parameters into a global diagnosis, how to use ambiguous test results, how to determine disease severity and prognosis, and how to monitor patients on treatment. This article describes how to incorporate available information into the diagnostic process, and where lack of concrete data should impose caution in patient management.

Among the many approaches for evaluating patients with pulmonary hypertension (PH), imaging plays a crucial role. The primary role of imaging is to identify the

and poorer prognosis than patients with idiopathic PAH (IPAH). Select patients with CTD-PAH may be candidates for lung transplantation, but results are less favorable than for IPAH because of comorbidities and complications specifically associated with CTD.

Many patients with congenital heart disease and systemic-to-pulmonary shunts develop pulmonary arterial hypertension (PAH), particularly if the cardiac defect is left unrepaired. A persistent increase in pulmonary blood flow may lead to obstructive arteriopathy and increased pulmonary vascular resistance, a condition that can lead to reversal of shunt and cyanosis (Eisenmenger syndrome). Cardiac catheterization is crucial to confirm diagnosis and facilitate treatment. Bosentan is the only medication to date to be compared with placebo in a randomized controlled trial specifically targeting congenital heart disease-associated PAH. Lung transplantation with repair of the cardiac defect or combined heart-lung transplantation is reserved for recalcitrant cases.

Pulmonary hypertension (PH) is characterized hemodynamically by significantly elevated pulmonary artery pressure, which if sustained can result in clinical deterioration due to progressive right-sided heart failure and death. Establishing the etiology of PH in a patient before treatment is imperative. Effective evidence-based therapeutic agents for treating PH have been developed. However, appropriately powered, randomized trials in PH associated with left-sided heart failure are sparse, and those that have been performed have shown no benefit or harm. An improved understanding of the pathophysiology, definition, and development of new therapies for treating PH associated with left-sided heart failure is urgently needed.

The pathophysiology of pulmonary hypertension (PH) in parenchymal lung diseases is partially related to hypoxic pulmonary vasoconstriction. PH treatment is controversial for these patients. This article focuses on group III PH, namely PH attributable to lung diseases and/or hypoxia. Group III includes chronic obstructive pulmonary disease and interstitial lung diseases, the most common parenchymal lung diseases associated with PH. It also includes sleep-disordered breathing and hypoventilation from any cause. Other parenchymal lung diseases associated with PH, namely sarcoidosis and systemic vasculitides (group V), are discussed. The data describing PH in specific parenchymal diseases are reviewed.

Chronic thromboembolic pulmonary hypertension (CTEPH) is a potentially life-threatening condition characterized by obstruction of pulmonary arterial vasculature by acute or recurrent thromboemboli with subsequent organization, leading to progressive pulmonary hypertension and right heart failure. Until relatively recently, CTEPH was a diagnosis made primarily at autopsy, but advances made in diagnostic modalities and surgical pulmonary endarterectomy techniques have made this disease treatable and even potentially curable. Although published guidelines are available, in the absence of randomized controlled trials regarding CTEPH there is a lack of standardization, and treatment options have to be individualized.

Exercise-Induced Pulmonary Hypertension 485

Eduardo Bossone and Robert Naeije

Exercise stress tests of the pulmonary circulation show promise for the detection of early or latent pulmonary vascular disease and may help us understand the clinical evolution and effects of treatments in patients with established disease. Exercise stresses the pulmonary circulation through increases in cardiac output and left atrial pressure. Recent studies have shown that exercise-induced increase in pulmonary artery pressure is associated with dyspnea-fatigue symptomatology, validating the notion of exercise-induced pulmonary hypertension. Exercise in established pulmonary hypertension has no diagnostic relevance, but may help in the understanding of changes in functional state and the effects of therapies.

HEART FAILURE CLINICS

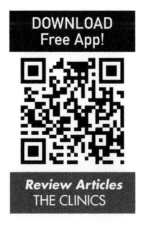

NOW AVAILABLE FOR YOUR iPhone and iPad

HEART FAILURE CLINICS

FORTHCOMING ISSUES

October 2013
Glucolipotoxicity and the Heart
Vasudevan A. Raghavan, MBBS, MD, and
Peter P. Toth, MD, PhD, Guest Editors

January 2013
Stress (Takotsubo) Cardiomyopathy
Eduardo Bossone, MD, PhD, and
Raimund Erbel, MD, Guest Editors

RECENT ISSUES

April 2012
Stage B, a Pre-cursor of Heart Failure, Part II
Jay N. Cohn, MD, and Gary S. Francis, MD,
Guest Editors

January 2012
Stage B Heart Failure, Part I
Jay N. Cohn, MD, and Gary S. Francis, MD,
Guest Editors

ISSUES OF RELATED INTEREST

Cardiology Clinics, May 2012 (Volume 30, Issue 2)
Assessment of Right Ventricular Failure
James A. Goldstein, MD, and Jonathan D. Rich, MD, Guest Editors

THE CLINICS ARE NOW AVAILABLE ONLINE!
Access your subscription at:
www.theclinics.com

NOW AVAILABLE FOR YOUR iPhone and iPad

Editorial

Treatment of Heart Failure in Pulmonary Arterial Hypertension—The Urgency of Getting This *Right*

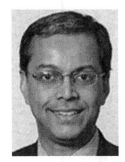 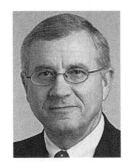

Ragavendra R. Baliga, MD, MBA   James B. Young, MD

Consulting Editors

The global burden[1] of pulmonary arterial hypertension (PAH) is unclear, but in France[2] the incidence and prevalence are 2.4 cases/million every year and 15 cases/million, respectively. In Scotland[3,4] the incidence and prevalence are 7.6 cases/million every year and 26 cases/million, respectively. These data suggest that the prevalence of pulmonary hypertension is higher than generally recognized. It is estimated that the burden in developing countries may be even greater because risk factors for PAH—such as sickle cell disease,[5] HIV, and schistosomiasis—are more prevalent. PAH has a 1-year incident annual mortality rate of 15%[6] and the 3-year survival rate, despite treatment with prostacyclin, endothelin antagonists, and phosphodiesterase-5 inhibitors, is only 58%.[7] The seven vasodilator drugs approved for therapy of PAH were approved not because of their mortality benefit but for their ability to improve exercise capacity for 3 to 4 months,[8] and recent data have shown that this ability to improve exercise capacity does not appear to retard the development of severe pulmonary vascular disease (**Figs. 1** and **2**) observed in the natural history of this syndrome.[9–11] The annual cost of these vasodilators

is currently estimated at $90,000 for inhaled iloprost and intravenous prostacyclin, $56,000 for bosentan, and $13,000 for sildenafil.[12] Of these agents, only intravenous prostacyclin has been demonstrated to improve survival.[13,14] There is an urgent and unsurpassed need to develop cost-effective therapies that substantially improve survival.

Although the pathophysiology of pulmonary hypertension has not been completely elucidated (**Fig. 3**), the natural history of patients with PAH is largely determined by comorbidities[3] and the underlying disease etiology. For example, PAH accompanying congenital heart disease has a better prognosis than idiopathic PAH (3-year survival 77% vs 35%).[15,16]

There are several promising targets[12] for new therapies, including modulation of endothelial function by regulating release of nitric oxide,[17] carbon monoxide,[18,19] and prostacyclin, and altering genetic components[20] of ion-channels, transporter genes, and bone morphogenetic protein receptor-2 (BMPR2). *BMPR2*, a cell surface protein belonging to the TGF-β receptor superfamily, is important in apoptosis, embryogenesis, and cellular proliferation and differentiation. It

Heart Failure Clin 8 (2012) xiii–xix
doi:10.1016/j.hfc.2012.05.002
1551-7136/12/$ – see front matter © 2012 Elsevier Inc. All rights reserved.

heartfailure.theclinics.com

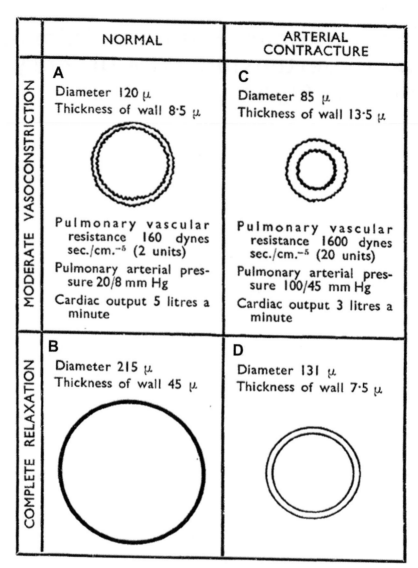

Fig. 1. Effect of arterial contracture on vascular resistance. (*A*) Normal small muscular artery. (*B*) The same artery completely relaxed. (*C*) The same artery after development of contracture. This moderate narrowing, if generalized, would increase pulmonary vascular resistance about 10-fold. There is no hypertrophy of arterial wall, cross-sectional area of media being the same in all four diagrams. (*D*) The same artery as in (*C*) completely relaxed, showing how resistance may be lowered despite organic arterial disease. (*From* Short DS. The arterial bed of the lung in pulmonary hypertension. Lancet 1957;270(6984):12–5; with permission.)

binds to a variety of cytokines, including TGF-β, bone morphogenetic protein (BMP), activin, and inhibin in the vascular smooth muscle cell. This results in inhibition of cell proliferation and promotes apoptosis. Therefore, when such signaling is absent, smooth muscle survival and proliferation are increased. In 50% of the familial cases of pulmonary arterial hypertension and 25% of sporadic cases, inactivating germline mutations in the *BMPR2* gene are found. In many families, even when the mutations in the coding regions of the *BMPR2* gene are absent, linkage to the *BMPR2* locus on chromosome 2q33 can be established, suggesting that other possible lesions such as gene rearrangements, large deletions, or insertions may be involved. Elucidation of the signaling pathway of BMP should provide novel therapies for PAH.

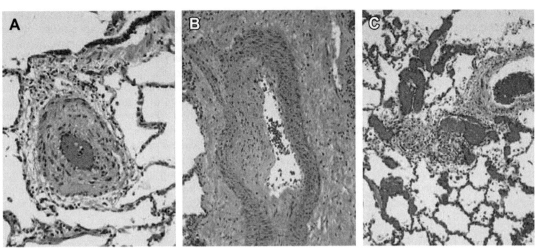

Fig. 2. Photomicrographs of pulmonary artery histologic lesions seen in cases of clinically unexplained pulmonary hypertension. (*A*) Medical hypertrophy with intimal proliferation. The vascular lumen is markedly reduced, contributing to the elevated resistance. (*B*) Eccentric intimal fibrosis. These are believed to be related to local thrombin deposition. (*C*) Plexiform lesion demonstrating obstruction in the arterial lumen, aneurysmal dilation, and proliferation of anastomosing vascular channels. Hematoxylin and eosin stains. (*A*) and (*B*), magnification, ×20; (*C*) magnification, ×4. (*From* Braunwald E, Bonow RO. Braunwald's heart disease: a textbook of cardiovascular medicine. 9th ed. Philadelphia: Saunders; 2011; with permission.)

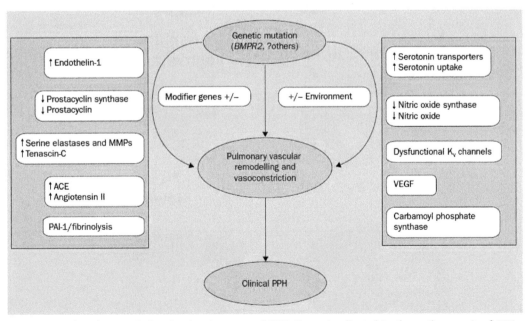

Fig. 3. Proposed pathogenesis for the development of PPH. Genes implicated in the pathogenesis of PPH are prostacyclin synthase, serotonin transporters, nitric oxide synthase, serine elastases, matrix metalloproteinases (MMPs), voltage-gated potassium (Kv) channels, angiotensin-converting enzyme (ACE), vascular endothelial growth factor (VEGF), carbamoyl phosphate synthase, and plasminogen activator inhibitor type 1 (PAI-1). Endothelin-1 production adds to the vasoconstriction in PPH, but whether this is secondary to changes in the above genes, a result of endothelial dysfunction, or a primary pathogenetic event is not clear. Pulmonary vascular remodeling results from the effects of genetics, modifying genes, and environment. (*From* Runo JR, Loyd JE. Primary pulmonary hypertension. Lancet 2003;361(9368):1533–44; with permission.)

Other treatment approaches might include modulating apoptosis and proliferation of vascular cells, reversing refractory vasoconstriction with *rho* kinase inhibition, and modulating right ventricular function by recruiting hibernating myocytes. The modulation of right ventricular function requires better understanding of the embryogenesis[21,22] (**Fig. 4**), and ventriculo-ventricular interaction and its relationship to myocardial mechanics (**Fig. 5**). The concertina-like mechanism of ventricular contraction that we recently proposed[23] is now considered an important mechanism for right ventricular contraction (**Fig. 6**).[24] The morphology of the right ventricle is designed to perfuse one organ, the lung, whereas the left ventricle is a high-pressure system built to perfuse to the entire body. In order to ensure that this hemodynamic equilibrium is maintained, the right ventricle has to adapt to changes "on the left side of the fence"[25] (the so-called "ventriculo-ventricular interaction") and to changes in the pulmonary microcirculation (the right ventricular-vascular interaction).[26] The superficial myocardial fibers of the right ventricle are circumferentially arranged and are in continuity with the fibers of the left ventricle, resulting in the movement of the right ventricular free wall toward the interventricular septum in systole (**Fig. 6**). In contrast, the deeper

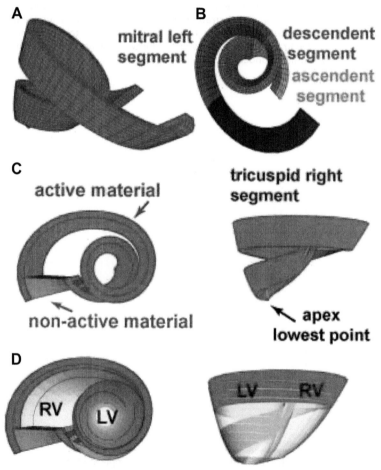

Fig. 4. Images of the double helical band model of the adult heart. The initial band shape and fitted volume shown from different points of view. (*A*) The double helical band. (*B*) The same band color-coded corresponding to physiologic segments. (*C*) The same band in different orientation, with labeled active and nonactive material, and the apex of the heart. (*D*) The fitted volumes for left ventricle (LV) and right ventricle (RV) are labeled on these pictures. (*From* Grosberg A, Gharib M. Physiology in phylogeny: modeling of mechanical driving forces in cardiac development. Heart Fail Clin 2008;4(3):247–59; with permission.)

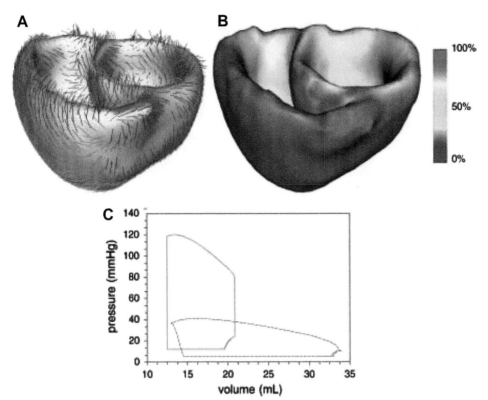

Fig. 5. (*A*) Anatomy of the right-ventricle overload patient with synthetic fiber orientations. (*B*) Contraction of the model: end-systole position; colors represent the contraction stress. (*C*) Pressure-volume loops, demonstrating right ventricle enlargement and regurgitations. (*From* Sermesant M, Peyrat JM, Chinchapatnam P, et al. Toward patient-specific myocardial models of the heart. Heart Fail Clin 2008;4(3):289–301; with permission.)

layers of the right ventricle are arranged such that in systole there is shortening of the right ventricular long axis. Contraction of the right ventricle in normal individuals is like a concertina with contraction beginning at the inflow region and progressing toward the outflow tract. This allows the right ventricle to adapt to volume changes while the left ventricle adapts to pressure changes at the same time. The interventricular septum, therefore, has to adapt as well and this has been described as the "motor" of interventricular adaptation.[27,28]

Ventricular-vascular interaction is also important in maintaining hemodynamic equilibrium.[26,29–31] Recent data suggest that elevations in systolic blood pressure are, in many situations, a result of central aortic vasculature increasing stiffness.[32] Similarly, it is increasingly apparent that pulmonary arterial hypertension can be the result of stiffness of the pulmonary artery and its branches, including the pulmonary microcirculation.[33–35] Newer

techniques to assess pulmonary microcirculation[36–39] should allow better data collection with respect to changes in the pulmonary vasculature in pulmonary hypertension, including changes in right ventriculo-arterial coupling.[26] These techniques should, in turn, promote the development of agents that "destiffen" or "loosen up" the pulmonary circulation.

The dismal mortality of pulmonary hypertension, not to mention the suffering of these dyspneic patients, heightens the importance of developing cost-effective therapies.[20] To discuss these challenges, Srinivas Murali, MD, and Raymond Benza, MD, from Allegheny University Hospital, have assembled a world-class team of experts in pulmonary hypertension. We hope that these scholarly articles result in the development of agents that will ameliorate the right heart dysfunction of pulmonary hypertension, which, in turn, will have an impact on this frustrating clinical problem. Given the poor prognosis of pulmonary

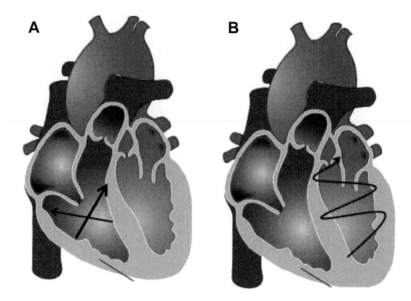

Fig. 6. Contrasting mechanisms of ventricular contraction. The RV is morphologically unique from the LV. It has a crescent-like shape and contracts with a peristaltic bellows-like action from apex to base. (*A*) The RV can accommodate large variations in venous return while maintaining a normal cardiac output. The bellows-like contraction results in a high ratio of RV volume change to RV free-wall surface area change, which allows it to eject a large volume of blood with little alteration in RV wall stretch. The relatively flat relationship between the right ventricular surface area and volume limits the use of the Frank-Starling mechanism to increase the strike volume. The LV has a spherical shape with a distinctly different multiplanar action of contraction that is more like the wringing of a towel. (*B*) The helical nature of the myocardial bands allows for a twisting motion to eject and reciprocal untwisting to fill rapidly. The twisting action tends to initiate from the apex and progresses toward the base allowing for forceful ejection of blood against high resistance. (*From* Rich S. Right ventricular adaptation and maladaptation in chronic pulmonary arterial hypertension. Cardiol Clin 2012;30(2):257–69; with permission.)

hypertension with right heart failure, we urgently must get going down the "right" path.

Ragavendra R. Baliga, MD, MBA
Division of Cardiovascular Medicine
The Ohio State University Medical Center
Columbus, OH, USA

James B. Young, MD
Lerner College of Medicine and
Endocrinology & Metabolism Institute
Cleveland Clinic
Cleveland, OH, USA

E-mail addresses:
Ragavendra.baliga@osumc.edu (R.R. Baliga)
youngj@ccf.org (J.B. Young)

REFERENCES

1. Rich S, Herskowitz A. Targeting pulmonary vascular disease to improve global health: pulmonary vascular disease: the global perspective. Chest 2010;137(Suppl 6):1S–5S.

2. Humbert M, Sitbon O, Chaouat A, et al. Pulmonary arterial hypertension in France: results from a national registry. Am J Respir Crit Care Med 2006;173(9):1023–30.

3. Carrington M, Murphy NF, Strange G, et al. Prognostic impact of pulmonary arterial hypertension: a population-based analysis. Int J Cardiol 2008; 124(2):183–7.

4. Peacock AJ, Murphy NF, McMurray JJ, et al. An epidemiological study of pulmonary arterial hypertension. Eur Respir J 2007;30(1):104–9.

5. Parent F, Bachir D, Inamo J, et al. A hemodynamic study of pulmonary hypertension in sickle cell disease. N Engl J Med 2011;365(1):44–53.

6. Thenappan T, Shah SJ, Rich S, et al. A USA-based registry for pulmonary arterial hypertension: 1982-2006. Eur Respir J 2007;30(6):1103–10.

7. Humbert M, Sitbon O, Chaouat A, et al. Survival in patients with idiopathic, familial, and anorexigen-associated pulmonary arterial hypertension in the modern management era. Circulation 2010;122(2): 156–63.

8. McLaughlin VV, McGoon MD. Pulmonary arterial hypertension. Circulation 2006;114(13):1417–31.

9. Short DS. The arterial bed of the lung in pulmonary hypertension. Lancet 1957;273(6984):12–5.

10. Achcar RO, Yung GL, Saffer H, et al. Morphologic changes in explanted lungs after prostacyclin therapy for pulmonary hypertension. Eur J Med Res 2006;11(5):203–7.

11. Rich S, Pogoriler J, Husain AN, et al. Long-term effects of epoprostenol on the pulmonary vasculature in idiopathic pulmonary arterial hypertension. Chest 2010;138(5):1234–9.

12. Archer SL, Weir EK, Wilkins MR. Basic science of pulmonary arterial hypertension for clinicians: new concepts and experimental therapies. Circulation 2010;121(18):2045–66.

13. Barst RJ, Rubin LJ, Long WA, et al. A comparison of continuous intravenous epoprostenol (prostacyclin) with conventional therapy for primary pulmonary hypertension. The Primary Pulmonary Hypertension Study Group. N Engl J Med 1996;334(5):296–302.

14. Kuhn KP, Byrne DW, Arbogast PG, et al. Outcome in 91 consecutive patients with pulmonary arterial hypertension receiving epoprostenol. Am J Respir Crit Care Med 2003;167(4):580–6.

15. Hopkins WE, Ochoa LL, Richardson GW, et al. Comparison of the hemodynamics and survival of adults with severe primary pulmonary hypertension or Eisenmenger syndrome. J Heart Lung Transplant 1996;15(1 Pt 1):100–5.

16. Berger RM, Beghetti M, Humpl T, et al. Clinical features of paediatric pulmonary hypertension: a registry study. Lancet 2012;379(9815):537–46.

17. Nathan C. Is iNOS beginning to smoke? Cell 2011; 147(2):257–8.

18. Zuckerbraun BS, Chin BY, Wegiel B, et al. Carbon monoxide reverses established pulmonary hypertension. J Exp Med 2006;203(9):2109–19.

19. Chandra S, Shah SJ, Thenappan T, et al. Carbon monoxide diffusing capacity and mortality in pulmonary arterial hypertension. J Heart Lung Transplant 2009;29(2):181–7.

20. Geraci MW, Bull TM, Tuder RM. Genomics of pulmonary arterial hypertension: implications for therapy. Heart Fail Clin 2010;6(1):101–14.

21. Grosberg A, Gharib M. Physiology in phylogeny: modeling of mechanical driving forces in cardiac development. Heart Fail Clin 2008;4(3):247–59.

22. Sermesant M, Peyrat JM, Chinchapatnam P, et al. Toward patient-specific myocardial models of the heart. Heart Fail Clin 2008;4(3):289–301.

23. Baliga RR, Young JB. The concertina pump. Heart Fail Clin 2008;4(3):xiii–xix.

24. Rich S. Right ventricular adaptation and maladaptation in chronic pulmonary arterial hypertension. Cardiol Clin 2012;30(2):257–69.

25. Tedford RJ, Hassoun PM, Mathai SC, et al. Pulmonary capillary wedge pressure augments right ventricular pulsatile loading. Circulation 2012; 125(2):289–97.

26. Sanz J, Garcia-Alvarez A, Fernandez-Friera L, et al. Right ventriculo-arterial coupling in pulmonary hypertension: a magnetic resonance study. Heart 2011;98(3):238–43.

27. Hoffman JI, Mahajan A, Coghlan C, et al. A new look at diastole. Heart Fail Clin 2008;4(3):347–60.

28. Narula J, Buckberg GD, Khandheria BK. It is not just a squeezebox! Heart Fail Clin 2008;4(3):xxi–xxii.

29. Kussmaul WG 3rd, Wieland J, Altschuler J, et al. Pulmonary impedance and right ventricular-vascular coupling during coronary angioplasty. J Appl Physiol 1993;74(1):161–9.

30. Kussmaul WG, Noordergraaf A, Laskey WK. Right ventricular-pulmonary arterial interactions. Ann Biomed Eng 1992;20(1):63–80.

31. Borlaug BA, Kass DA. Ventricular-vascular interaction in heart failure. Heart Fail Clin 2008;4(1):23–6.

32. Baliga RR, Young JB. "Stiff central arteries" syndrome: does a weak heart really stiff the kidney? Heart Fail Clin 2008;4(4):ix–xii.

33. Gan CT, Lankhaar JW, Westerhof N, et al. Noninvasively assessed pulmonary artery stiffness predicts mortality in pulmonary arterial hypertension. Chest 2007;132(6):1906–12.

34. Sanz J, Kariisa M, Dellegrottaglie S, et al. Evaluation of pulmonary artery stiffness in pulmonary hypertension with cardiac magnetic resonance. JACC Cardiovasc Imaging 2009;2(3):286–95.

35. Stevens GR, Garcia-Alvarez A, Sahni S, et al. RV dysfunction in pulmonary hypertension is independently related to pulmonary artery stiffness. JACC Cardiovasc Imaging 2012;5(4):378–87.

36. Salehi Ravesh M, Brix G, Laun FB, et al. Quantification of pulmonary microcirculation by dynamic contrast-enhanced magnetic resonance imaging: Comparison of four regularization methods. Magn Reson Med 2012. DOI:10.1002/mrm.2422.

37. Farkas L, Kolb M. Pulmonary microcirculation in interstitial lung disease. Proc Am Thorac Soc 2011; 8(6):516–21.

38. Kang KW, Chang HJ, Kim YJ, et al. Cardiac magnetic resonance imaging-derived pulmonary artery distensibility index correlates with pulmonary artery stiffness and predicts functional capacity in patients with pulmonary arterial hypertension. Circ J 2011;75(9):2244–51.

39. Ibrahim el SH, Shaffer JM, White RD. Assessment of pulmonary artery stiffness using velocity-encoding magnetic resonance imaging: evaluation of techniques. Magn Reson Imaging 2011;29(7):966–74.

Preface
Pulmonary Hypertension

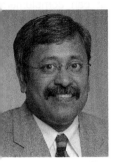 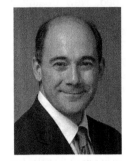

Srinivas Murali, MD   Raymond L. Benza, MD
Guest Editors

Pulmonary hypertension is defined as a group of diseases characterized by a progressive increase in pulmonary vascular load, leading to a marked increase in pulmonary artery pressure, right ventricular failure, and premature death. This condition can develop in association with a diverse group of diseases, and because its occurrence consistently portends an ominous outcome, it has generated considerable attention from scientists and clinicians alike. Knowledge of the pathophysiology and treatment of pulmonary hypertension has expanded rapidly over the past decade. A number of seminal discoveries in molecular biology and genetics have vastly improved the understanding of disease mechanisms and revolutionized the approach to treatment of this deadly disease. At the same time, clinical observations from large registries have provided insight into pathogenesis, thus drawing science and clinical practice toward one another.

The goal of this issue of *Heart Failure Clinics* is to provide a comprehensive overview of the current state of knowledge in pulmonary hypertension, and provide key points along the way to help develop a framework for patient management. The issue begins with an article on classification of pulmonary hypertension that was originally developed at a 1973 meeting organized by the World Health Organization and has since undergone three revisions, most recently in 2008. As the understanding of the biology evolves, another revision may be forthcoming at the next meeting scheduled in 2013.

The genetics of pulmonary arterial hypertension and the potential application of pharmacogenomics to help offset the heterogeneity of clinical treatment responses and individualize treatment strategies are discussed in the next article. The

serious adverse effects of some of the therapies and the high cost of drugs make it imperative that patient-specific treatments become the foundation of clinical care in this disease.

The article on diagnosis examines not only how to screen asymptomatic patients at high risk for developing pulmonary hypertension but also the guideline-driven diagnostic algorithm for the patient who presents with symptoms. Included in this article are dilemmas that clinicians frequently encounter when presented with patients who have mixed characteristics and do not precisely fit into a single category in the current classification system. The diagnostic challenge in these patients poses serious management issues, as in many cases prescribed treatments are not covered by the Center for Medicaid and Medicare Services and commercial insurers.

Imaging of the right ventricle, which is the affected organ in pulmonary hypertension, is critical to the diagnosis and prognosis. The imaging tools available to the clinician have continued to evolve and have clearly enhanced the accuracy of diagnosis and the reliability of predicting prognosis. Some of these tools, such as cardiac magnetic resonance imaging, are too sophisticated and unfortunately not readily available in all communities. Another challenge is the inappropriate and incomplete use of echocardiography, which is readily available to all clinicians. This results in the wrong diagnosis and often the wrong treatment prescription, which can result in considerable harm to the patient. The medical community bears the responsibility to apply the imaging tools appropriately in order to enable the correct diagnosis and treatment decisions.

Heart Failure Clin 8 (2012) xxi–xxii
doi:10.1016/j.hfc.2012.05.001
1551-7136/12/$ – see front matter © 2012 Elsevier Inc. All rights reserved.

heartfailure.theclinics.com

Since the availability of the first disease-specific treatment for patients with pulmonary arterial hypertension in 1996, eight more such therapies have received approval by the Food and Drug Administration, and a few more are under review. The strategy is to recommend the right initial monotherapy for each patient, set treatment goals, and monitor response. Sequential combination of drugs is the next step, and several clinical trials are underway to explore the degree of incremental benefit from combining therapies. The benefits of combination therapy right from the outset in treatment-naïve patients are also under investigation. Molecular biology has identified several new potential therapeutic targets, all of which hold considerable promise. It is conceivable that pulmonary arterial hypertension may have over a dozen disease-specific therapies in the next 3 years. Clinical pathways that are evidence-based and allow for the right combination of drugs in each patient are necessary to achieve maximum benefit at an optimal cost.

Assessing prognosis to allow for timely intervention in an effort to modify disease progression is discussed in a separate article. A number of surrogates for predicting prognosis have now been identified, and the clinician's task is to integrate all of this information to achieve the best clinical outcomes.

The right ventricle undergoes both adaptive and maladaptive remodeling in pulmonary hypertension. Evaluating this response reliably and developing targeted therapies that improve right ventricular structure and function remain a significant gap in the management of these patients. The heterogeneous behavior of the right ventricle in the different forms of pulmonary hypertension is poorly understood. This probably accounts for the observed differences in prognosis and outcome.

Pulmonary hypertension associated with connective tissue diseases carries a significantly worse prognosis, and standard disease-specific treatments have limited effectiveness. This article explains that inflammation may play a particularly pivotal role in the pathogenesis and this lends itself to targeted anti-inflammatory therapy, which is currently under investigation.

Many children with congenital heart disease survive to adulthood and develop pulmonary hypertension. Some with uncorrected shunts develop Eisenmenger's physiology and have marked limitation of exercise tolerance. The principles of management, drug treatments, and transplantation are discussed in detail in this article.

Left heart disease is the most common cause of pulmonary hypertension in the United States. To date, none of the nine disease-specific drugs that are used in pulmonary arterial hypertension are approved by the Food and Drug Administration for the treatment of left heart disease patients. In fact, some of these drugs, such as endothelin receptor antagonists and prostanoids, increase morbidity and mortality and should not be prescribed. New treatments that can complement the management of left heart dysfunction are sorely needed.

The article on pulmonary parenchymal disease highlights the role of hypoxia-mediated pulmonary vasoconstriction and inflammation in the pathogenesis. Treatment with disease-specific therapy in both obstructive and restrictive lung disease has not shown sustained reliable benefit.

Chronic thromboembolic pulmonary hypertension is potentially curable with surgical endarterectomy in carefully selected patients. As described in this article, the critical importance of clinical suspicion and proper diagnosis cannot be overemphasized. Results with disease-specific medical therapies are inconsistent.

The final article on exercise-induced pulmonary hypertension examines the normal physiology of the pulmonary circulation and its response to exercise in both health and disease. Exercise hemodynamic studies can shed important diagnostic information and aid therapeutic decisions, particularly in challenging patients.

We want to sincerely thank all the contributors for providing up-to-date texts that are both informative and substantive to the reader. We are confident that this issue will aid physicians and other health professionals in understanding the complex pathophysiologic mechanisms that are the basis for the current state of clinical practice in pulmonary hypertension. Our understanding of this complex condition is evolving rapidly and it remains to be seen if basic science and translational research will allow us to reverse the disease effectively in the not so distant future.

We are indebted to our wives, Marie (Murali) and Edwina (Benza), and our children, Vijay, Sara, and Rani (Murali), and Evan (Benza) for providing us with perspective and balance. We also thank Barbara Cohen-Kligerman for her administrative and editorial assistance.

Srinivas Murali, MD
Raymond L. Benza, MD

Cardiovascular Institute
Allegheny General Hospital
320 East North Avenue
Pittsburgh, PA 15212, USA

E-mail addresses:
SMURALI@wpahs.org (S. Murali)
RBENZA@wpahs.org (R.L. Benza)

Classification of Pulmonary Hypertension

Dana McGlothlin, MD

KEYWORDS

- Pulmonary hypertension • Hemodynamics • Pulmonary arterial hypertension • WHO classification

KEY POINTS

- Pulmonary hypertension (PH) can develop in association with many different diseases and risk factors, and its presence is nearly always associated with reduced survival.
- Medical management of PH depends largely on its underlying etiology.
- The combination of clinical and hemodynamic classifications of PH provides a framework for the diagnostic evaluation of PH to establish a final clinical diagnosis, which guides therapy.

INTRODUCTION

Pulmonary hypertension (PH) is a condition of many causes in which there is an elevation in pulmonary artery pressure (PAP) that results from an increase in:

1. Resistance to blood flow within the pulmonary arteries (ie, pulmonary vascular resistance [PVR])
2. Pulmonary blood flow
3. Pulmonary venous pressure from left-sided heart failure (LHF)
4. A combination of any of these 3 elements.

There is growing interest in PH among many medical specialists including cardiologists, pulmonologists, and rheumatologists, likely because of the current availability of specific drugs approved to treat a group of rare conditions defined as pulmonary arterial hypertension (PAH). The similarity between the terms "pulmonary hypertension" and "pulmonary arterial hypertension" has led to confusion and ambiguity in both clinical practice and the medical literature. Therefore, it is important to clarify the different hemodynamic definitions and the clinical classification of PH that, along with a complete diagnostic evaluation, lead to a final clinical diagnosis. The proper clinical diagnosis of PH is important because management of PH is dependent upon the underlying etiology and therapies that are effective in treating PAH may be detrimental when used inappropriately to treat other causes of PH.

HEMODYNAMIC CLASSIFICATION OF PULMONARY HYPERTENSION

PH is defined hemodynamically by invasive right heart catheterization (RHC) as a mean pulmonary artery pressure (mPAP) greater than 25 mm Hg. Formerly, PH was also diagnosed if the mPAP reached greater than 30 mm Hg during exercise; however, the exercise criterion was eliminated during the fourth World Symposium on PH because it was not supported by published data, and healthy individuals can reach higher levels of PAP.[1,2]

In hemodynamic terms, PH related to increased PVR of 3.0 Wood units (WU) or more without pulmonary capillary wedge pressure (PCWP) elevation (PCWP ≤15 mm Hg) is referred to as precapillary PH because the location of pressure elevation lies proximal to the pulmonary capillary bed within the pulmonary arteries (**Table 1**).[3] Postcapillary PH (also known as pulmonary venous, passive, or congestive PH) is the hemodynamic consequence of resulting from any cause of LHF. In pure postcapillary PH, the elevated left atrial pressure (LAP) is passively transmitted backward

Division of Cardiology, UCSF Medical Center, 505 Parnassus Avenue, Box 0124, San Francisco, CA 94143-0124, USA
E-mail address: mcglothl@medicine.ucsf.edu

Heart Failure Clin 8 (2012) 301–317
doi:10.1016/j.hfc.2012.04.013
1551-7136/12/$ – see front matter © 2012 Elsevier Inc. All rights reserved.

Table 1
Hemodynamic definitions of pulmonary hypertension (PH)

Definition	Hemodynamic Characteristics	WHO Clinical Groups[13]
PH	mPAP >25 mm Hg CO normal, reduced, or high[a]	All
Precapillary PH	PCWP/LVEDP ≤15 mm Hg TPG ≥12–15 mm Hg	1. PAH 3. PH due to lung disease and/or hypoxemia 4. CTEPH 5. PH with unclear or multifactorial mechanisms[b]
Postcapillary PH	PCWP/LVEDP >15 mm Hg, PVR ≤3 WU TPG <12 mm Hg	2. PH owing to LHD
Mixed PH Reactive[c] Nonreactive/fixed[d]	PCWP/LVEDP >15 mm Hg, PVR >3 WU TPG ≥12–15 mm Hg	2. PH owing to LHD

All values measured at rest.
Abbreviations: CO, cardiac output; CTEPH, chronic thromboembolic PH; LHD, left heart disease; LVEDP, left ventricular end-diastolic pressure; mPAP, mean pulmonary artery pressure; PAH, pulmonary arterial hypertension; PCWP, pulmonary capillary wedge pressure; PH, pulmonary hypertension; PVR, pulmonary vascular resistance; TPG, transpulmonary gradient; WHO, World Health Organization; WU, Wood Units.
   [a] High CO can be present in cases of portal hypertension (POPH; portopulmonary hypertension), hyperthyroidism, anemia, sepsis, systemic-to-pulmonary shunts (pulmonary circulation only), and so forth.
   [b] With some excepts, most cases of WHO Group 5 PH cause pre-capillary PH.
   [c] PVR and TPG reverse with vasodilators and/or normalization of PCWP/LVEDP.
   [d] PVR and TPG remain elevated despite normalization of PCWP/LVEDP with vasodilators, diuretics, and/or ventricular assist devices.

into the pulmonary veins and arteries, leading to elevated PAP, and it is characterized by a PCWP greater than 15 mm Hg with normal PVR and transpulmonary gradient (TPG) (TPG = mPAP − PCWP). Commonly the pulmonary arterial diastolic pressure will then also fall within 5 mm Hg or less of the left ventricular end-diastolic pressure (LVEDP). Upon reduction of the PCWP with diuretics and systemic vasodilators in patients with postcapillary PH, the PAP also decreases proportionately, and therefore, with normalization of the PCWP, the mPAP and PVR usually normalize.

Mixed PH (ie, mixed pre- and postcapillary PH), otherwise known in the literature as "reactive" PH, results from the presence of chronic pulmonary venous hypertension in the setting of LHF, which then leads to pulmonary arterial vasoconstriction and vascular remodeling.[3–8] This type of PH is characterized by an increased PCWP greater than 15 mm Hg (often >18 mm Hg), PVR to 3.0 WU or more, and a TPG of 12 to 15 mm Hg or greater.[9–12] The condition is often described in patients with mitral or aortic valve disease requiring surgery or in patients with advanced heart failure being considered for heart transplantation. In these cases, the elevation in mPAP is out of proportion to the degree of PCWP elevation, hence the popular term "PH out of proportion to left heart disease" that is also often used to

describe this condition. Although concomitant causes of pulmonary vascular disease (eg, sleep-disordered breathing, pulmonary disorders, chronic pulmonary embolism) should be sought in such situations, most cases are ultimately attributable to chronic untreated pulmonary venous hypertension. Mixed PH may be described as vasoreactive if normalization of the left ventricular (LV) filling pressure (PCWP) with diuretics and vasodilators (or an LV assist device) also reduces the TPG to less than 12 mm Hg and PVR to less than 3 WU, or else a "fixed" component to the PH may be deemed if the TPG and PVR do not normalize accordingly. Rarely, increased pulmonary blood flow from a systemic-to-pulmonary shunt or high cardiac output state (eg, anemia, sepsis, thyrotoxicosis) leads to PH without an elevation in PCWP or PVR.[3]

PAH represents a type of PH that it is classified clinically by the World Health Organization (WHO) as Group 1 of 5 in the updated 2008 Dana Point classification of PH.[13] The other WHO Groups of PH, discussed later, include PH owing to left heart disease (WHO Group 2 PH), whether associated with purely postcapillary or mixed PH; WHO Group 3 PH, in which PH is related to lung disease and/or hypoxemia; WHO Group 4 PH, which is chronic thromboembolic pulmonary hypertension (CTEPH); and, PH associated with unclear multifactorial

(WHO Group 5 PH). WHO Groups 1, 3, and 4 PH are each hemodynamically characterized as pre-capillary PH by RHC because they all involve diseases that increase PVR, and the LV filling pressure (PCWP and/or LVEDP) is normal. WHO Group 5 PH involves miscellaneous or multifactorial causes of PH that also, with rare exception (eg, sarcoid infiltrative cardiomyopathy), do not cause left-sided heart disease and therefore the PCWP is typically normal. Thus, WHO Group 2 PH from LHF can easily be distinguished hemodynamically with heart catheterization by the presence of elevated PCWP and/or LVEDP, and the accurate measurement of LV filling pressure becomes the most critical aspect defining the nature of PH.

CLINICAL CLASSIFICATION OF PULMONARY HYPERTENSION

The clinical classification system for PH continues to evolve as our understanding of the pathologic basis of the various diseases that underlie the syndrome improves. The classification of PH has undergone a series of changes since it was first proposed in 1973.[14]

The initial classification designated only 2 categories: primary pulmonary hypertension (PPH) or secondary PH, depending on the presence or absence of identifiable causes or risk factors. Twenty-five years later (1998), the second World Symposium on PH developed the Evian classification that included 5 groups of PH, which were categorized based on similar histopathologic, pathophysiologic, and clinical features including responsiveness to pulmonary vasodilator therapy.[15] This classification system allowed clinical trials to occur among patients with PPH who had shared underlying pathogenesis.

In 2003, the third World Symposium was held in Venice, Italy. The resulting Venice classification notably omitted the term PPH in favor of the terms idiopathic PAH (IPAH) when there was no identifiable cause of PAH; familial PAH (FPAH) when there was a family history of PAH; and associated PAH (APAH) when an underlying cause of PAH such as connective tissue disease was present.[16]

The most current clinical classification was developed in 2008 during the fourth World Symposium on PH in Dana Point, California, which resulted in a revision of the Venice classification (**Box 1**).[13] During this meeting, the term familial PAH was replaced by the term heritable PAH (HPAH) because germline mutations in the bone morphogenetic protein receptor type 2 (*BMPR2*) gene, which is responsible for approximately 70% of FPAH cases, have also been identified in 11% to 40% of IPAH patients without a family

history, and therefore it can be inherited. In addition, in 30% of familial cases of PAH, no genetic mutation has been identified. HPAH includes IPAH patients who have germline mutations known to be associated with PAH as well as familial PAH with or without identified associated genetic mutations.

It is important to note that it is not uncommon for an individual with PH to have more than one etiological factor, which prevents their classification into a single WHO PH Group, and highlights the need for a complete diagnostic evaluation which includes right and sometimes left heart catheterization in addition to a thorough noninvasive workup so that all contributing factors to the PH can be identified and managed.

Pulmonary Arterial Hypertension (WHO Group 1 PH)

PAH has an estimated prevalence of 15 cases per million,[17] whereas the prevalence of idiopathic PAH is estimated to be approximately 6 cases per million.[17] Women are more often affected than men, with female to male ratios ranging from 1.5:1 to 4.1:1.[18,19] Age of onset is typically in the fourth to fifth decade based on findings from the REVEAL registry.[18] Subgroups of PAH include idiopathic and heritable cases, drugs and toxins, PAH associated with connective tissue disease (CTD), human immunodeficiency virus (HIV) infection, portal hypertension, congenital heart disease (CHD), schistosomiasis, and chronic hemolytic anemia. WHO Group 1 PH also includes persistent PH of the newborn, pulmonary veno-occlusive disease (PVOD), and pulmonary capillary hemangiomatosis (PCH).

PAH has been the major focus of the classification and therapeutic clinical trials of PH since the first classification in 1973. To date, the majority of randomized controlled trials of all the currently available therapeutic drugs for PH (prostanoids, endothelin receptor antagonists, and phosphodiesterase-5 inhibitors) have been performed in patients with PAH as opposed to other WHO PH groups, and these PH-specific therapies are currently only approved by the Food and Drug Administration (FDA) to treat patients with WHO Group 1 PH (PAH).

Idiopathic PAH

In the past, the term PAH was used to describe patients with idiopathic or familial PAH, and all other causes of PH were considered to be secondary PH. However, these terms have been abandoned in favor of more clinically meaningful terms. IPAH represents a sporadic and very rare disease for which no identifiable cause or risk factor exists. It is a diagnosis made by excluding

---

Box 1
Clinical classification of pulmonary hypertension (Dana Point, 2008)

1. Pulmonary arterial hypertension (PAH)

    1.1. Idiopathic PAH (IPAH)

    1.2. Heritable

        1.2.1. *BMPR2*

        1.2.2. ALK, endoglin (with or without hereditary hemorrhagic telangiectasia

        1.2.3. Unknown

    1.3. Drug and toxin induced

    1.4. Associated with:

        1.4.1. Connective tissue diseases

        1.4.2. Human immunodeficiency virus infection

        1.4.3. Portal hypertension

        1.4.4. Congenital heart diseases

        1.4.5. Schistosomiasis

        1.4.6. Chronic hemolytic anemia

    1.5. Persistent pulmonary hypertension of the newborn

1'. Pulmonary veno-occlusive disease (PVOD) and/or pulmonary capillary hemangiomatosis (PCH)

2. Pulmonary hypertension owing to left heart disease

    2.1. Systolic dysfunction

    2.2. Diastolic dysfunction

    2.3. Valvular disease

3. Pulmonary hypertension owing to lung diseases and/or hypoxemia

    3.1. Chronic obstructive pulmonary disease

    3.2. Interstitial lung disease

    3.3. Other pulmonary diseases with mixed restrictive and obstructive pattern

    3.4. Sleep-disordered breathing

    3.5. Alveolar hypoventilation disorders

    3.6. Chronic exposure to high altitude

    3.7. Developmental abnormalities

4. Chronic thromboembolic pulmonary hypertension (CTEPH)

5. Pulmonary hypertension with unclear multifactorial mechanisms

    5.1. Hematologic disorders: myeloproliferative disorders, splenectomy

    5.2. Systemic disorders: sarcoidosis, pulmonary Langerhans cell histiocytosis: lymphangioleiomyomatosis, neurofibromatosis, vasculitis

    5.3. Metabolic disorders: glycogen storage disease, Gaucher disease, thyroid disorders

    5.4. Other: tumoral obstruction, fibrosing mediastinitis, chronic renal failure on dialysis

From Simonneau G, et al. Updated clinical classification of pulmonary hypertension. J Am Coll Cardiol 2009; 54(Suppl 1):S43–54; with permission.

---

all other risk factors and conditions associated with PH via a thorough evaluation. The prevalence of IPAH is 5.9 cases per million, accounting for approximately 40% of cases of PAH.[17]

Heritable PAH
The subgroup of HPAH includes familial cases of PAH and/or patients with germline mutations associated with PAH.[20,21] Several germline mutations

have been identified in familial cases of PAH. The most common involves the bone morphogenetic protein receptor type 2 (BMPR2) gene, a member of the transforming growth factor (TGF)-β signaling family. BMPR2 gene mutations are found in 58% to 74% of patients with FPAH.[22–24] In addition, sporadic mutations in the BMPR2 gene are present in 11% to 40% of patients with otherwise IPAH.[25,26] BMPR2 mutations have rarely been identified in patients with PAH associated with CHD or use of the diet drug fenfluramine. Inheritance is autosomal dominant with incomplete penetrance (only 20% of patients with BMPR2 mutations develop PAH) and genetic anticipation, whereby future generations in familial cases tend to develop clinical disease at a younger age. Recently it has been suggested that cases of HPAH associated with BMPR2 mutations represent a subgroup with less acute vasoreactivity and more severe disease.[22] In addition, women tend to be affected more frequently than men, although sex does not appear to be associated with outcome.[27]

BPMR2 mutations are not the only heritable mutations identified in patients with PAH. Rarely, mutations of the actinin receptor–like kinase type 1 (ALK-1) and endoglin, both members of the TGF-β signaling family, have been identified in patients with PAH mostly associated with hereditary hemorrhagic telangiectasia (HHT). These patients tend to present earlier than those with BMPR2 mutations, and have a more severe clinical course.[24]

Drug-induced and toxin-induced PAH
Several drugs and toxins have been identified as risk factors for the development of PAH. These risk factors, defined as any factor or condition that is suspected to play a predisposing or facilitating role in the development of the disease, are categorized as definite, very likely, possible, or unlikely, based on the strength of their association with PH and their probable causal role. The updated Dana Point classification[13] categorized aminorex, fenfluramine, dexfenfluramine, and toxic rapeseed oil as definite risk factors, whereas amphetamines, L-tryptophan, and methamphetamines were considered likely risk factors, and cocaine, phenylpropanolamine, St. John's wort, certain chemotherapeutic agents, and selective serotonin receptor reuptake inhibitors (SSRIs) were considered possible risk factors for the development of PAH. Oral contraceptives, estrogen, and cigarette smoking are unlikely to play a causative role in PAH. The epidemiologic association between PAH and aminorex fumarate was first observed in the 1960s, and was followed by associations between the disease and fenfluramine in the 1990s in France.[28]

The risk of PAH following exposure to dexfenfluramine seems to increase with total exposure to the drug and can occur following short exposure.[28] Despite the earlier findings, fenfluramine and dexfenfluramine were widely used in the 1990s for weight control. Because of reports of the development of valvular abnormalities following their use, they were withdrawn from the United States market in 1997.[29] The exact cause of anorexigen-associated PAH is unclear, but may be due to altered serotonin metabolism and increased levels of plasma serotonin.[30] The Surveillance of Pulmonary Hypertension in America (SOPHIA) study found no increased risk for developing PAH with the use of SSRIs, other antidepressants, and anxiolytics[29]; however, a study of SSRI use in pregnant women showed an increased risk of the offspring developing persistent PH of the newborn, which suggests SSRIs are a possible risk factor for PAH, at least in association with pregnancy.[31] Illicit drugs, including methamphetamines and cocaine, have also been associated with PAH.[32] Although the incidence is uncertain, methamphetamine-induced PH poses a significant public health risk, as methamphetamine use has rapidly increased throughout the world since the 1990s. Methamphetamine is cheap and easy to make, and is the most commonly used illicit drug among high-school students.[33] In a retrospective analysis of patients treated at a tertiary care center for PAH, almost 30% of patients diagnosed with idiopathic PAH reported stimulant usage, primarily methamphetamines.[34]

Associated PAH
Connective tissue disease PAH has been associated with nearly every autoimmune disease; however the highest risk of PAH is found among patients with the scleroderma spectrum of diseases (SSc), particularly with limited cutaneous systemic sclerosis and CREST syndrome (Calcinosis, Raynaud, Esophageal dysfunction, Sclerodactyly, Telangiectasias). In early studies of patients with CTD, including SSc, Doppler echocardiography without confirmation by RHC probably led to an overestimation of the prevalence of PAH.[35] Subsequent prospective studies using screening echocardiography followed by diagnostic RHC for confirmation of PAH have found that the prevalence of PAH in patients with SSc is between 5% and 12%.[17,36–39] Systemic lupus erythematosus (SLE)[40–42] and mixed CTD[42] are associated with PAH less frequently than SSc; however, PAH also develops in patients with other types of CTD, including Sjögren syndrome,[43] rheumatoid arthritis,[44] and polymyositis.[45] Chronic inflammation may play a role, and macrophages,

T and B lymphocytes, and dendritic cells have been identified surrounding plexiform lesions.[46]

It is important to recognize that PAH is not the only cause of PH in patients with SSc. Patients with SSc are also at risk for the development of interstitial lung disease (ILD), which is a frequent cause of PH (WHO Group 3 PH).[47] In addition, PAH and PH due to ILD from SSc may coexist in these patients. Moreover, LV diastolic heart failure related to myocardial fibrosis in patients with SSc can lead to pulmonary venous hypertension (WHO Group 2 PH). Therefore, distinguishing between the relative contribution of each disease process in the development of PH is important in guiding appropriate therapy, as vasodilator therapies have not been well studied in SSc patients with PH related to ILD or diastolic heart failure, and they could be harmful.

HIV infection PAH is a well-established complication of HIV infection that was first recognized in 1987.[48–51] The prevalence of HIV-associated PAH is estimated to be 0.5% and it has not changed with the introduction of highly antiretroviral therapies.[52,53] In contrast to IPAH, the male to female ratio is lower, approximately 1.5:1, and the average age of diagnosis is 33 years.[54] Patients with HIV tend to present with worse functional class than do other patients with PAH, and they tend to have more rapid symptomatic progression.[54] Although the mechanism for its development is unclear, the clinical, hemodynamic, and histologic characteristics of HIV-associated PAH are similar to those of IPAH.[51,55] Neither the virus nor viral DNA have been found in pulmonary endothelial cells, and therefore an indirect mechanism of action through second messengers such as cytokines, growth factors, endothelin, or viral proteins is suspected.[50,56–59] Of importance, there is no clear association with HIV viral load or CD4 cell count and the development of PAH or its progression.[49]

Portopulmonary hypertension PAH associated with portal hypertension, better known as portopulmonary hypertension (POPH), can be distinguished from other forms of PAH by the presence of PAH in association with elevated portal pressure as measured by a hepatic venous pressure gradient greater than 5 mm Hg or the presence of esophageal varices.[60] Although cirrhosis is not necessary for the diagnosis, cirrhotic liver disease is the most common underlying etiology.[60] Prospective studies have found that 2% to 9% of patients with portal hypertension have elevated PAP.[61–63] In the French Registry of PAH, 10% of cases of PAH were due to POPH.[17]

Characteristically, patients with POPH have increased or preserved cardiac output (CO) despite elevated mPAP and PVR, although CO may decrease as the disease becomes advanced. It must be noted that POPH is not the only potential cause of PH in patients with advanced liver disease. Such patients are also at risk for PH because of high CO state from systemic vasodilation or pulmonary venous hypertension related to fluid overload and/or underlying LV diastolic dysfunction. The PVR may be elevated or normal in these cases. Therefore, an RHC is mandatory for the definitive diagnosis of POPH. in the US-based Registry to Evaluate Early and Long-term Pulmonary Arterial Hypertension Disease Management (REVEAL Registry), POPH was associated with poorer survival compared with patients with IPAH and FPAH, despite having better hemodynamics at diagnosis.[64]

Congenital heart disease Approximately 5% to 10% of patients with congenital systemic-to-pulmonary shunts develop PAH, and the prevalence of CHD-associated PAH (CHD-PAH) in Europe and North America ranges between 1.6 and 12.5 cases per million adults.[65–67] The clinical classification of congenital heart defects outlined in **Box 2** may be useful to distinguish between several distinct clinical phenotypes.[13] PAH typically develops in the presence of large systemic-to-pulmonary shunts, such as ventricular septal defects (VSD), atrial septal defects (ASD), anomalous pulmonary venous drainage, patent ductus arteriosus, and other, more complex CHDs. Patients with large VSDs tend to develop PAH at an earlier age than do patients with interatrial communications.[67] Over time, pulmonary pressures can gradually increase to systemic levels and the shunt flow can reverse, leading to central cyanosis and Eisenmenger syndrome (ES), which represents the most advanced form of CHD-PAH. ES occurs in 25% to 58% of patients with CHD-PAH.[68,69]

Schistosomiasis Before the updated Dana Point classification, PAH associated with schistosomiasis was categorized in Group 4, PH related to chronic thrombotic and/or embolic disease, because embolic obstruction of the pulmonary arteries by *Schistosoma* eggs was thought to be the primary mechanism responsible for the development of PH. More recently, however, studies have indicated that PAH associated with schistosomiasis can have similar histopathologic features, including plexiform lesions, and clinical presentation as in IPAH, and for that reason it is now subcategorized within Group 1 PH. It is now

---

Box 2
Anatomic-pathophysiologic classification of congenital systemic-to-pulmonary shunts associated with PAH

1. Type

  1.1. Simple pretricuspid shunts

    1.1.1. Atrial septal defect (ASD)

      1.1.1.1. Ostium secundum

      1.1.1.2. Sinus venosus

      1.1.1.3. Ostium primum

    1.1.2. Total or partial unobstructed anomalous pulmonary venous return

  1.2. Simple posttricuspid shunts

    1.2.1. Ventricular septal defect (VSD)

    1.2.2. Patent ductus arteriosus

  1.3. Combined shunts (describe combination and define predominant defect)

  1.4. Complex congenital heart disease

    1.4.1. Complete atrioventricular septal defect

    1.4.2. Truncus arteriosus

    1.4.3. Single-ventricle physiology with unobstructed pulmonary blood flow

    1.4.4. Transposition of the great arteries with VSD (without pulmonary stenosis) and/or patent ductus arteriosus

    1.4.5. Other

2. Dimension (specify for each defect if >1 congenital heart defect)

  2.1. Hemodynamic (specify Qp/Qs)[a]

    2.1.1. Restrictive (pressure gradient across the defect)

    2.1.2. Nonrestrictive

  2.2. Anatomic

    2.2.1. Small to moderate (ASD $\leq$2.0 cm and VSD $\leq$1.0 cm)

    2.2.2. Large (ASD $\geq$2.0 cm and VSD $\geq$1.0 cm)

3. Direction of shunt

  3.1. Predominantly systemic to pulmonary

  3.2. Predominantly pulmonary to systemic

  3.3. Bidirectional

4. Associated cardiac and extracardiac abnormalities

5. Repair status

  5.1. Unoperated

  5.2. Palliated (specify type of operation[s], age at surgery)

  5.3. Repaired (specify type of operation[s], age at surgery)

[a] Ratio of pulmonary (Qp) to systemic (Qs) blood flow.

From Simonneau G, et al. Updated clinical classification of pulmonary hypertension. J Am Coll Cardiol 2009;54(Suppl 1):S43–54; with permission.

---

better understood that the development of PAH related to schistosomiasis may be multifactorial and related to vascular inflammation from impacted *Schistosoma* eggs, as well as potentially by the coexistence of POPH, which is a common consequence of this disease.[70] Pulmonary embolic obstruction by *Schistosoma* eggs appears to play a minor role in the development of PH in these patients. Data from a recent hemodynamic study of patients with hepatosplenic schistosomiasis showed that the prevalence of PAH in these patients was 4.6%, whereas 3% of the patients had pulmonary venous hypertension.[71] These findings reinforce the need for a diagnostic RHC in patients with schistosomiasis and suspected PH. More than 200 million people are infected with schistosomiasis, with the vast majority of cases in Africa,[72] making schistosomiasis possibly the most common cause of PH worldwide.[70]

Chronic hemolytic anemia PAH has been reported in patients with chronic hemolytic anemias, including sickle cell disease (SCD), thalassemia, paroxysmal nocturnal hemoglobinuria, hereditary spherocytosis, malaria, and others.[73,74] The exact mechanism(s) involved in the development of PAH in these patients is unclear. Among patients with chronic hemolytic anemias, SCD-associated PAH (SCD-PAH) has been described most frequently with histologic findings that are similar to those in patients with IPAH. Hemolysis may result in a nitric-oxide deficient state through free hemoglobin scavenging of nitric oxide and through release of erythrocyte arginase, which limits L-arginine, a substrate for nitric oxide synthesis.[75] In common with other causes of PAH, endothelin levels are also increased.[76] Hypoxic mediated vasoconstriction and direct injury to the pulmonary vascular bed during sickle crises may also play a role in SCD-PAH.[74] Splenectomy, which is used to treat certain hemolytic disorders, has also been associated with the development of PH in these patients. It is also important to note that PAH is not the only type of PH in patients with chronic hemolytic anemias. Such patients may develop a high CO state from anemia and/or LV diastolic heart failure with pulmonary venous hypertension as the cause of PH. Studies of PAH in patients with SCD initially using echocardiography without hemodynamic confirmation found that prevalence varies significantly between 9% and 32% depending on the tricuspid regurgitant jet velocity criteria used.[77] A recent prospective study of SCD patients who were screened for PH by echocardiography revealed that 27% of patients had a tricuspid regurgitant jet velocity of 2.5 m per second (corresponding to a RVSP of 25 mm Hg plus the RAP) or more; however, the prevalence of PH as confirmed on catheterization was only 6%. Among the 24 patients with confirmed PH, PAH was found in 46% patients whereas pulmonary venous hypertension was present in 54%.[78] These results highlight the need for an invasive hemodynamic study for confirmation and proper diagnosis of PH in SCD patients who are suspected of having PAH.

Persistent pulmonary hypertension of the newborn

Persistent PH of the newborn (PPHN) is characterized by severe hypoxemia shortly after birth, absence of cyanotic CHD, and suprasystemic PH with right-to-left shunting across the ductus arteriosus and/or foramen ovale.[79,80] In utero, several factors determine the normally high PVR that results in a suprasystemic PAP. However, abnormal conditions may arise antenatally, during, or soon after birth, resulting in the failure of the PVR to decrease normally as the circulation evolves from a fetal to a postnatal state. The PVR may remain elevated because of pulmonary hypoplasia as seen with congenital diaphragmatic hernia, maldevelopment of the pulmonary arteries as seen in meconium aspiration syndrome, or maladaption of the pulmonary vascular bed as occurs with perinatal asphyxia.

Primary pulmonary capillary hemangiomatosis and pulmonary veno-occlusive disease

Although classified as a subgroup of PAH, PCH and PVOD are distinguished from other subgroups of PAH by the presence of pathologic obstruction within the pulmonary veins in addition to the pulmonary arteries that can lead to the development of pulmonary edema in the absence of LHF. In the REVEAL registry, PVOD and PCH accounted for less than 0.5% of patients with PAH, but their prevalence is unknown because of the rarity of the disease and the difficulty of making an antemortem diagnosis.[18] Both diseases appear to occur with equal frequency in men and women. PCH tends to present in patients aged 20 to 40 years, and PVOD can present in any decade of life.[81] Pathologic findings in PVOD include fibrotic obliteration of the preseptal pulmonary venules and thrombotic occlusion of small postcapillary vessels,[82] whereas PCH tends to be associated with tumorigenic proliferation of the capillaries. PVOD and PCH share similar pathologic features in the pulmonary parenchyma, including pulmonary hemosiderosis, interstitial edema, and lymphatic dilation, as well as intimal thickening and medial hypertrophy in the small pulmonary arteries, although plexiform arteriopathy is typically absent.[82] The etiologic basis for PVOD and PCH is unclear; however, they both have similar clinical presentation, histopathologic features in the pulmonary arteries, and risk factors (scleroderma spectrum of disease, HIV infection, anorexigen exposure, and *BMPR2* gene mutations) that are typical of associated PAH subgroups.[82–84] On the other hand, there are several important differences with PVOD and PCH that are notable. First, clinical features that can distinguish these entities from PAH include the presence of pulmonary rales and digital clubbing on examination; ground-glass opacities, interlobular septal thickening, and mediastinal adenopathy on chest computed tomography (CT); and severely reduced lung diffusion capacity for carbon monoxide (DLCO) and partial pressure of arterial oxygen. Second, and probably more importantly, the prognosis with PVOD and PCH is worse in comparison with PAH, and patients with PVOD/PCH can develop pulmonary edema and clinical deterioration in response to pulmonary vasodilator therapies. For these reasons, in the Dana Point classification PVOD/PCH are not completely separated from PAH, but are designated as Group 1'.[13]

Pulmonary Hypertension Owing to Left Heart Disease

LHF is by far the most common cause of PH, being responsible for greater than 80% of all cases.[4,13,85–88] Whether it is caused by LV systolic or diastolic dysfunction, or left-sided valvular heart disease (mitral or aortic regurgitation or stenosis), the presence of PH usually confers a poor prognosis, and the hallmark of PH due to LHF (PH-LHF) is elevated LAP.[10,89–93]

The prevalence of PH-LHF among patients with chronic heart failure from LV systolic dysfunction (HF with reduced LV ejection fraction [HFrEF]) is approximately 60% to 70% whereas PH may be present in more than 80% of patients with LV diastolic dysfunction (HF with preserved LV ejection fraction [HFpEF]), and it is more common among the elderly.[88,92,94–96] Patients with LV systolic dysfunction have reduced contractility of the left ventricle with attendant declines in LV ejection fraction (LVEF). Causes of HFrEF include coronary artery disease and myocardial infarction, familial or idiopathic dilated cardiomyopathy (IDCM), myocarditis, and exposure to certain drugs or toxins. In patients with HFpEF, the left ventricle's capacity to fill during diastole is impaired while the LVEF remains above 50%. Major causes of HFpEF include hypertension, ischemia, fibrosis, infiltrative/restrictive disease, hypertrophic cardiomyopathy, and pericardial disease. Significant mitral or aortic stenosis and/or regurgitation can also lead to LHF and pulmonary venous hypertension. In clinical practice, more than one of these disease processes are often present in a particular case of PH related to LHF.

In the setting of chronically elevated left-sided filling pressures, pulmonary vascular remodeling can occur such that the PVR and transpulmonary gradient increase out of proportion to the degree of PCWP and/or LVEDP elevation. In such cases,

the TPG is greater than the normal 10 mm Hg or less (usually 12–15 mm Hg or greater).[97] Chronically elevated endothelin levels leading to pulmonary arterial medial hypertrophy and obliterative arteriopathy may play a role in the pathogenesis of this type of PH.[98] This hemodynamic profile with an elevated mPAP, elevated PCWP and/or LVEDP, and elevated PVR and TPG is variably described in the literature as "PH out of proportion to left heart disease," "mixed" PH, or "reactive" PH. Moreover, when the PVR fails to decrease to less than 3 WU with acute pulmonary vasodilators, the PH may be described as "fixed" or "nonreactive." In each of these instances, however, the underlying etiology of PH is left-sided heart disease, and it is not considered to be PAH.

Pulmonary Hypertension Owing to Lung Diseases and/or Hypoxia

The predominant cause of PH in this category is inadequate oxygenation of arterial blood as a result of parenchymal lung disease, impaired ventilation and/or disordered respiratory mechanics, or residence at high altitude. Specific examples of this type of PH include severe chronic obstructive pulmonary disease (COPD), ILD (including pulmonary fibrosis that is idiopathic or related to CTD, hypersensitivity pneumonitis, or obliterative bronchiolitis), other pulmonary diseases with mixed restrictive and obstructive pattern, sleep-disordered breathing, alveolar hypoventilation disorders (eg, obesity-hypoventilation syndrome), chronic exposure to high altitude, and developmental disorders.

PH occurs frequently in patients with advanced lung disease such as COPD and ILD, with some case series reporting a prevalence of PH above 50%, depending on the population studied in addition to the diagnostic methods and criteria.[99–106] In the majority of cases the increase in mPAP is modest (<35–40 mm Hg), the CO is typically preserved, and only in exceptional cases is the PVR greater than 480 dyne/s/cm^5).[100] Numerous studies have indicated that even mild forms of PH may be clinically significant in patients with COPD as well as in patients with pulmonary fibrosis, as they are associated with worse oxygenation, decreased exercise capacity, and poorer prognosis.[101,107–110]

Of the parenchymal lung diseases, ILD most commonly results in PH through capillary destruction and hypoxic vasoconstriction.[111,112] Patients with CTD, in particular those with SSc of CTD, are at increased risk for the development of ILD and secondary PH. Occasionally such patients will develop coexistent pulmonary vascular disease (PAH), and it is important to distinguish as much as possible between PAH and PH related to ILD, because none of the current therapies for PAH have been shown to be safe and effective in treating PH related to ILD. Moreover, in some cases (particularly with systemically administered pulmonary vasodilators) they can be deleterious by increasing perfusion to poorly ventilated lung units and increasing ventilation-perfusion mismatching, resulting in worsened hypoxia.[113] On the other hand, in addition to specific treatment of the underlying ILD, oxygen is a pulmonary vasodilator that is the mainstay of therapy for WHO Group 3 PH. Indeed, long-term oxygen therapy (16 or 24 h/d) improves survival in patients with COPD.[114,115]

Diagnostically it can be challenging to distinguish PAH from PH related to ILD, particularly in patients with scleroderma or other CTD, because they can develop PAH, ILD, with secondary PH, or concomitant disorders. For practical purposes, because alveolar volumes on spirometry and body plethysmography are determined by the underlying lung disease and are not significantly affected by concomitant PH, coexistent pulmonary vascular disease is suggested in patients with ILD in whom the degree of reduced DLCO is out of proportion to the reduction in lung volume, as suggested by a forced vital capacity to DLCO ratio of 1.4 or more.[116]

Although typically considered to be associated with precapillary PH, obstructive sleep apnea (OSA) can also be caused by and is associated with LHF, and can therefore coexist with pulmonary venous hypertension.[117,118] There are no clear estimates of the prevalence of PH in OSA, but OSA is common in the general population and likely to increase with increasing rates of obesity and heart failure.[119]

Prolonged exposure to high altitudes can also lead to PH, chronic mountain sickness, and in some cases fatal pulmonary edema.[120,121] The precise pathophysiology of high altitude–related PH is unclear, but contributing factors likely include hypoventilation, hypoxia-mediated pulmonary vasoconstriction, and free radical–mediated reduction in nitric oxide.[122,123]

Chronic Thromboembolic Pulmonary Hypertension

In the Venice classification of PH, Group 4 PH was very heterogeneous and included obstruction of pulmonary arterial vessels by thromboemboli, tumors, or foreign bodies, but the clinical presentation, radiographic features, and therapeutic management were unique to each etiology. For this reason, the Dana Point classification of WHO Group 4 PH includes only patients with CTEPH. Approximately 2% to 4% of patients develop CTEPH after an acute pulmonary embolism despite anticoagulation, which represents a relatively frequent cause of PH.[124,125] CTEPH is diagnosed if a patient has evidence of PH 6 months after pulmonary embolism is diagnosed.[126] Thrombolysis given for acute pulmonary embolism and right ventricular dysfunction can decrease the incidence of CTEPH[127]; however, patients who develop CTEPH often have a honeymoon period after an acute pulmonary embolism during which symptoms are absent despite the onset of PH, and many patients (approximately one-quarter) do not have an antecedent history of clinically overt pulmonary embolism.[128] The diagnosis is often overlooked[129] because the clues to the condition are subtle, which helps to explain why the median time from symptom onset to diagnosis was more than 14 months in a large, international registry.[128] The condition is usually detected when worsening PH and right ventricular dysfunction lead to dyspnea, exercise intolerance, fatigue, hypoxemia, and progressive right ventricular failure. In addition to pulmonary arterial mural thrombi, webbing, bands, and obliteration of the larger pulmonary vessels, patients with CTEPH may also have pathologic changes in nonoccluded pulmonary artery segments, including medial hypertrophy and intimal hyperplasia that is indistinguishable from PAH.[130,131] Survival with CTEPH is poor and depends on the hemodynamic severity of disease; however, successful removal of obstructive, whitish, hardened thromboembolic material with pulmonary thromboendarterectomy (PTE) surgery can markedly improve hemodynamic measures of mPAP, PVR, and CO with reversal of right ventricular failure, improved exercise tolerance, and survival.[132,133] Unfortunately, not all pulmonary emboli are amenable to removal with surgery, as only lesions in the proximal vessels can be surgically accessed. In a large, international registry that included 679 consecutive patients, nearly one-third of patients were nonoperable (36% nonoperable vs 63% operable).[128] It is highly recommended that patients with symptomatic CTEPH be referred for evaluation at a specialized center with expertise in PTE surgery, because PTE can be potentially curative, with much better survival compared with medical treatment, and because 30-day mortality after PTE surgery is significantly better in the most experienced centers (less than 5% vs 10% elsewhere).[126,132,134]

Pulmonary Hypertension with Multiple Unclear Mechanisms

This category of PH consists of several forms of PH for which the etiology is unclear or multifactorial.

Hematologic disorders such as chronic myeloproliferative disorders (eg, myeloid metaplasia with myelofibrosis, polycythemia vera, essential thrombocythemia, myelodysplastic syndromes, and chronic myeloid leukemia) and postsplenectomy state can cause PH by various mechanisms.[135] High CO, obstruction of pulmonary arteries by circulating megakaryocytes, CTEPH, POPH, congestive heart failure, and splenectomy can all play a role in the development of PH in these patients. PH after splenectomy, whether auto or surgical, can develop as a result of CTEPH due to abnormal postsplenectomy erythrocyte activities or abnormal platelet activation and the development of a primarily distal CTEPH disease that is nonoperable.[128,136,137] However, several cases of disease indistinguishable from PAH with intimal fibrosis, medial hypertrophy, and plexiform lesions in the pulmonary vasculature have been described in association with postsplenectomy.[138,139]

Systemic disorders associated with the development of PH include sarcoidosis, pulmonary Langerhans cell histiocytosis, and neurofibromatosis type 1 (also known as von Recklinghausen disease). PH has been diagnosed in 1% to 28% of patients with sarcoidosis, a common granulomatous disease, and the possible pathophysiologic mechanism(s) of developing PH in these patients includes fibrotic pulmonary disease with capillary destruction and chronic hypoxemia, granulomatous involvement of the pulmonary veins mimicking PVOD, congestive heart failure from sarcoid infiltrative cardiomyopathy, extrinsic compression of the pulmonary arteries from bulky hilar and mediastinal adenopathy, and more rarely, POPH.[103,140–143] Pulmonary Langerhans cell histiocytosis, an uncommon infiltrative lung disease associated with pulmonary parenchymal destruction, has been associated with PH from chronic hypoxemia and/or abnormal pulmonary mechanics; however, the PH can be severe in end-stage disease, for which histopathologic findings have demonstrated diffuse pulmonary vascular remodeling similar to PAH with intimal fibrosis and medial hypertrophy.[144,145] Lymphangioleiomyomatosis, which is a rare multisystem disorder affecting mostly women that is associated with lung destruction, lymphatic abnormalities, and abdominal tumors, uncommonly leads to PH predominantly via chronic hypoxemia and capillary destruction caused by cystic lesions.[146,147] The autosomal dominant disease neurofibromatosis type 1, or von Recklinghausen

disease, which is characterized by cutaneous fibromas and café-au-lait skin lesions and occasional systemic vasculopathy, can cause PH; however, the mechanism is unclear. The neurofibromatosis type 1 gene has been shown to modulate protein kinase B, which is an important regulator of cell proliferation. Lung fibrosis and CTEPH are thought to be the predominant pathologic mechanism for the development of PH in these patients; however, medial and/or intimal hypertrophy and fibrosis with narrowing of pulmonary arteries and veins on histologic examination have been identified and may also play a role.[148–152] Rare cases of PH with a clinical presentation similar to PAH in patients with antineutrophil cytoplasmic antibodies–associated vasculitis have been reported; however, histologic data are not available.[153]

Metabolic disorders, such as type Ia glycogen storage disease (a rare autosomal recessive disorder caused by a deficiency of glucose-6-phosphatase), Gaucher disease, and thyroid disease, have been associated with a risk for developing PH. In each of these disorders, the pathophysiology of PH is either unclear or related to multiple potential underlying mechanisms.[13] PH has been found by echocardiography in greater than 40% of patients with thyroid diseases (both hyperthyroidism and hypothyroidism) in a prospective study, and given a reported 49% prevalence of autoimmune thyroid disease among 63 patients with PAH, an immunogenetic susceptibility link is suggested.[154–158]

The last subgroup includes miscellaneous conditions that have been linked to the development of PH. Patients receiving long-term hemodialysis for end-stage renal disease have PH relatively frequently, with prevalence estimated to be up to 40%. There are several potential pathophysiologic mechanisms responsible for the development of PH in these patients, including the consequences of chronic or dynamic volume overload from inadequate hemodialysis, often with underlying LV diastolic and/or systolic dysfunction and neurohormonal activation, leading to purely passive PH, reactive pulmonary vasoconstriction, and/or pulmonary vascular remodeling.[159,160] In addition, patients with arteriovenous fistulas can develop PH related to high CO and often concomitant anemia. Pulmonary artery obstruction due to progressive growth of tumor, often pulmonary artery sarcomas, within the central pulmonary arteries along with thrombosis can lead to PH and is often rapidly fatal. This condition can be confused with CTEPH; however, CT and magnetic resonance imaging can be used to differentiate between tumor and thrombosis. Metastatic tumor microemboli are rare but can lead to rapidly progressive and fatal PH. Patients with this condition usually have a history of cancer (typically breast, lung, or gastric carcinomas) and are hypoxic on presentation, with clear lung fields on imaging and no evidence of pulmonary emboli on CT pulmonary angiography. Ventilation-perfusion scanning often shows abnormalities of perfusion, including diffusely heterogeneous perfusion abnormalities without segmental or subsegmental defects or multiple subsegmental ventilation-perfusion mismatches.[161,162] Pulmonary microvascular blood aspiration via a pulmonary artery catheter in the wedge position with cytologic analysis for tumor cells can be diagnostic in these cases. Mediastinal fibrosis, often derived from fungal infections such as histoplasmosis or tuberculosis, can lead to compression of the pulmonary arteries and veins and cause severe PH.[163–165]

SUMMARY

PH can develop in association with many different diseases and risk factors, and its presence is nearly always associated with reduced survival. Medical management of PH is largely dependent on its underlying etiology, and the combination of clinical and hemodynamic classifications of PH provides a framework for the diagnostic evaluation of PH to establish a final clinical diagnosis, and to guide therapy. The classification system for PH will continue to evolve as our understanding of the different pathologic mechanisms that underlie the syndrome increases.

REFERENCES

1. Kovacs G, Berghold A, Scheidl S, et al. Pulmonary arterial pressure during rest and exercise in healthy subjects: a systematic review. Eur Respir J 2009; 34(4):888–94.
2. Naeije R, Melot C, Niset G, et al. Mechanisms of improved arterial oxygenation after peripheral chemoreceptor stimulation during hypoxic exercise. J Appl Phys 1993;74(4):1666–71.
3. Chatterjee K, De Marco T, Alpert JS. Pulmonary hypertension: hemodynamic diagnosis and management. Arch Intern Med 2002;162(17): 1925–33.
4. Oudiz RJ. Pulmonary hypertension associated with left-sided heart disease. Clin Chest Med 2007; 28(1):233–41, x.
5. Capomolla S, Febo O, Guazzotti G, et al. Invasive and non-invasive determinants of pulmonary hypertension in patients with chronic heart failure. J Heart Lung Transplant 2000;19(5):426–38.
6. Drazner MH, Hamilton MA, Fonarow G, et al. Relationship between right and left-sided filling pressures in 1000 patients with advanced heart failure. J Heart Lung Transplant 1999;18(11):1126–32.
7. Drazner MH, Prasad A, Ayers C, et al. The relationship of right- and left-sided filling pressures in patients with heart failure and a preserved ejection fraction. Circ Heart Fail 2010;3(2):202–6.
8. Enriquez-Sarano M, Rossi A, Seward JB, et al. Determinants of pulmonary hypertension in left ventricular dysfunction. J Am Coll Cardiol 1997; 29(1):153–9.
9. Costard-Jackle A, Fowler MB. Influence of preoperative pulmonary artery pressure on mortality after heart transplantation: testing of potential reversibility of pulmonary hypertension with nitroprusside is useful in defining a high risk group. J Am Coll Cardiol 1992;19(1):48–54.
10. Abramson SV, Burke JF, Kelly JJ Jr, et al. Pulmonary hypertension predicts mortality and morbidity in patients with dilated cardiomyopathy. Ann Intern Med 1992;116(11):888–95.
11. Zener JC, Hancock EW, Shumway NE, et al. Regression of extreme pulmonary hypertension after mitral valve surgery. Am J Cardiol 1972;30(8):820–6.
12. Braunwald E, Braunwald NS, Ross J Jr, et al. Effects of mitral-valve replacement on the pulmonary vascular dynamics of patients with pulmonary hypertension. N Engl J Med 1965;273:509–14.
13. Simonneau G, Robbins IM, Beghetti M, et al. Updated clinical classification of pulmonary hypertension. J Am Coll Cardiol 2009;54(Suppl 1):S43–54.
14. Hatano S, Strasser T. Primary pulmonary hypertension. Report on a WHO meeting. Geneva (Switzerland): World Health Organization; 1975.
15. Fishman AP. Clinical classification of pulmonary hypertension. Clin Chest Med 2001;22(3):385–91, vii.
16. Simonneau G, Galiè N, Rubin LJ, et al. Clinical classification of pulmonary hypertension. J Am Coll Cardiol 2004;43(12 Suppl S):5S–12S.
17. Humbert M, Sitbon O, Chaouat A, et al. Pulmonary arterial hypertension in France: results from a national registry. Am J Respir Crit Care Med 2006;173(9):1023–30.
18. Badesch DB, Raskob GE, Elliott CG, et al. Pulmonary arterial hypertension: baseline characteristics from the REVEAL Registry. Chest 2010;137(2): 376–87.
19. Rich S, Dantzker DR, Ayres SM, et al. Primary pulmonary hypertension. A national prospective study. Ann Intern Med 1987;107(2):216–23.
20. Chaouat A, Coulet F, Favre C, et al. Endoglin germline mutation in a patient with hereditary haemorrhagic telangiectasia and dexfenfluramine associated pulmonary arterial hypertension. Thorax 2004;59(5): 446–8.
21. Trembath RC. Mutations in the TGF-beta type 1 receptor, ALK1, in combined primary pulmonary hypertension and hereditary haemorrhagic telangiectasia, implies pathway specificity. J Heart Lung Transplant 2001;20(2):175.

22. Sztrymf B, Coulet F, Girerd B, et al. Clinical outcomes of pulmonary arterial hypertension in carriers of BMPR2 mutation. Am J Respir Crit Care Med 2008;177(12):1377–83.

23. Rosenzweig EB, Morse JH, Knowles JA. Clinical implications of determining BMPR2 mutation status in a large cohort of children and adults with pulmonary arterial hypertension. J Heart Lung Transplant 2008;27:668–74.

24. Girerd B, Montani D, Coulet F, et al. Clinical outcomes of pulmonary arterial hypertension in patients carrying an ACVRL1 (ALK1) mutation. Am J Respir Crit Care Med 2010;181(8):851–61.

25. Machado RD, Aldred MA, James V, et al. Mutations of the TGF-beta type II receptor BMPR2 in pulmonary arterial hypertension. Hum Mutat 2006;27(2): 121–32.

26. Thomson JR, Machado RD, Pauciulo MW, et al. Sporadic primary pulmonary hypertension is associated with germline mutations of the gene encoding BMPR-II, a receptor member of the TGF-beta family. J Med Genet 2000;37(10):741–5.

27. Girerd B, Montani D, Eyries M, et al. Absence of influence of gender and BMPR2 mutation type on clinical phenotypes of pulmonary arterial hypertension. Respir Res 2010;11:73.

28. Abenhaim L, Moride Y, Brenot F, et al. Appetite-suppressant drugs and the risk of primary pulmonary hypertension. International Primary Pulmonary Hypertension Study Group. N Engl J Med 1996; 335(9):609–16.

29. Walker AM, Langleben D, Korelitz JJ, et al. Temporal trends and drug exposures in pulmonary hypertension: an American experience. Am Heart J 2006;152(3):521–6.

30. Simonneau G, Fartoukh M, Sitbon O, et al. Primary pulmonary hypertension associated with the use of fenfluramine derivatives. Chest 1998;114(Suppl 3): 195S–9S.

31. Chambers CD, Hernandez-Diaz S, Van Marter LJ, et al. Selective serotonin-reuptake inhibitors and risk of persistent pulmonary hypertension of the newborn. N Engl J Med 2006;354(6):579–87.

32. Schaiberger PH, Kennedy TC, Miller FC, et al. Pulmonary hypertension associated with long-term inhalation of "crank" methamphetamine. Chest 1993;104(2):614–6.

33. Wu LT, Schlenger WE, Galvin DM. Concurrent use of methamphetamine, MDMA, LSD, ketamine, GHB, and flunitrazepam among American youths. Drug Alcohol Depend 2006;84(1):102–13.

34. Chin KM, Channick RN, Rubin LJ. Is methamphetamine use associated with idiopathic pulmonary arterial hypertension? Chest 2006;130(6):1657–63.

35. Wigley FM, Lima JA, Mayes M, et al. The prevalence of undiagnosed pulmonary arterial hypertension in subjects with connective tissue disease at the secondary health care level of community-based rheumatologists (the UNCOVER study). Arthritis Rheum 2005;52(7):2125–32.

36. Hachulla E, Gressin V, Guillevin L, et al. Early detection of pulmonary arterial hypertension in systemic sclerosis: a French nationwide prospective multicenter study. Arthritis Rheum 2005; 52(12):3792–800.

37. Mukerjee D, St George D, Coleiro B, et al. Prevalence and outcome in systemic sclerosis associated pulmonary arterial hypertension: application of a registry approach. Ann Rheum Dis 2003; 62(11):1088–93.

38. Avouac J, Airò P, Meune C, et al. Prevalence of pulmonary hypertension in systemic sclerosis in European Caucasians and metaanalysis of 5 studies. J Rheumatol 2010;37(11):2290–8.

39. Condliffe R, Kiely DG, Peacock AJ, et al. Connective tissue disease-associated pulmonary arterial hypertension in the modern treatment era. Am J Respir Crit Care Med 2009;179(2):151–7.

40. Asherson RA. Pulmonary hypertension in systemic lupus erythematosus. J Rheumatol 1990;17(3):414–5.

41. Tanaka E, Harigai M, Tanaka M, et al. Pulmonary hypertension in systemic lupus erythematosus: evaluation of clinical characteristics and response to immunosuppressive treatment. J Rheumatol 2002;29(2):282–7.

42. Jais X, Launay D, Yaici A, et al. Immunosuppressive therapy in lupus- and mixed connective tissue disease-associated pulmonary arterial hypertension: a retrospective analysis of twenty-three cases. Arthritis Rheum 2008;58(2):521–31.

43. Launay D, Hachulla E, Hatron PY, et al. Pulmonary arterial hypertension: a rare complication of primary Sjogren syndrome: report of 9 new cases and review of the literature. Medicine (Baltimore) 2007;86(5):299–315.

44. Dawson JK, Goodson NG, Graham DR, et al. Raised pulmonary artery pressures measured with Doppler echocardiography in rheumatoid arthritis patients. Rheumatology (Oxford) 2000;39(12):1320–5.

45. Bunch TW, Tancredi RG, Lie JT. Pulmonary hypertension in polymyositis. Chest 1981;79(1):105–7.

46. Le Pavec J, Humbert M, Mouthon L, et al. Systemic sclerosis-associated pulmonary arterial hypertension. Am J Respir Crit Care Med 2010;181(12): 1285–93.

47. Launay D, Mouthon L, Hachulla E, et al. Prevalence and characteristics of moderate to severe pulmonary hypertension in systemic sclerosis with and without interstitial lung disease. J Rheumatol 2007; 34(5):1005–11.

48. Kim KK, Factor SM. Membranoproliferative glomerulonephritis and plexogenic pulmonary arteriopathy in a homosexual man with acquired immunodeficiency syndrome. Hum Pathol 1987;18(12):1293–6.

49. Degano B, Guillaume M, Savale L, et al. HIV-associated pulmonary arterial hypertension: survival and prognostic factors in the modern therapeutic era. AIDS 2010;24(1):67–75.

50. Almodovar S, Cicalini S, Petrosillo N, et al. Pulmonary hypertension associated with HIV infection: pulmonary vascular disease: the global perspective. Chest 2010;137(Suppl 6):6S–12S.

51. Mehta NJ, Khan IA, Mehta RN, et al. HIV-Related pulmonary hypertension: analytic review of 131 cases. Chest 2000;118(4):1133–41.

52. Opravil M, Pechère M, Speich R, et al. HIV-associated primary pulmonary hypertension. A case control study. Swiss HIV Cohort Study. Am J Respir Crit Care Med 1997;155(3):990–5.

53. Sitbon O, Lascoux-Combe C, Delfraissy JF, et al. Prevalence of HIV-related pulmonary arterial hypertension in the current antiretroviral therapy era. Am J Respir Crit Care Med 2008;177(1):108–13.

54. Cicalini S, Almodovar S, Grilli E, et al. Pulmonary hypertension and human immunodeficiency virus infection: epidemiology, pathogenesis, and clinical approach. Clin Microbiol Infect 2011;17(1):25–33.

55. Petitpretz P, Brenot F, Azarian R, et al. Pulmonary hypertension in patients with human immunodeficiency virus infection. Comparison with primary pulmonary hypertension. Circulation 1994;89(6):2722–7.

56. Humbert M, Monti G, Fartoukh M, et al. Platelet-derived growth factor expression in primary pulmonary hypertension: comparison of HIV seropositive and HIV seronegative patients. Eur Respir J 1998; 11(3):554–9.

57. Kanmogne GD, Primeaux C, Grammas P. HIV-1 gp120 proteins alter tight junction protein expression and brain endothelial cell permeability: implications for the pathogenesis of HIV-associated dementia. J Neuropathol Exp Neurol 2005;64(6):498–505.

58. Kim J, Ruff M, Karwatowska-Prokopczuk E, et al. HIV envelope protein gp120 induces neuropeptide Y receptor-mediated proliferation of vascular smooth muscle cells: relevance to AIDS cardiovascular pathogenesis. Regul Pept 1998;75–76:201–5.

59. Rusnati M, Presta M. HIV-1 Tat protein and endothelium: from protein/cell interaction to AIDS-associated pathologies. Angiogenesis 2002;5(3):141–51.

60. Le Pavec J, Souza R, Herve P, et al. Portopulmonary hypertension: survival and prognostic factors. Am J Respir Crit Care Med 2008;178(6):637–43.

61. Krowka M. Portopulmonary hypertension. Semin Respir Crit Care Med 2012;33(1):17–25.

62. Hadengue A, Benhayoun MK, Lebrec D, et al. Pulmonary hypertension complicating portal hypertension: prevalence and relation to splanchnic hemodynamics. Gastroenterology 1991;100(2):520–8.

63. Krowka MJ, Swanson KL, Frantz RP, et al. Portopulmonary hypertension: results from a 10-year screening algorithm. Hepatology 2006;44(6):1502–10.

64. Krowka MJ, Miller DP, Barst RJ, et al. Portopulmonary hypertension: a report from the US-based REVEAL registry. Chest 2012;141(4):906–15.

65. Kidd L, Driscoll DJ, Gersony WM, et al. Second natural history study of congenital heart defects. Results of treatment of patients with ventricular septal defects. Circulation 1993;87(Suppl 2):I38–51.

66. Steele PM, Fuster V, Cohen M, et al. Isolated atrial septal defect with pulmonary vascular obstructive disease–long-term follow-up and prediction of outcome after surgical correction. Circulation 1987; 76(5):1037–42.

67. Diller GP, Gatzoulis MA. Pulmonary vascular disease in adults with congenital heart disease. Circulation 2007;115(8):1039–50.

68. Galie N, Manes A, Palazzini M, et al. Management of pulmonary arterial hypertension associated with congenital systemic-to-pulmonary shunts and Eisenmenger's syndrome. Drugs 2008;68(8):1049–66.

69. Duffels MG, Engelfriet PM, Berger RM, et al. Pulmonary arterial hypertension in congenital heart disease: an epidemiologic perspective from a Dutch registry. International journal of cardiology 2007;120(2):198–204.

70. dos Santos Fernandes CJ, Jardim CV, Hovnanian A, et al. Survival in schistosomiasis-associated pulmonary arterial hypertension. J Am Coll Cardiol 2010; 56(9):715–20.

71. Lapa M, Dias B, Jardim C, et al. Cardiopulmonary manifestations of hepatosplenic schistosomiasis. Circulation 2009;119(11):1518–23.

72. Steinmann P, Keiser J, Bos R, et al. Schistosomiasis and water resources development: systematic review, meta-analysis, and estimates of people at risk. Lancet Infect Dis 2006;6(7):411–25.

73. Barnett CF, Hsue PY, Machado RF. Pulmonary hypertension: an increasingly recognized complication of hereditary hemolytic anemias and HIV infection. JAMA 2008;299(3):324–31.

74. Machado RF, Gladwin MT. Pulmonary hypertension in hemolytic disorders: pulmonary vascular disease: the global perspective. Chest 2010;137(Suppl 6): 30S–8S.

75. Morris CR, Kato GJ, Poljakovic M, et al. Dysregulated arginine metabolism, hemolysis-associated pulmonary hypertension, and mortality in sickle cell disease. JAMA 2005;294(1):81–90.

76. Ergul S, Brunson CY, Hutchinson J, et al. Vasoactive factors in sickle cell disease: in vitro evidence for endothelin-1-mediated vasoconstriction. Am J Hematol 2004;76(3):245–51.

77. Gladwin MT, Sachdev V, Jison ML, et al. Pulmonary hypertension as a risk factor for death in patients with sickle cell disease. N Engl J Med 2004; 350(9):886–95.

78. Parent F, Bachir D, Inamo J, et al. A hemodynamic study of pulmonary hypertension in sickle cell disease. N Engl J Med 2011;365(1):44–53.

79. Ostrea EM, Villanueva-Uy ET, Natarajan G, et al. Persistent pulmonary hypertension of the newborn: pathogenesis, etiology, and management. Paediatr Drugs 2006;8(3):179–88.

80. Stayer SA, Liu Y. Pulmonary hypertension of the newborn. Best Pract Res Clin Anaesthesiol 2010; 24(3):375–86.

81. Montani D, O'Callaghan DS, Savale L, et al. Pulmonary veno-occlusive disease: recent progress and current challenges. Respir Med 2010;104(Suppl 1): S23–32.

82. Montani D, Price LC, Dorfmuller P, et al. Pulmonary veno-occlusive disease. Eur Respir J 2009;33(1): 189–200.

83. Lantuejoul S, Sheppard MN, Corrin B, et al. Pulmonary veno-occlusive disease and pulmonary capillary hemangiomatosis: a clinicopathologic study of 35 cases. Am J Surg Pathol 2006;30(7):850–7.

84. Johnson SR, Patsios D, Hwang DM, et al. Pulmonary veno-occlusive disease and scleroderma associated pulmonary hypertension. J Rheumatol 2006;33(11):2347–50.

85. Guazzi M, Arena R. Pulmonary hypertension with left-sided heart disease. Nature reviews. Cardiology 2010;7(11):648–59.

86. Guglin M, Khan H. Pulmonary hypertension in heart failure. J Card Fail 2010;16(6):461–74.

87. Hoeper MM, Barberà JA, Channick RN, et al. Diagnosis, assessment, and treatment of non-pulmonary arterial hypertension pulmonary hypertension. J Am Coll Cardiol 2009;54(Suppl 1):S85–96.

88. Lam CS, Roger VL, Rodeheffer RJ, et al. Pulmonary hypertension in heart failure with preserved ejection fraction: a community-based study. J Am Coll Cardiol 2009;53(13):1119–26.

89. Bursi F, McNallan SM, Redfield MM, et al. Pulmonary pressures and death in heart failure: a community study. J Am Coll Cardiol 2012;59(3):222–31.

90. Kalogeropoulos AP, Vega JD, Smith AL, et al. Pulmonary hypertension and right ventricular function in advanced heart failure. Congest Heart Fail 2011;17(4):189–98.

91. Ben-Dor I, Goldstein SA, Pichard AD, et al. Clinical profile, prognostic implication, and response to treatment of pulmonary hypertension in patients with severe aortic stenosis. Am J Cardiol 2011; 107(7):1046–51.

92. Cappola TP, Felker GM, Kao WH, et al. Pulmonary hypertension and risk of death in cardiomyopathy: patients with myocarditis are at higher risk. Circulation 2002;105(14):1663–8.

93. Kjaergaard J, Akkan D, Iversen KK, et al. Prognostic importance of pulmonary hypertension in patients with heart failure. Am J Cardiol 2007; 99(8):1146–50.

94. Ghio S, Gavazzi A, Campana C, et al. Independent and additive prognostic value of right ventricular systolic function and pulmonary artery pressure in patients with chronic heart failure. J Am Coll Cardiol 2001;37(1):183–8.

95. Grigioni F, Potena L, Galiè N, et al. Prognostic implications of serial assessments of pulmonary hypertension in severe chronic heart failure. J Heart Lung Transplant 2006;25(10):1241–6.

96. Khush KK, Tasissa G, Butler J, et al. Effect of pulmonary hypertension on clinical outcomes in advanced heart failure: analysis of the Evaluation Study of Congestive Heart Failure and Pulmonary Artery Catheterization Effectiveness (ESCAPE) database. Am Heart J 2009;157(6):1026–34.

97. Dadfarmay S, Berkowitz R, Kim B, et al. Differentiating pulmonary arterial and pulmonary venous hypertension and the implications for therapy. Congest Heart Fail 2010;16(6):287–91.

98. Moraes DL, Colucci WS, Givertz MM. Secondary pulmonary hypertension in chronic heart failure: the role of the endothelium in pathophysiology and management. Circulation 2000;102(14):1718–23.

99. Behr J, Ryu JH. Pulmonary hypertension in interstitial lung disease. Eur Respir J 2008;31(6):1357–67.

100. Chaouat A, Naeije R, Weitzenblum E. Pulmonary hypertension in COPD. Eur Respir J 2008;32(5): 1371–85.

101. Lettieri CJ, Nathan SD, Barnett SD, et al. Prevalence and outcomes of pulmonary arterial hypertension in advanced idiopathic pulmonary fibrosis. Chest 2006;129(3):746–52.

102. Scharf SM, Iqbal M, Keller C, et al. Hemodynamic characterization of patients with severe emphysema. Am J Respir Crit Care Med 2002;166(3):314–22.

103. Shorr AF, Helman DL, Davies DB, et al. Pulmonary hypertension in advanced sarcoidosis: epidemiology and clinical characteristics. Eur Respir J 2005;25(5):783–8.

104. Shorr AF, Wainright JL, Cors CS, et al. Pulmonary hypertension in patients with pulmonary fibrosis awaiting lung transplant. Eur Respir J 2007;30(4): 715–21.

105. Thabut G, Dauriat G, Stern JB, et al. Pulmonary hemodynamics in advanced COPD candidates for lung volume reduction surgery or lung transplantation. Chest 2005;127(5):1531–6.

106. Weitzenblum E, Moyses B, Methlin G. Relationship between pulmonary artery mean pressure and the vertical gradient of perfusion in chronic respiratory diseases. Respiration 1984;46(4):337–41.

107. Cottin V, LePavec J, Prévot G, et al. Pulmonary hypertension in patients with combined pulmonary fibrosis and emphysema syndrome. Eur Respir J 2010;35(1):105–11.

108. Cottin V, Nunes H, Brillet PY, et al. Combined pulmonary fibrosis and emphysema: a distinct underrecognised entity. Eur Respir J 2005;26(4): 586–93.

109. Hamada K, Nagai S, Tanaka S, et al. Significance of pulmonary arterial pressure and diffusion capacity of the lung as prognosticator in patients with idiopathic pulmonary fibrosis. Chest 2007; 131(3):650–6.

110. Weitzenblum E, Hirth C, Ducolone A, et al. Prognostic value of pulmonary artery pressure in chronic obstructive pulmonary disease. Thorax 1981;36(10):752–8.

111. Patel NM, Lederer DJ, Borczuk AC, et al. Pulmonary hypertension in idiopathic pulmonary fibrosis. Chest 2007;132(3):998–1006.

112. Todd NW, Lavania S, Park MH, et al. Variable prevalence of pulmonary hypertension in patients with advanced interstitial pneumonia. J Heart Lung Transplant 2010;29(2):188–94.

113. Stolz D, Rasch H, Linka A, et al. A randomised, controlled trial of bosentan in severe COPD. Eur Respir J 2008;32(3):619–28.

114. Group NOTT. Continuous or nocturnal oxygen therapy in hypoxemic chronic obstructive lung disease: a clinical trial. Nocturnal Oxygen Therapy Trial Group. Ann Intern Med 1980;93(3):391–8.

115. Party BMRC. Long term domiciliary oxygen therapy in chronic hypoxic cor pulmonale complicating chronic bronchitis and emphysema. Report of the Medical Research Council Working Party. Lancet 1981;1(8222):681–6.

116. Steen VD, Graham G, Conte C, et al. Isolated diffusing capacity reduction in systemic sclerosis. Arthritis Rheum 1992;35(7):765–70.

117. Minai OA, Ricaurte B, Kaw R, et al. Frequency and impact of pulmonary hypertension in patients with obstructive sleep apnea syndrome. Am J Cardiol 2009;104(9):1300–6.

118. Kasai T, Bradley TD. Obstructive sleep apnea and heart failure: pathophysiologic and therapeutic implications. J Am Coll Cardiol 2011;57(2):119–27.

119. Young T, Palta M, Dempsey J, et al. The occurrence of sleep-disordered breathing among middle-aged adults. N Engl J Med 1993;328(17): 1230–5.

120. Hackett PH, Roach RC. High-altitude illness. N Engl J Med 2001;345(2):107–14.

121. Maignan M, Rivera-Ch M, Privat C, et al. Pulmonary pressure and cardiac function in chronic mountain sickness patients. Chest 2009;135(2):499–504.

122. Bailey DM, Dehnert C, Luks AM, et al. High-altitude pulmonary hypertension is associated with a free radical-mediated reduction in pulmonary nitric oxide bioavailability. J Physiol 2010;588(Pt 23): 4837–47.

123. Penaloza D, Arias-Stella J. The heart and pulmonary circulation at high altitudes: healthy highlanders and chronic mountain sickness. Circulation 2007;115(9): 1132–46.

124. Becattini C, Agnelli G, Pesavento R, et al. Incidence of chronic thromboembolic pulmonary hypertension after a first episode of pulmonary embolism. Chest 2006;130(1):172–5.

125. Pengo V, Lensing AW, Prins MH, et al. Incidence of chronic thromboembolic pulmonary hypertension after pulmonary embolism. N Engl J Med 2004; 350(22):2257–64.

126. Piazza G, Goldhaber SZ. Chronic thromboembolic pulmonary hypertension. N Engl J Med 2011; 364(4):351–60.

127. Kline JA, Steuerwald MT, Marchick MR, et al. Prospective evaluation of right ventricular function and functional status 6 months after acute submassive pulmonary embolism: frequency of persistent or subsequent elevation in estimated pulmonary artery pressure. Chest 2009;136(5):1202–10.

128. Pepke-Zaba J, Delcroix M, Lang I, et al. Chronic thromboembolic pulmonary hypertension (CTEPH): results from an international prospective registry. Circulation 2011;124(18):1973–81.

129. Dentali F, Donadini M, Gianni M, et al. Incidence of chronic pulmonary hypertension in patients with previous pulmonary embolism. Thromb Res 2009; 124(3):256–8.

130. Moser KM, Braunwald NS. Successful surgical intervention in severe chronic thromboembolic pulmonary hypertension. Chest 1973;64(1):29–35.

131. Hoeper MM, Mayer E, Simonneau G, et al. Chronic thromboembolic pulmonary hypertension. Circulation 2006;113(16):2011–20.

132. Jamieson SW, Kapelanski DP, Sakakibara N, et al. Pulmonary endarterectomy: experience and lessons learned in 1,500 cases. Ann Thorac Surg 2003;76(5):1457–62 [discussion: 1462–4].

133. Lewczuk J, Piszko P, Jagas J, et al. Prognostic factors in medically treated patients with chronic pulmonary embolism. Chest 2001;119(3):818–23.

134. Mayer E, Jenkins D, Lindner J, et al. Surgical management and outcome of patients with chronic thromboembolic pulmonary hypertension: results from an international prospective registry. J Thorac Cardiovasc Surg 2011;141(3):702–10.

135. Dingli D, Utz JP, Krowka MJ, et al. Unexplained pulmonary hypertension in chronic myeloproliferative disorders. Chest 2001;120(3):801–8.

136. Jais X, Ioos V, Jardim C, et al. Splenectomy and chronic thromboembolic pulmonary hypertension. Thorax 2005;60(12):1031–4.

137. Bonderman D, Wilkens H, Wakounig S, et al. Risk factors for chronic thromboembolic pulmonary hypertension. Eur Respir J 2009;33(2):325–31.

138. Guilpain P, Montani D, Damaj G, et al. Pulmonary hypertension associated with myeloproliferative disorders: a retrospective study of ten cases. Respiration 2008;76(3):295–302.

139. Hoeper MM, Niedermeyer J, Hoffmeyer F, et al. Pulmonary hypertension after splenectomy? Ann Intern Med 1999;130(6):506–9.

140. Bourbonnais JM, Samavati L. Clinical predictors of pulmonary hypertension in sarcoidosis. Eur Respir J 2008;32(2):296–302.

141. Gluskowski J, Hawrylkiewicz I, Zych D, et al. Pulmonary haemodynamics at rest and during exercise in patients with sarcoidosis. Respiration 1984;46(1):26–32.

142. Handa T, Nagai S, Miki S, et al. Incidence of pulmonary hypertension and its clinical relevance in patients with sarcoidosis. Chest 2006;129(5):1246–52.

143. Nunes H, Humbert M, Capron F, et al. Pulmonary hypertension associated with sarcoidosis: mechanisms, haemodynamics and prognosis. Thorax 2006;61(1):68–74.

144. Dauriat G, Mal H, Thabut G, et al. Lung transplantation for pulmonary Langerhans' cell histiocytosis: a multicenter analysis. Transplantation 2006;81(5):746–50.

145. Fartoukh M, Humbert M, Capron F, et al. Severe pulmonary hypertension in histiocytosis X. Am J Respir Crit Care Med 2000;161(1):216–23.

146. Harari S, Simonneau G, De Juli E, et al. Prognostic value of pulmonary hypertension in patients with chronic interstitial lung disease referred for lung or heart-lung transplantation. J Heart Lung Transplant 1997;16(4):460–3.

147. Taveira-DaSilva AM, Hathaway OM, Sachdev V, et al. Pulmonary artery pressure in lymphangioleiomyomatosis: an echocardiographic study. Chest 2007;132(5):1573–8.

148. Aoki Y, Kodama M, Mezaki T, et al. von Recklinghausen disease complicated by pulmonary hypertension. Chest 2001;119(5):1606–8.

149. Engel PJ, Baughman RP, Menon SG, et al. Pulmonary hypertension in neurofibromatosis. Am J Cardiol 2007;99(8):1177–8.

150. Samuels N, Berkman N, Milgalter E, et al. Pulmonary hypertension secondary to neurofibromatosis: intimal fibrosis versus thromboembolism. Thorax 1999;54(9):858–9.

151. Simeoni S, Puccetti A, Chilosi M, et al. Type 1 neurofibromatosis complicated by pulmonary artery hypertension: a case report. J Med Invest 2007;54(3–4):354–8.

152. Stewart DR, Cogan JD, Kramer MR, et al. Is pulmonary arterial hypertension in neurofibromatosis type 1 secondary to a plexogenic arteriopathy? Chest 2007;132(3):798–808.

153. Launay D, Souza R, Guillevin L, et al. Pulmonary arterial hypertension in ANCA-associated vasculitis. Sarcoidosis Vasc Diffuse Lung Dis 2006;23(3):223–8.

154. Chu JW, Kao PN, Faul JL, et al. High prevalence of autoimmune thyroid disease in pulmonary arterial hypertension. Chest 2002;122(5):1668–73.

155. Ferris A, Jacobs T, Widlitz A, et al. Pulmonary arterial hypertension and thyroid disease. Chest 2001;119(6):1980–1.

156. Kokturk N, Demir N, Demircan S, et al. Pulmonary veno-occlusive disease in a patient with a history of Hashimoto's thyroiditis. Indian J Chest Dis Allied Sci 2005;47(4):289–92.

157. Li JH, Safford RE, Aduen JF, et al. Pulmonary hypertension and thyroid disease. Chest 2007;132(3):793–7.

158. Merce J, Ferras S, Oltra C, et al. Cardiovascular abnormalities in hyperthyroidism: a prospective Doppler echocardiographic study. Am J Med 2005;118(2):126–31.

159. Nakhoul F, Yigla M, Gilman R, et al. The pathogenesis of pulmonary hypertension in haemodialysis patients via arterio-venous access. Nephrol Dial Transplant 2005;20(8):1686–92.

160. Yigla M, Nakhoul F, Sabag A, et al. Pulmonary hypertension in patients with end-stage renal disease. Chest 2003;123(5):1577–82.

161. Dot JM, Sztrymf B, Yaici A, et al. Pulmonary arterial hypertension due to tumor emboli. Rev Mal Respir 2007;24(3 Pt 1):359–66 [in French].

162. McCabe JM, Bhave PD, McGlothlin D, et al. Running from her past: a case of rapidly progressive dyspnea on exertion. Circulation 2011;124(21):2355–61.

163. Davis AM, Pierson RN, Loyd JE. Mediastinal fibrosis. Semin Respir Infect 2001;16(2):119–30.

164. Goodwin RA, Nickell JA, Des Prez RM. Mediastinal fibrosis complicating healed primary histoplasmosis and tuberculosis. Medicine 1972;51(3):227–46.

165. Loyd JE, Tillman BF, Atkinson JB, et al. Mediastinal fibrosis complicating histoplasmosis. Medicine 1988;67(5):295–310.

Genetics and Pharmacogenomics in Pulmonary Arterial Hypertension

Benjamin P. Smith, MD[a], D. Hunter Best, BS, PhD[b,c],
C. Gregory Elliott, MD[d,e],*

KEYWORDS

- Genetics • Pharmacogenomics • Pulmonary arterial hypertension

KEY POINTS

- With the discoveries that mutations with the *BMPR2*, *ACVRL1*, and *ENG* genes lead to the phenotypic expression of PAH, there have been advances in our understanding of PAH pathogenesis.
- There is variability in phenotypic expression of PAH causing mutations among family members due to incomplete penetrance, genetic anticipation, and possibly environmental factors.
- The presence of mutations within the *BMPR2* and *ACVRL1* genes are associated with a less favorable clinical response to therapy (acute vasoreactivity), and an overall poorer prognosis.
- Continued advances in molecular and genetic analysis may help us to further our understanding of both the pathophysiology of PAH, as well as the development of patient specific, disease modifying therapies.

INTRODUCTION TO PAH

Pulmonary arterial hypertension (PAH) remains an uncommon disease in the general population, but a disease with significant morbidity and mortality nonetheless. The natural history of PAH includes increases in pulmonary vascular resistance (PVR) and mean pulmonary artery pressure (mPAP), leading to either sudden cardiac death or death from progressive right ventricular failure.[1] Effective therapies are available, although no therapy provides a cure.

PAH is a clinical diagnosis, which cannot be made accurately without obtaining hemodynamic measurements by right heart catheterization (RHC). The current hemodynamic definition of PAH is an mPAP 25 mm Hg or greater; a pulmonary capillary wedge pressure 15 mm Hg or less; and a PVR greater than 3 Wood units.[2] At the time of a diagnostic RHC, acute vasoreactivity testing should be

Disclosure: BPS is a Co-Investigator on an Intermountain Research & Medical Foundation grant. DHB has nothing to disclose except his employment with ARUP. CGE is employed by Intermountain Healthcare (IHC Health Services). In the last 12 months IHC Health Services has received compensation for clinical trial contracts (on which Dr Elliott is the Principal Investigator) from Actelion, United Therapeutics, and Gilead. CGE is currently the Principal Investigator on an Intermountain Research & Medical Foundation grant and in the past 12 months, has served as a consultant to Bayer Pharmaceuticals and received an honorarium, plus reimbursement for travel expenses. CGE also served on the Data and Safety Monitoring Board for Pfizer. CGE has also received honoraria for his service on the REVEAL Steering Committee, which is supported by Actelion.

[a] Division of Pulmonary and Critical Care Medicine, University of Utah, Maxwell Wintrobe Research Building, 26 North Medical Drive, Room 743, Salt Lake City, UT 84132, USA; [b] Department of Pathology, University of Utah School of Medicine, 500 Chipeta Way, Salt Lake City, UT 84108-1221, USA; [c] Genetics Division, Associated Regional and University Pathologists (ARUP), 500 Chipeta Way, Salt Lake City, UT 84108-1221, USA; [d] Department of Internal Medicine, University of Utah, 30 North 1900 East, Salt Lake City, UT 84132, USA; [e] Department of Medicine, Intermountain Medical Center, 5121 South Cottonwood Street, #307, Murray, UT 84107, USA
* Corresponding author. Department of Medicine, Intermountain Medical Center, 5121 South Cottonwood Street, #307, Murray, UT 84107.
E-mail address: greg.elliott@imail.org

Heart Failure Clin 8 (2012) 319–330
doi:10.1016/j.hfc.2012.04.008
1551-7136/12/$ – see front matter © 2012 Elsevier Inc. All rights reserved.

performed for most patients with PAH. A positive vasodilator response identifies a small subgroup of patients who have an excellent prognosis when treated with high doses of calcium channel blockers such as diltiazem or nifedipine.[3,4] The hemodynamic definition of a positive acute vasoreactivity test includes a reduction in mPAP of at least 10 mm Hg to an absolute mPAP less than 40 mm Hg, with a preserved or increased cardiac output.[5]

The most recent clinical classification of pulmonary hypertension from the Fourth World Symposium on Pulmonary Hypertension includes 5 major diagnostic subgroups, with group 1 encompassing PAH (**Box 1**). Within group 1, the diagnoses include idiopathic PAH (IPAH) (formerly referred to as primary pulmonary hypertension [PPH]), heritable PAH (HPAH), and PAH associated with a variety of circumstances (APAH) (eg, drug-induced and toxin-induced, congenital heart diseases, connective tissue diseases, portal hypertension, and human immunodeficiency virus [HIV] infection).[6] The Fourth World Symposium on Pulmonary Hypertension revised group 1 to include the subcategory HPAH. This subcategory includes PAH cases with either more than 1 family member diagnosed with PAH or the presence of an identifiable germline mutation within the transforming growth factor β (TGF-β) signaling family known to be associated with familial cases of PAH.[7–9] When considering a link between genetic markers, the development of PAH, and disease behavior, it is within group 1 pulmonary hypertension that the work has begun.

PREVALENCE OF HPAH

The prevalence of HPAH remains unknown. Twelve of 187 (6.4%) patients in the US National Institutes of Health (NIH) PPH Registry had 1 or more family members affected with PPH.[10] These results are similar to those found in the national PAH registry in France, which reported 9.0% of 290 enrolled patients without APAH having familial PAH (FPAH).[11] The REVEAL Registry (Registry to Evaluate Early and Long Term PAH Disease Management) is the largest registry of World Health Organization (WHO) group 1 patients to date, with 2525 adult patients meeting traditional hemodynamic criteria for PAH. In this registry, investigators diagnosed FPAH in 5.5% of 1234 patients who did not have APAH and 3% of the total cohort diagnosed with group 1 PAH.[12] These reports likely underestimate proportions of HPAH because of small family pedigrees, fragmented families, unknown medical histories, incomplete penetrance, and the lack of regular testing for genetic mutations known to be linked with PAH. When genetic testing is performed, the proportion of

patients with sporadic PAH or IPAH who carry a germline mutation known to be associated with PAH is approximately 25%.[13] When genetic testing is combined with family histories, the estimated prevalence of HPAH among patients with PAH seems closer to 15% (**Fig. 1**).

Introduction to the Genetics and Inheritance of PAH

The first familial case of PPH was described by Dresdale in 1954,[14] when he reported PPH in a mother, her sister, and her son. By 1984, Loyd and colleagues[15] described 14 families with 2 or more members affected by PPH. There was vertical transmission between generations in 10 of the 14 families. Furthermore, there was an example of disease transmission from a father to son, and a grandfather to a granddaughter through a father, which excluded X-linked inheritance. Together these pedigrees suggested an autosomal-dominant mode of inheritance.

INCOMPLETE PENETRANCE

The transmission of PPH through 9 individuals who were without evidence of disease was another important observation from the pedigrees assembled by Loyd.[15] These obligate carriers of a disease-causing gene without PPH suggested that incomplete genetic penetrance also characterizes FPAH (**Fig. 2**). It seems that the lifetime risk of developing PAH is only 10% to 20% for carriers of disease-causing mutations.[16]

The reason for incomplete penetrance among HPAH pedigrees is not well understood. The only clear predilection for the development of PAH within families is female gender. The idea of a second hit is a popular concept that is not unlike that regarding the development of many malignancies. The concept suggests an interplay between a genetic predisposition and either an environmental stimulus or another genetic abnormality that leads to clinical expression of the disease. What this second hit may be is not clear.

GENETIC ANTICIPATION

The earlier onset of more severe disease in successive generations was identifiable in previous pedigree analyses as well (see **Fig. 2**).[15] Based on analyses of pedigrees it appeared that family members affected with PAH in each successive generation had a life expectancy approximately 10 years shorter than the previous generation. The concept of genetic anticipation in FPAH has been scrutinized, in the belief that an ascertainment bias exists in the evaluation of familial cases because of a heightened awareness

---

Box 1
Updated Clinical Classification of Pulmonary Hypertension (Dana Point, 2008)

1. Pulmonary arterial hypertension (PAH)

    1.1. Idiopathic PAH

    1.2. Heritable

        1.2.1. BMPR2

        1.2.2. ALK1, endoglin (with or without hereditary hemorrhagic telangiectasia)

        1.2.3. Unknown

    1.3. Drug- and toxin-induced

    1.4. Associated with

        1.4.1. Connective tissue diseases

        1.4.2. HIV infection

        1.4.3. Portal hypertension

        1.4.4. Congenital heart diseases

        1.4.5. Schistosomiasis

        1.4.6. Chronic hemolytic anemia

    1.5. Persistent pulmonary hypertension of the newborn

    1.6. Pulmonary veno-occlusive disease (PVOD) and/or pulmonary capillary hemangiomatosis (PCH)

2. Pulmonary hypertension owing to left heart disease

    2.1. Systolic dysfunction

    2.2. Diastolic dysfunction

    2.3. Valvular disease

3. Pulmonary hypertension owing to lung diseases and/or hypoxia

    3.1. Chronic obstructive pulmonary disease

    3.2. Interstitial lung disease

    3.3. Other pulmonary diseases with mixed restrictive and obstructive pattern

    3.4. Sleep-disordered breathing

    3.5. Alveolar hypoventilation disorders

    3.6. Chronic exposure to high altitude

    3.7. Developmental abnormalities

4. Chronic thromboembolic pulmonary hypertension (CTEPH)

5. Pulmonary hypertension with unclear multifactorial mechanisms

    5.1. Hemtologic disorders: myeloproliferative disorders, splenectomy

    5.2. Systemic disorders: sarcoidosis, pulmonary Langerhans cell histiocytosis: lymphangioleiomyomatosis, neurofibromatosis, vasculitis

    5.3. Metabolic disorders: glycogen storage disease, Gaucher disease, thyroid disorders

    5.4. Others: tumoral obstruction, fibrosing mediastinitis, chronic renal failure on dialysis

From Simonneau G, Robbins IM, Beghetti M, et al. Updated clinical classification of pulmonary hypertension. J Am Coll Cardiol 2009;54(Suppl 1):S45; with permission.

---

of the disease within an affected family. There was an attempt to control for this potential bias in a study of 60 pairs of an affected parent and child. When the age of death was compared among consecutive generations, it was confirmed that there was an earlier age of death.[17]

Other disorders display genetic anticipation, including Huntington disease, myotonic dystrophy

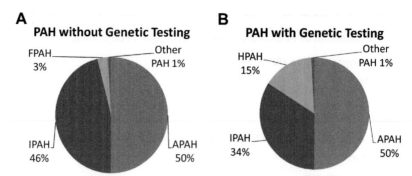

A
PAH without Genetic Testing

FPAH 3% — Other PAH 1%
IPAH 46%
APAH 50%

B
PAH with Genetic Testing

HPAH 15% — Other PAH 1%
IPAH 34%
APAH 50%

Fig. 1. WHO group 1 PAH classification. (*A*) WHO group 1 classification from the REVEAL Registry. Using family histories only, FPAH represents approximately 3% of patients with PAH. (*B*) When using genetic testing in cases of sporadic or IPAH, approximately 25% of patients have a germline mutation known to be associated with PAH, making the prevalence of HPAH a larger proportion of patients with PAH. Other PAH, pulmonary capillary hemangiomatosis, pulmonary hypertension of the newborn, pulmonary veno-occlusive disease. ([*A*] *Modified form* Badesch DB, Raskob GE, Elliott CG, et al. Pulmonary arterial hypertension: baseline characteristics from the REVEAL Registry. Chest 2010;137(2):379, with permission; and [*B*] *Data from* Thomson JR, Machado RD, Pauciulo MW, et al. Sporadic primary pulmonary hypertension is associated with germline mutations of the gene encoding BMPR-II, a receptor member of the TGF-beta family. J Med Genet 2000;37(10):741–5.)

type 1, and spinocerebellar ataxia. In these disorders, an association of genetic anticipation with trinucleotide repeat expansions (TRE) has been identified.[18] The magnitude of a TRE can lead to the phenotypic expression of a disease with such non-Mendelian inheritance patterns. However, with respect to HPAH, there is no obvious molecular cause for the apparent genetic anticipation.

COMMON ANCESTRY

Investigators also considered the possibility that many patients diagnosed with sporadic PPH may have unrecognized familial PPH.[19] A study of 7 patients with sporadic PPH identified in Utah as part of the NIH PPH Registry successfully showed coancestry, which was unlikely to have been a chance occurrence.[20] A subsequent report

FAMILY 5 n = 71

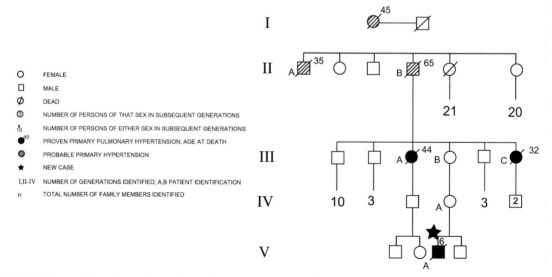

O	FEMALE
□	MALE
Ø	DEAD
⊙	NUMBER OF PERSONS OF THAT SEX IN SUBSEQUENT GENERATIONS
⬧	NUMBER OF PERSONS OF EITHER SEX IN SUBSEQUENT GENERATIONS
●	PROVEN PRIMARY PULMONARY HYPERTENSION; AGE AT DEATH
⊘	PROBABLE PRIMARY HYPERTENSION
★	NEW CASE
I,II-IV	NUMBER OF GENERATIONS IDENTIFIED; A,B PATIENT IDENTIFICATION
n	TOTAL NUMBER OF FAMILY MEMBERS IDENTIFIED

Fig. 2. This family pedigree shows incomplete penetrance. Family member V-A died of PPH. It was later discovered that the grandmother (III-B) had PPH. This situation makes the mother (IV-A) an obligate carrier of the familial gene. This pedigree also shows genetic anticipation. Starting with family member II-B, deaths secondary to PPH in subsequent generations occurred at earlier ages. (Pedigree from family 5.) (*From* Loyd JE, Primm RK, Newman JH. Familial primary pulmonary hypertension: clinical patterns. Am Rev Respir Dis 1984;129(1):194–7; with permission.)

uncovered a kindred affected by familial PPH that spanned 7 generations and involved 5 subfamilies initially not known to be related.[21] This kindred included 12 affected members who were initially believed to have sporadic PPH and 7 affected members whose conditions were first misdiagnosed as other cardiopulmonary diseases.

THE DISCOVERY OF MUTATIONS IN THE BONE MORPHOGENETIC PROTEIN RECEPTOR TYPE 2 GENE

Investigators at Vanderbilt and Columbia Universities assembled familial PPH pedigrees, identified affected and unaffected individuals, and collected DNA samples. By the 1990s, enough DNA samples from these patients had been stored to provide the power necessary for a genome-wide search for a familial PPH locus. In 1997, 2 independent teams performed linkage studies using microsatellite DNA probes and identified a PPH gene locus on chromosome 2q31-32.[22,23] Three years later, the same teams of investigators independently characterized mutations in a gene within this chromosomal locus among familial cases of PPH. The gene identified encoded the protein bone morphogenetic protein receptor type II (BMPRII), a member of the TGF-β superfamily of receptors.[7,8] Since that time, mutations have been identified in activin receptor-like kinase 1 (ACVRL1) and endoglin (ENG) genes, both members of the TGF-β superfamily, associated with the development of hereditary hemorrhagic telangectasia (HHT) and PAH.[9] Even with these discoveries, there remains up to 30% of patients with FPAH without an identified genetic abnormality.[24,25]

Also in the year 2000, 50 unrelated, sporadic cases of PPH were analyzed for the presence of mutations in BMPR2. Eleven novel heterozygous mutations in BMPR2 were discovered in 13 of 50 patients, suggesting a common genetic pathway in both familial and some sporadic cases of PAH.[13] The current understanding of BMPR2 germline mutations in IPAH cases is that 10% to 40% of such cases have a detectable mutation.[13,25,26] However, in some of these cases, the mutation is a de novo mutation.[13,27]

BMPRII STRUCTURE AND FUNCTION

The BMPRII receptor consists of 4 functional domains: an N-terminal ligand binding domain, a single transmembrane region, a serine/threonine-kinase, and a cytoplasmic domain. BMPRII functions as a receptor for a group of cytokines known as bone morphogenetic proteins (BMPs), the signaling pathway of which affects cellular function in a tissue-specific manner. BMPs may influence cellular proliferation, migration, differentiation, and apoptosis, as well as extracellular matrix secretion and deposition.[16] Within the pulmonary circulation, it is thought that the BMPRII pathway leads to inhibition of cellular proliferation, especially within pulmonary arterial smooth muscle cells.[28]

METHODOLOGY OF DETECTING BMPR2 MUTATIONS

Originally, BMPR2 clinical testing included Sanger sequencing of the patient's DNA for the entire coding region of the gene (exons 1–13), as well as the intron/exon boundaries, allowing screening for mutations that can lead to aberrant gene splicing. Then in 2005, Cogan and colleagues[29] reported that approximately 30% of familial patients with PAH who were negative for BMPR2 mutations by sequence analysis had large deletions or duplications in the BMPR2 gene. This study showed the limitations of solely performing DNA sequencing, and as a result, Southern blotting and mRNA analysis by reverse-transcriptase polymerase chain reaction (RT-PCR) were incorporated into PAH clinical testing protocols. By the inclusion of this methodology, laboratories were able to detect large gene rearrangements and further increase the sensitivity of the test. However, these methods can be labor intensive and costly, and therefore are not ideal for the clinical setting. Recent technological advances have seen the replacement of the Southern blotting/RT-PCR protocols with multiplex ligation-dependent probe amplification (MLPA).[30] MLPA is a simple technique that allows detection of large deletions or duplications in a gene directly from a DNA sample in a rapid and cost-effective manner.[30] With the addition of MLPA to PAH testing protocols, laboratories are able to offer BMPR2 mutation testing in a more timely fashion compared with the standard combination of DNA sequencing and Southern blotting.

MUTATION HETEROGENEITY OF BMPR2

A total of 298 mutations have been identified throughout the BMPR2 gene, with the exception of exon 13.[16] All types of mutations have been described, with approximately two-thirds of mutations (203 of 298) predicting premature truncation of the protein. Of the premature truncation mutations, 29% are nonsense mutations (85 of 298), 24% are frameshift mutations (73 of 298), 9% are splice-site mutations (26 of 298), and 6% are of the duplication/deletion variety (19 of 298).[16] Regardless of the exon mutation site or the type of mutation, the result is haploinsufficiency of the BMPRII signaling pathway, and a failure of antiproliferative effects within the pulmonary vasculature (**Fig. 3**).[27,28]

BMPR2 MUTATIONS IN OTHER FORMS OF PAH
Anorexigen-associated PAH

In cases of anorexigen-associated PAH, the exact mechanism responsible for the development of PAH remains unknown. Approximately 1 in 10,000 people exposed to fenfluramine derivatives developed PAH, and attempts were made to uncover a link between BMPR2 mutations and the development of PAH in such patients. Humbert and colleagues[31] examined 33 unrelated patients with anorexigen-associated PAH and 2 affected sisters

and found 3 mutations in BMPR2 that predicted alterations in the BMPRII protein structure in the 33 unrelated cases (9%), and a fourth mutation among the 2 sisters. Despite these findings, it seems that a germline mutation in BMPR2 establishing a genetic predisposition is not a frequent enough occurrence to propose that exposure to fenfluramine derivatives provided a second hit leading to the development of PAH. However, when compared with mutation-negative patients, those patients with a BMPR2 mutation and anorexigen exposure had a shorter duration of fenfluramine exposure before the onset of symptoms.[31] This finding, along with the higher prevalence of both BMPR2 mutations and PAH among the population exposed to fenfluramine when compared with the general population, suggests that in some cases the development of PAH may have been a result of a genetic (BMPR2) and environmental (fenfluramine) interaction.

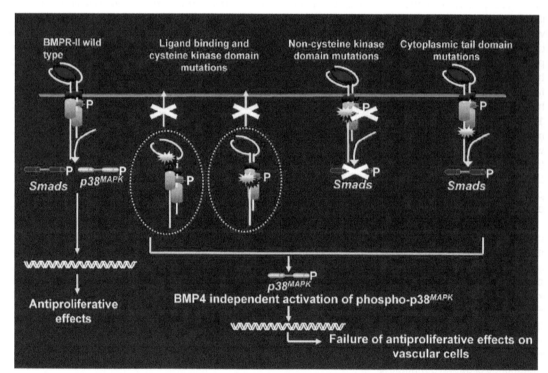

Fig. 3. The wild-type BMPR2 function leads to phosphorylation of the Smad and p38MAPK pathways with antiproliferative effects. Some mutations that occur may lead to nonsense mediated messenger RNA decay and failure to express protein. There may also be mutations in the ligand binding domain, the kinase domain, that lead to either a lack of trafficking to the cell surface or loss of function. The mechanism in which BMPR2 mutants disrupt signaling is heterogeneous and mutation specific. The result, whether the protein never reaches the cell surface or fails to activate the Smad pathway, is haploinsufficiency. A feature common to all mutations is a gain of function involving p38MAPK activation. This imbalance between the Smad and p38MAPk pathway is believed to lead to increased cellular proliferation and contributes to the pathologic lesions seen in PAH. (*From* Humbert M, Morrell NW, Archer SL, et al. Cellular and molecular pathobiology of pulmonary arterial hypertension. J Am Coll Cardiol 2004;43(12 Suppl S):20S; with permission.)

Congenital Systemic to Pulmonary Shunts

TGF-β receptors have pivotal roles in cardiac embryogenesis and vascular development. Roberts and colleagues[32] explored the potential relationship of PAH and genetic mutations within BMPR2 in 40 adults and 66 children with PAH associated with congenital heart disease (CHD) (APAH-CHD). BMPR2 mutations were found in 6% of cases from this mixed cohort and consisted of mutations in the extracellular ligand binding domain, the kinase domain, and the cytoplasmic tail domain. The observed frequency of BMPR2 mutations in patients with APAH-CHD when compared with the general population suggests a potential pathophysiologic role of BMPR2 mutations in the development of APAH-CHD; however, the evidence does not support a fundamental mechanism for most patients with APAH-CHD.

Connective tissue diseases, HIV infection, and portal hypertension

PAH is also associated with connective tissue diseases (APAH-CTD), infection with HIV, and portal hypertension. Although one-third of patients with the scleroderma spectrum of disease develop PAH, 2 small studies have failed to show BMPR2 mutations among patients with APAH-CTD.[33,34] An equally small study examined PAH associated with HIV infection and failed to identify BMPR2 mutations.[35] Furthermore, there are no reports of BMPR2 mutations associated with portopulmonary hypertension. However, investigators have associated portopulmonary hypertension with single nucleotide polymorphisms (SNPs) in genes related to estrogen signaling and cell growth regulation.[36]

Mutations in the activin receptor-like kinase-1 gene in PAH

One year after the discovery of the role of BMPR2 mutations in PAH, a study was conducted to identify other potential genetic components of PAH.[9] The investigators of this study noted that patients suffering from the autosomal-dominant genetic disorder HHT sometimes present with PAH.[9] These investigators identified 10 patients suffering from both HHT and PAH and screened them for mutations in the BMPR2 gene as well as the activin receptor-like kinase-1 (ACVRL1) gene, and reported that patients suffering from both HHT and PAH commonly had mutations in the ACVRL1 (formerly ALK1) gene. Additional studies on 14 probands with clinical symptoms of both HHT and PAH identified 8 novel ACVRL1 missense mutations.[37]

ALK-1 Protein Structure and Function

The protein produced by the ACVRL1 gene is called ALK-1 (also known as serine/threonine-protein kinase receptor R3). The ALK-1 protein comprises 3 main functional domains: an extracellular domain, a transmembrane domain, and an intracellular domain.[38–40] In the wild-type cell, the extracellular domain mainly functions in ligand binding but it is also involved in complex formation with type II TGF-β receptor (TRβII).[38,40,41]

Associated pathophysiology of ALK-1

Mutations in the ACVRL1 gene are primarily associated with HHT, an autosomal-dominant vascular dysplasia characterized by the presence of arteriovenous malformations, recurrent epistaxis, and mucocutaneous telangiectasias.[42,43] More recently, mutations in this gene have been implicated in the development of pulmonary hypertension (with or without symptoms of HHT).[9,37,43,44] Although more than 100 ACVRL1 mutations have been described that result in the development of HHT, only a select few have been associated with PAH.[9,16,37,43,44] The bulk of PAH-causing ACVRL1 mutations are missense mutations that occur in ALK-1 functional domains (ie, the kinase domain).[16] Functional studies using ALK-1 mutant constructs suggest that disruption of receptor complex trafficking is the primary cause of the vascular phenotype observed in these patients.[37,43]

Clinical outcomes in patients with PAH with ACVRL1 mutations

Although rare, the role of ACVRL1 mutations in PAH has been the focus of several studies.[9,37,43,44] In each of these studies, it has been noted that the disease onset in ACVRL1 mutation carriers occurs at a young age and that disease characteristics seem to be severe compared with mutation-negative patients with PAH. Perhaps the most striking findings were reported by Girerd and colleagues,[44] who performed ACVRL1 and BMPR2 mutation analysis on 379 of the 388 patients in the French PAH network. These investigators identified 93 BMPR2 mutation-positive patients and 9 ACVRL1 mutation-positive patients and an additional 23 ACVRL1 mutation-positive patients with PAH from previous publications. The investigators compared ACVRL1 mutation-positive patients with PAH to BMPR2 mutation-positive patients and found that patients harboring ACVRL1 mutations were significantly younger at diagnosis and at death than BMPR2-positive patients. Together these findings suggest that disease is more severe in patients with PAH with ACVRL1 mutations and these patients have an overall poorer prognosis when compared with all other groups of patients with PAH.

Mutations in the Endoglin Gene in PAH

Shortly after the discovery that *ACVRL1* mutations were involved in the development of PAH, investigators examined the endoglin gene (*ENG*), as a potential genetic cause of PAH. Harrison and colleagues[37] performed DNA sequencing for the *BMPR2*, *ACVRL1*, and *ENG* genes on a cohort of 11 patients suffering from HPAH and showed an *ENG* frameshift mutation in 2 of the 11 patients, suggesting that *ENG* mutations can cause PAH. In a subsequent study of 18 children with a clinical diagnosis of PAH, 1 child harbored an intronic splicing mutation in the *ENG* gene.[43]

ENG STRUCTURE AND FUNCTION

The protein produced by the *ENG* gene is also known as ENG (or endoglin) and is a transmembrane glycoprotein that is expressed predominantly on endothelial cells.[45,46] The ENG protein contains 3 main functional domains: a cytoplasmic domain, involved in regulating dimerization and protein trafficking activity, a transmembrane domain, and an extracellular domain, which is important in the interactions of the protein with other signaling proteins.[45,46] Like ALK-1, ENG is a member of the TGF-β superfamily of receptors that interact with both type I and type II TGF-β signaling receptors to control cellular responses to TGF-β.[45] However, unlike many receptors in this superfamily, ENG is not capable of binding a ligand unless it is already bound to a TGF-β signaling receptor.[45] Recently, functional studies have suggested that wild-type ENG is important in angiogenesis, and that mutations in the *ENG* gene likely result in haploinsufficiency. The remaining wild-type protein is not capable of maintaining proper angiogenesis, vascular malformations, inappropriate proliferation of endothelial cells, and the disease phenotype observed in patients with HHT.[47]

GENETIC SCREENING

Two consensus guidelines recommend that physicians offer genetic testing and professional genetic counseling to relatives of patients with HPAH.[2,48] In addition, the investigators of these guidelines have recommended that patients with IPAH be advised about the availability of genetic testing and counseling because of the possibility that they carry a disease-causing mutation. In either circumstance, the identification of a disease-causing mutation may be useful for early disease recognition and for family planning.

Clinical monitoring of *BMPR2* mutation carriers remains an inexact science with respect to which test(s) to perform and the frequency of testing. The American College of Cardiology Foundation and the American Heart Association expert consensus[2] task force on pulmonary hypertension recommended that *BMPR2* mutation carriers should be screened annually by echocardiography and that an RHC should be performed if an echocardiogram showed evidence of PAH.[2] The American College of Chest Physicians expert consensus group also recommended Doppler echocardiography for asymptomatic patients at high risk, without stating at what time intervals echocardiography should be repeated. Several centers offer genetic testing and counseling approved by the Clinical Laboratory Improvement Amendments for patients with PAH and their family members.

Physicians, patients with PAH, and their family members have not embraced these guidelines for several reasons. First, genetic testing is expensive ($1000–$3000 to analyze the first proband; and $300–$500 to test other family members for a known family-specific mutation). Second, the psychological impact of either a positive test (anxiety and depression) or a negative test (survivor guilt) is important for some individuals, and test results may affect other family members who do not wish to know their mutational status. Third, concerns over discrimination remain, despite the passage of the Genetic Information Non-discrimination Act (GINA, HR493). Although GINA protects against discrimination by insurers and employers, there are some gaps in GINA protections (eg, when applying for life, disability or long-term insurance; or when employed by a business with fewer than 15 employees).

PHARMACOGENETICS OF PAH

A patient's clinical response to disease-specific therapy is complex, involving the severity of the patient's disease, other comorbidities, appropriateness of the prescribed therapy, and patient compliance. It has been stated that approximately 30% of patients benefit from a given medication, whereas another 30% of patients show no benefit at all. Furthermore, 30% of patients are noncompliant with their medication, and the remaining 10% experience only side effects from the medication.[49] This unpredictable response means that a given therapy has the potential to be ineffective, harmful, or to allow progression of untreated illness. In an ideal scenario, medical therapy would be tailored to an individual, with a predictable response that included maximum benefit and no harm.

Pharmacogenetics (the science of effects of single gene variants on drug efficacy and toxicity) and pharmacogenomics (the science of multiple interacting gene variants on drug efficacy and toxicity) both offer the promise of pharmacotherapy uniquely targeted to individual patients.[49] Although physicians have always individualized treatment, the hope is that knowledge of the patient's genes would advance the safety and efficacy of medical therapeutics. Such an advance would be welcome for physicians who treat PAH, because therapeutic responses and drug toxicities are unpredictable for individual patients (**Fig. 4**).[50]

For a given medication to have its desired effect, several steps may be required. A medication may need to be absorbed across a membrane, transported via carrier proteins to a cellular target, interact with cell-specific receptors, and then be eliminated from the body. These steps often involve various enzymatic activities, which may be altered by genetic polymorphisms. Advances in pharmacogenetics in terms of variable pharmacokinetics, bioavailability, and metabolism of several medications, such as warfarin, phenytoin, some cardiovascular drugs, and antipsychotics, have occurred already. These discoveries stem from an understanding of the genetic variability seen in multiple enzymatic pathways, like the cytochrome P450 enzymes.[49] Although many polymorphisms exist in relevant biologic pathways,

(eg, endothelin[51]) little is known about the pharmacogenetics of PAH-specific therapies.

WARFARIN DOSING

Warfarin is often used as an adjuvant therapy in patients with PAH. The cytochrome P450 isoform CYP2C9 and the vitamin K epoxide reductase complex subunit 1 (VKORC1) are the enzymes primarily responsible for warfarin oxidative metabolism.[52] Two common SNP within the CYP2C9 gene have been shown to be associated with reduced enzymatic metabolism of warfarin and lower dose requirements. When compared with the wild-type allele, SNP *2 results in 14% to 20% lower warfarin dose requirements, and SNP *3 is associated with a 21% to 49% reduction in warfarin dose.[53] In addition, 10 VKORC1 polymorphisms have been described that are associated with variable warfarin dose requirements.[52]

Algorithms that incorporate knowledge of a patient's genotype for CYP2C9 or VKORC1 have led to more accurate dosing at the time of warfarin initiation.[52,53] Anderson and colleagues[52] used knowledge of SNPs within CYP2C9 and VKORC1 for purposes of warfarin initiation and management, and compared this method with standard prescription practices. Pharmacogenetic-guided therapy decreased the number of dose adjustments, although total adverse events and serious clinical events were not different between prescribing practices.[52]

CALCIUM CHANNEL BLOCKERS AND VASOREACTIVITY

Because of the favorable prognostic implications and survival benefit, it is important to determine whether or not a patient displays acute vasoreactivity in response to a pulmonary vasodilator agent during a diagnostic RHC. Using the current definition for vasoreactivity, approximately 10% of patients with IPAH have a positive acute vasoreactivity test, which predicts an approximate 95% 5-year survival in response to prolonged oral calcium channel blocker therapy.[3,4]

It is possible that genetic tests can identify a marker that can identify patients with PAH who are not candidates for calcium channel blocker monotherapy. Elliott and colleagues[54] evaluated 52 patients with IPAH and 15 patients with FPAH. Twenty-seven of 67 patients were found to have a nonsynonymous BMPR2 mutation. Using the current definition of acute vasoreactivity, these investigators showed that 3.7% of patients with PAH with a nonsynonymous BMPR2 mutation were vasoreactive compared with 35% of patients

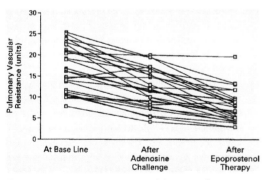

Fig. 4. Long-term epoprostenol improved symptoms and hemodynamics for 26 of 27 patients. On average, PVR declined by 53%. However, individual responses to epoprostenol varied. Genetic differences may underlie the variation in individual response to PAH-specific medications like epoprostenol. (*From* McLaughlin VV, Genthner DE, Panella MM, et al. Reduction in pulmonary vascular resistance with long-term epoprostenol (prostacyclin) therapy in primary pulmonary hypertension. N Engl J Med 1998;338(5):276; with permission.)

without a nonsynonymous *BMPR2* mutation. Similar results were subsequently found in a cohort of 147 children and adults with IPAH and FPAH, in whom again the presence of *BMPR2* mutations was associated with nonvasoreactivity (4% vs 33%).[55] In addition, Sztrymf and colleagues[56] examined 379 patients with either IPAH or FPAH. The patients with *BMPR2* mutations were unlikely to be acutely vasoreactive at diagnostic RHC. The small number of patients who were positive for an *ACVRL1* mutation were also universally nonvasoreactive when compared with patients with PAH who were not carriers of an *ACVRL1* mutation.[44] Thus, the presence of a mutation in the TGF-β superfamily of receptors seems to identify a population of patients with PAH for whom calcium channel blockers are ineffective.

SUMMARY

With the discoveries that mutations within the *BMPR2*, *ACVRL1*, and *ENG* genes lead to the phenotypic expression of PAH, there have been advances in our understanding of PAH pathogenesis. Furthermore, there is variability in the phenotypic expression of PAH causing mutations among family members due to incomplete penetrance, genetic anticipation, and possibly environmental factors. The presence of mutations within the *BMPR2* and *ACVRL1* genes are associated with a less favorable clinical response to therapy (acute vasoreactivity), and an overall poorer prognosis. However, continued advances in molecular and genetic analysis may help us to further our understanding of both the pathobiology of PAH, as well as the development of patient specific, disease modifying therapies.

REFERENCES

1. Rubin LJ. Primary pulmonary hypertension. Chest 1993;104(1):236–50.
2. McLaughlin VV, Archer SL, Badesch DB, et al. ACCF/AHA 2009 expert consensus document on pulmonary hypertension: a report of the American College of Cardiology Foundation Task Force on Expert Consensus Documents and the American Heart Association: developed in collaboration with the American College of Chest Physicians, American Thoracic Society, Inc., and the Pulmonary Hypertension Association. Circulation 2009; 119(16):2250–94.
3. Rich S, Kaufmann E, Levy PS. The effect of high doses of calcium-channel blockers on survival in primary pulmonary hypertension. N Engl J Med 1992;327(2):76–81.
4. Sitbon O, Humbert M, Jais X, et al. Long-term response to calcium channel blockers in idiopathic pulmonary arterial hypertension. Circulation 2005; 111(23):3105–11.
5. Badesch DB, Abman SH, Ahearn GS, et al. Medical therapy for pulmonary arterial hypertension: ACCP evidence-based clinical practice guidelines. Chest 2004;126(Suppl 1):35S–62S.
6. Simonneau G, Robbins IM, Beghetti M, et al. Updated clinical classification of pulmonary hypertension. J Am Coll Cardiol 2009;54(1 Suppl 1):S43–54.
7. Deng Z, Morse JH, Slager SL, et al. Familial primary pulmonary hypertension (gene PPH1) is caused by mutations in the bone morphogenetic protein receptor-II gene. Am J Hum Genet 2000;67(3): 737–44.
8. Lane KB, Machado RD, Pauciulo MW, et al. Heterozygous germline mutations in BMPR2, encoding a TGF-beta receptor, cause familial primary pulmonary hypertension. The International PPH Consortium. Nat Genet 2000;26(1):81–4.
9. Trembath RC, Thomson JR, Machado RD, et al. Clinical and molecular genetic features of pulmonary hypertension in patients with hereditary hemorrhagic telangiectasia. N Engl J Med 2001;345(5):325–34.
10. Rich S, Dantzker DR, Ayres SM, et al. Primary pulmonary hypertension: a national prospective study. Ann Intern Med 1987;107(2):216–23.
11. Humbert M, Sitbon O, Chaouat A, et al. Pulmonary arterial hypertension in France: results from a national registry. Am J Respir Crit Care Med 2006;173(9):1023–30.
12. Badesch DB, Raskob GE, Elliott CG, et al. Pulmonary arterial hypertension: baseline characteristics from the REVEAL Registry. Chest 2010;137(2):376–87.
13. Thomson JR, Machado RD, Pauciulo MW, et al. Sporadic primary pulmonary hypertension is associated with germline mutations of the gene encoding BMPR-II, a receptor member of the TGF-beta family. J Med Genet 2000;37(10):741–5.
14. Dresdale DT, Michtom RJ, Schultz M. Recent studies in primary pulmonary hypertension, including pharmacodynamic observations on pulmonary vascular resistance. Bull N Y Acad Med 1954;30(3):195–207.
15. Loyd JE, Primm RK, Newman JH. Familial primary pulmonary hypertension: clinical patterns. Am Rev Respir Dis 1984;129(1):194–7.
16. Machado RD, Eickelberg O, Elliott CG, et al. Genetics and genomics of pulmonary arterial hypertension. J Am Coll Cardiol 2009;54(1 Suppl 1):S32–42.
17. Loyd J, Butler M, Foroud T, et al. Genetic anticipation and abnormal gender ratio at birth in familial primary pulmonary hypertension. Am J Respir Crit Care Med 1995;152(1):93–7.
18. Ashley CT Jr, Warren ST. Trinucleotide repeat expansion and human disease. Annu Rev Genet 1995;29: 703–28.

19. Newman JH, Loyd JE. Familial pulmonary hypertension. In: Fishman AP, editor. The pulmonary circulation: normal and abnormal. Philadelphia: University of Pennsylvania Press; 1990. p. 301–13.

20. Elliott CG, Alexander G, Leppert M, et al. Coancestry in apparently sporadic primary pulmonary hypertension. Chest 1995;108:973–7.

21. Newman JH, Wheeler L, Lane KB, et al. Mutation in the gene for bone morphogenetic protein receptor II as a cause of primary pulmonary hypertension in a large kindred. N Engl J Med 2001;345(5): 319–24.

22. Nichols WC, Koller DL, Slovis B, et al. Localization of the gene for familial primary pulmonary hypertension to chromosome 2q31-32. Nat Genet 1997; 15(3):277–80.

23. Morse JH, Jones AC, Barst RJ, et al. Mapping of familial primary pulmonary hypertension locus (PPH1) to chromosome 2q31-q32. Circulation 1997;95(12):2603–6.

24. Cogan JD, Pauciulo MW, Batchman AP, et al. High frequency of BMPR2 exonic deletions/duplications in familial pulmonary arterial hypertension. Am J Respir Crit Care Med 2006;174(5):590–8.

25. Aldred MA, Vijayakrishnan J, James V, et al. BMPR2 gene rearrangements account for a significant proportion of mutations in familial and idiopathic pulmonary arterial hypertension. Hum Mutat 2006; 27(2):212–3.

26. Machado RD, Aldred MA, James V, et al. Mutations of the TGF-beta type II receptor BMPR2 in pulmonary arterial hypertension. Hum Mutat 2006;27(2): 121–32.

27. Machado RD, Pauciulo MW, Thomson JR, et al. BMPR2 haploinsufficiency as the inherited molecular mechanism for primary pulmonary hypertension. Am J Hum Genet 2001;68(1):92–102.

28. Humbert M, Morrell NW, Archer SL, et al. Cellular and molecular pathobiology of pulmonary arterial hypertension. J Am Coll Cardiol 2004;43(12 Suppl S):13S–24S.

29. Cogan JD, Vnencak-Jones CL, Phillips JA 3rd, et al. Gross BMPR2 gene rearrangements constitute a new cause for primary pulmonary hypertension. Genet Med 2005;7(3):169–74.

30. Schouten JP, McElgunn CJ, Waaijer R, et al. Relative quantification of 40 nucleic acid sequences by multiplex ligation-dependent probe amplification. Nucleic Acids Res 2002;30(12):e57.

31. Humbert M, Deng Z, Simonneau G, et al. BMPR2 germline mutations in pulmonary hypertension associated with fenfluramine derivatives. Eur Respir J 2002;20(3):518–23.

32. Roberts KE, McElroy JJ, Wong WP, et al. BMPR2 mutations in pulmonary arterial hypertension with congenital heart disease. Eur Respir J 2004;24(3): 371–4.

33. Morse J, Barst R, Horn E, et al. Pulmonary hypertension in scleroderma spectrum of disease: lack of bone morphogenetic protein receptor 2 mutations. J Rheumatol 2002;29(11):2379–81.

34. Tew MB, Arnett FC, Reveille JD, et al. Mutations of bone morphogenetic protein receptor type II are not found in patients with pulmonary hypertension and underlying connective tissue diseases. Arthritis Rheum 2002;46(10):2829–30.

35. Nunes H, Humbert M, Sitbon O, et al. Prognostic factors for survival in human immunodeficiency virus-associated pulmonary arterial hypertension. Am J Respir Crit Care Med 2003;167(10):1433–9.

36. Roberts KE, Fallon MB, Krowka MJ, et al. Genetic risk factors for portopulmonary hypertension in patients with advanced liver disease. Am J Respir Crit Care Med 2009;179(9):835–42.

37. Harrison RE, Flanagan JA, Sankelo M, et al. Molecular and functional analysis identifies ALK-1 as the predominant cause of pulmonary hypertension related to hereditary haemorrhagic telangiectasia. J Med Genet 2003;40(12):865–71.

38. Attisano L, Carcamo J, Ventura F, et al. Identification of human activin and TGF beta type I receptors that form heteromeric kinase complexes with type II receptors. Cell 1993;75(4):671–80.

39. Wu X, Robinson CE, Fong HW, et al. Cloning and characterization of the murine activin receptor like kinase-1 (ALK-1) homolog. Biochem Biophys Res Commun 1995;216(1):78–83.

40. Favaro JP, Wiley K, Blobe GC. Alk1. UCSD-Nature Molecule Pages 2005. Available at: http://www.signaling-gateway.org/molecule/. Accessed April 17, 2012.

41. ten Dijke P, Yamashita H, Ichijo H, et al. Characterization of type I receptors for transforming growth factor-beta and activin. Science 1994; 264(5155):101–4.

42. Abdalla SA, Letarte M. Hereditary haemorrhagic telangiectasia: current views on genetics and mechanisms of disease. J Med Genet 2006; 43(2):97–110.

43. Harrison RE, Berger R, Haworth SG, et al. Transforming growth factor-beta receptor mutations and pulmonary arterial hypertension in childhood. Circulation 2005;111(4):435–41.

44. Girerd B, Montani D, Coulet F, et al. Clinical outcomes of pulmonary arterial hypertension in patients carrying an ACVRL1 (ALK1) mutation. Am J Respir Crit Care Med 2010;181(8):851–61.

45. Llorca O, Trujillo A, Blanco FJ, et al. Structural model of human endoglin, a transmembrane receptor responsible for hereditary hemorrhagic telangiectasia. J Mol Biol 2007;365(3):694–705.

46. Ray B, Blobe GC. Endoglin UCSD-Nature Molecule Pages 2005. Available at: http://www.signaling-gateway.org/molecule/. Accessed April 17, 2012.

47. Shovlin CL. Hereditary haemorrhagic telangiectasia: pathophysiology, diagnosis and treatment. Blood Rev 2010;24(6):203–19.

48. Badesch DB, Abman SH, Simonneau G, et al. Medical therapy for pulmonary arterial hypertension: updated ACCP evidence-based clinical practice guidelines. Chest 2007;131(6):1917–28.

49. Maitland-van der Zee AH, de Boer A, Leufkens HG. The interface between pharmacoepidemiology and pharmacogenetics. Eur J Pharmacol 2000; 410(2–3):121–30.

50. Murali S. Pulmonary arterial hypertension. Curr Opin Crit Care 2006;12(3):228–34.

51. Ghofrani HA, Barst RJ, Benza RL, et al. Future perspectives for the treatment of pulmonary arterial hypertension. J Am Coll Cardiol 2009;54(Suppl 1): S108–17.

52. Anderson JL, Horne BD, Stevens SM, et al. Randomized trial of genotype-guided versus standard warfarin dosing in patients initiating oral anticoagulation. Circulation 2007;116(22):2563–70.

53. Gage BF, Eby C, Milligan PE, et al. Use of pharmacogenetics and clinical factors to predict the maintenance dose of warfarin. Thromb Haemost 2004; 91(1):87–94.

54. Elliott CG, Glissmeyer EW, Havlena GT, et al. Relationship of BMPR2 mutations to vasoreactivity in pulmonary arterial hypertension. Circulation 2006; 113(21):2509–15.

55. Rosenzweig EB, Morse JH, Knowles JA, et al. Clinical implications of determining BMPR2 mutation status in a large cohort of children and adults with pulmonary arterial hypertension. J Heart Lung Transplant 2008;27(6):668–74.

56. Sztrymf B, Coulet F, Girerd B, et al. Clinical outcomes of pulmonary arterial hypertension in carriers of BMPR2 mutation. Am J Respir Crit Care Med 2008;177(12):1377–83.

Diagnostic Dilemmas in Pulmonary Hypertension

Robert P. Frantz, MD*, Michael D. McGoon, MD

KEYWORDS

- Pulmonary hypertension • Diagnosis • Pulmonary arterial hypertension

KEY POINTS

- Pulmonary hypertension (PH) is commonly detected in patients being evaluated for dyspnea or other symptoms, and is also found incidentally on echocardiography performed for various reasons. Algorithms for the evaluation and classification of PH are well described and useful, but many patients have mixed characteristics that present a dilemma for the clinician. In these instances, the clinician must think carefully about the underlying pathophysiology, and apply considerable judgment in coming to decisions regarding treatment.
- Most patients with PH have associated left heart disease or parenchymal lung disease. Whether specific treatment of PH in these patients is associated with clinical or prognostic benefit is largely unknown.
- Screening for PH is justified in patients with connective tissue disease, a family history of pulmonary arterial hypertension (PAH), and in dyspneic patients with HIV.
- Exercise hemodynamics in dyspneic patients with normal resting hemodynamics may be useful in detecting occult heart failure with preserved ejection fraction, and may detect early pulmonary arterial vasculopathy. However, performance and interpretation of exercise hemodynamics requires considerable skill, is subject to great variability among centers, and requires additional investigation.
- Goal-directed treatment of PAH is strongly recommended. However, the specific treatment goals and understanding of prognostic implications continue to evolve.

INTRODUCTION

Evaluation of patients with symptoms or risks of pulmonary hypertension (PH) has become increasingly well defined. The basic process of assessing patients with PH has been codified to provide physicians with guidelines to ensure a comprehensive and productive workup. The goals of evaluation are to detect whether PH is likely to be present and, if so, to confirm the diagnosis, elucidate the contributory clinical substrates, and determine the most appropriate approach to treatment. The importance

Financial Disclosures: Dr Frantz's institution has received research funding from Medtronic, Inc, Actelion Pharmaceuticals, Ltd, United Therapeutics Corporation, and Gilead Sciences, Inc. He has served on advisory boards for United Therapeutics Corporation, Actelion Pharmaceuticals, Ltd, and Gilead Sciences, Inc. Any honoraria for these activities have streamed to Mayo Foundation research accounts in keeping with institutional policy for investigators. Dr McGoon's institution has received research funding from Medtronic, Inc, and Gilead Sciences, Inc He currently serves on advisory, steering, and/or endpoint/DSMB committees for Actelion Pharmaceuticals, Ltd, Gilead Sciences, Inc, Lung Rx, LLC, and GlaxoSmithKline. He is Chair of the REVEAL Registry (funded by Actelion Pharmaceuticals, Ltd). He has received honoraria for speaking at conferences supported by Actelion Pharmaceuticals, Ltd and Gilead Sciences, Inc. The authors' institution receives pulmonary arterial hypertension–related research funding from Actelion Pharmaceuticals, Ltd, Gilead Sciences, Inc, Medtronic, Inc, Pfizer Inc, United Therapeutics Corporation, Novartis Pharmaceuticals Corporation, SHAPE Medical Systems, Inc, and Bayer HealthCare Pharmaceuticals.
Division of Cardiovascular Diseases and Internal Medicine, Mayo Clinic, 200 1st Street Southwest, Rochester, MN 55905, USA
* Corresponding author.
E-mail address: frantz.robert@mayo.edu

Heart Failure Clin 8 (2012) 331–352
doi:10.1016/j.hfc.2012.04.006
1551-7136/12/$ – see front matter © 2012 Elsevier Inc. All rights reserved.

of thorough and accurate diagnosis is based on the recognition that PH is a devastating illness, which, if inadequately assessed and treated, is progressively symptomatic and ultimately fatal. A clear evidence-based and consensus-driven diagnostic strategy is mandated by the expectation that it will facilitate optimal outcomes.

Diagnostic guidelines (**Fig. 1**) consist of recommendations based on evidence and concepts that have evolved from formal research and observations that apply to general populations.[1–3] One important goal of PH diagnostic evaluation is to be able to place the patient into one of the five accepted diagnostic groups (group I, pulmonary arterial hypertension [PAH]; group II, PH owing to left heart disease; group III, PH with lung disease/hypoxemia; group IV, chronic thromboembolic PH [CTEPH]; group V, PH with unclear multifactorial mechanisms). This framework is critically valuable to the clinician in characterizing patients. In reality, many patients have features from multiple groups, particularly across groups I, II, and III. Patients falling outside of group I have been meticulously excluded from randomized trials of PAH therapy that targeted patients in group I. PAH therapies are generally not approved for treatment of PH associated with groups II or III.

Given the expense and uncertainty regarding risk/benefit, the clinician dedicated to relieving suffering of patients with overlap characteristics is left with little guidance from the literature aside from the simplistic "evidence is not available" mantra. Therefore, individual patients continue to present unique problems that may not be fully covered by universal guidelines and thus require decision-making based on ambiguous, controversial, conflicting, or even nonexistent data. Under these circumstances, it may be useful to consider less codified approaches to classification and management, which are based on logic, observation, experience, and common sense. This paper addresses some of the dilemmas that emerge during the evaluation of patients with suspected or established PH, including those with overlapping classification features, and suggests ways in which the dilemmas might be resolved. The hope is that the incisive clinician will be assisted in conceptualizing the issues, and motivated to adequately characterize and apply understanding of individual patient pathophysiology, thereby improving treatment of real-world patients. For the purposes of discussion, three phases of the diagnostic process are considered: screening, evaluation of symptomatic suspected PH, and follow-up reassessment.

SCREENING

Compelling evidence shows that the presence of PH is usually diagnosed at a late point in the disease, even after symptoms have developed,[4–6] and that an earlier awareness of the presence of PH would lead to more expeditious initiation of therapy with presumably better outcomes.[7] A further inference of this line of reasoning is that identification of the earliest stage of PH before the emergence of overt symptoms could provide the most benefit. Although no direct evidence shows that the initiation of presymptomatic treatment

Fig. 1. Three recently published diagnostic algorithms. (*A*) A simple diagnostic algorithm for the evaluation of PH.[1] This flow diagram indicates key tests and the diagnostic purpose for obtaining them but does not show what conclusions or actions should be pursued based on test results. Abnl, abnormality; CHD, congenital heart disease; ECG, electrocardiogram; htn, hypertension; LFTs, liver function tests; PFTs, pulmonary function tests; RA, rheumatoid arthritis; RAE, right atrial enlargement; RH, right heart; RVE, right ventricular enlargement; RVSP, right ventricular systolic pressure; SLE, systemic lupus erythematosus; VHD, valvular heart disease. (*From* McLaughlin VV, McGoon MD. Pulmonary arterial hypertension. Circulation 2006;114(13):1417–31; with permission.) (*B*) These general guidelines distinguish between pivotal and contingent tests but also do not suggest ways in which the evidence in the test results guide decision making.[2] Pivotal tests are required for a definitive diagnosis and baseline characterization. Contingent tests are recommended to elucidate or confirm results of the pivotal tests, and need only be performed in the appropriate clinical context. 6MWT, 6-min walk test; ABGs, arterial blood gases; ANA, antinuclear antibody serology; Cath, catheterization; CHD, congenital heart disease; CPET, cardiopulmonary exercise test; CTD, connective tissue disease; CXR, chest radiograph; ECG, electrocardiogram; Echo, echocardiogram; Exam, examination; HIV, human immunodeficiency virus screening; Htn, hypertension; LFT, liver function test; PE, pulmonary embolism; PFT, pulmonary function test; PH, pulmonary hypertension; RA, rheumatoid arthritis; RAE, right atrial enlargement; RH Cath, right heart catheterization; RV, right ventricular; RVE, right ventricular enlargement; RVSP, right ventricular systolic pressure; SLE, systemic lupus erythematosus; TEE, transesophageal echocardiography; VHD, valvular heart disease; V/Q scan, ventilation-perfusion scintigram. (*From* McLaughlin VV, Archer SL, Badesch DB, et al. ACCF/AHA 2009 expert consensus document on pulmonary hypertension: a report of the American College of Cardiology Foundation Task Force on Expert Consensus Documents and the American Heart Association: developed in collaboration with the American College of Chest Physicians, American Thoracic Society, Inc., and the Pulmonary Hypertension Association. Circulation 2009; 119(16):2250–94; with permission.)

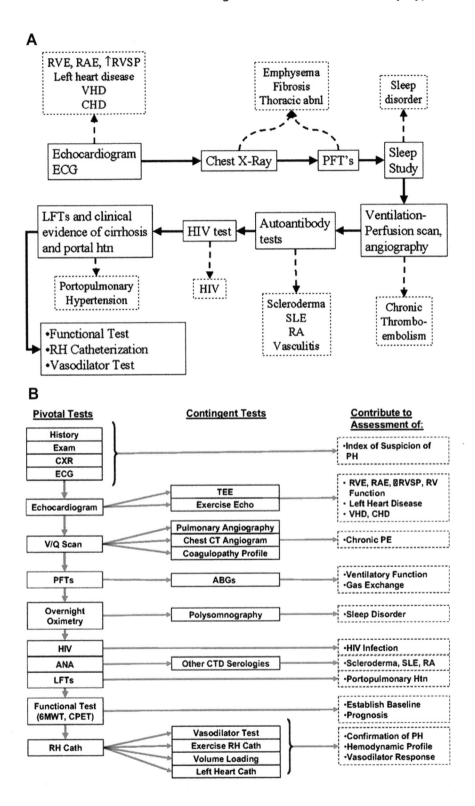

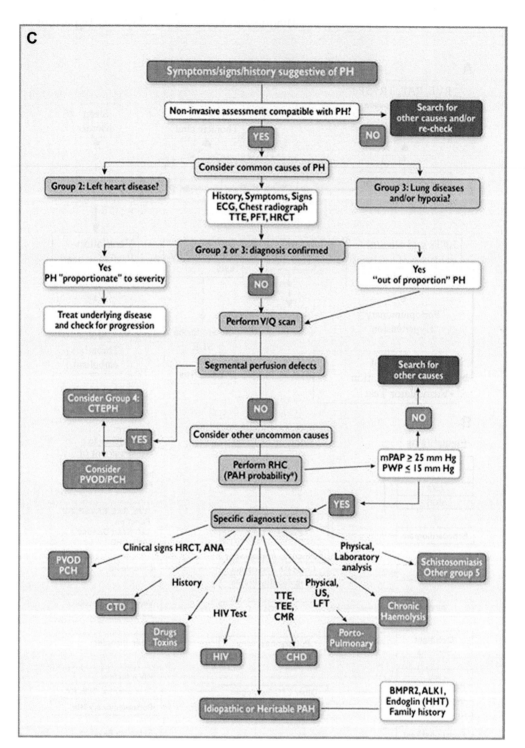

Fig. 1. (*C*) This diagnostic algorithm includes basic dichotomous decision points that determine further evaluation.[3] ALK-1, activin-receptor-like kinase; ANA, antinuclear antibodies; BMPR2, bone morphogenetic protein receptor 2; CHD, congenital heart disease; CMR, cardiac magnetic resonance; CTD, connective tissue disease; CTEPH, chronic thromboembolic pulmonary hypertension; ECG, electrocardiogram; Group, clinical group; HHT, hereditary hemorrhagic telangiectasia; HRCT, high-resolution computed tomography; LFT, liver function tests; mPAP, mean pulmonary arterial pressure; PAH, pulmonary arterial hypertension; PCH, pulmonary capillary hemangiomatosis; PFT, pulmonary function test; PH, pulmonary hypertension; PVOD, pulmonary veno-occlusive disease; PWP, pulmonary wedge pressure; RHC, right heart catheterization; TEE, transesophageal echocardiography; TTE, transthoracic echocardiography; US, ultrasonography; V/Q scan, ventilation/perfusion lung scan. (*From* Galie N, Hoeper MM, Humbert M, et al. Guidelines for the diagnosis and treatment of pulmonary hypertension: the Task Force for the Diagnosis and Treatment of Pulmonary Hypertension of the European Society of Cardiology (ESC) and the European Respiratory Society (ERS), endorsed by the International Society of Heart and Lung Transplantation (ISHLT). Eur Heart J 2009;30(20):2493–537; with permission.)

improves outcomes, particularly because most pharmacologic strategies are potentially toxic themselves, a general consensus is that early diagnosis is desirable if only to trigger more focused follow-up and higher sensitivity to subtle symptoms or diminution of exercise capacity.

However, the relative infrequency of PH in the general population, and the need for specific testing to justifiably suspect PH, makes a population-wide screening strategy undesirable from a socioeconomic perspective and clinically unfeasible. The dilemma arises as to whether specific characteristics in some populations cause sufficient risk of having subclinical PH or of developing it in the foreseeable future that patients should be systematically screened periodically for its presence. These populations have been identified and recommendations have been advanced.

In Whom

A screening strategy is predicated on several convergent issues: (1) that distinct high-risk patient populations can be defined, (2) that the prevalence of the disease in the high-risk population reaches a threshold level that makes the pretest likelihood of evaluation sufficiently high to yield reasonable predictive accuracy, and (3) that treatment for PH in a high-risk group is available and yields a beneficial outcome.

Patients with potentially high-risk are those who have clinical substrates associated with PH. These populations are well recognized and are represented in the classification of PH most recently developed by the 4th World Symposium on Pulmonary Arterial Hypertension (**Box 1**).[8] Thus, clinically identifiable and distinct subgroups exist, in keeping with predicate 1, although not every population meets the other two predicates.

Patient populations for whom screening has been recommended tend to have a prevalence of PH greater than 4%. This finding represents a substantially larger background risk than exists in the general population, in which the prevalence of PAH is approximately 16 per million (0.0016%). These populations include individuals with a known bone morphogenetic protein receptor 2 mutation (approximately 10% chance of developing phenotypic PAH) or who come from kindreds with two or more individuals with PAH (approximately 5% chance of developing PAH); those who have scleroderma (about 8% prevalence of invasively documented PAH[9,10] and an incidence of 0.61 cases per 100 patient-years[11]); or patients with portal hypertension who are undergoing evaluation for orthotopic liver transplantation (1%–6% prevalence of PAH[12–15]). These groups meet the criteria of predicate 2. In addition,

clinical studies have provided data that treatment with pulmonary vasomodulating medications is efficacious in providing partial benefit in terms of functional status, activity tolerance, and/or survival in these patients.[16]

Patients for whom the risk does not justify routine screening in the absence of preexisting signs or symptoms of PH include those with HIV infection (prevalence of 0.5%[17,18]), recognized toxic exposures (30 per million or 0.005% among those who took fenfluramine derivatives for more than 3 months),[19] or past acute pulmonary thromboembolism (cumulative incidence in large studies of 0.57% over 34 months to 3.8% over 2 years,[20,21] although small studies suggested a higher incidence of up to 8.8% within 1 year[22]). These groups do not meet the criteria of predicate 2, even though, if discovered, specific treatment (vasomodulating drugs or pulmonary thromboendarterectomy) may be considered.

Although the presence of PH in patients with sickle cell anemia has been reported to occur in as many as 32% of patients, this relies on a liberal definition of PH based on a tricuspid regurgitant velocity of 2.5 m/s (an estimated right ventricular systolic pressure of 35 mm Hg) as measured with Doppler echocardiography. Although this is associated with a lower survival, the causal relationship remains controversial and the effect of treatment is unknown and may be deleterious. These patients therefore may not meet criteria for screening, but currently the consensus is to screen them for PAH.[2]

Although the prevalence of PAH among patients with congenital heart disease (CHD) is not accurately known, it is undoubtedly high, with estimates of Eisenmenger syndrome developing in 20% to 50% of large ventricular septal defects, 20% of patent ductus arteriosus, and 10% of large atrial septal defects.[23,24] In reality, CHD is either diagnosed before significant PAH develops and is operated on if feasible, or it is discovered during the evaluation of symptoms.

Patients with left-sided heart disease or hypoxemic lung disease may have secondary PH, as reflected by group 2 or 3 classifications, respectively.[8] Although patients with these underlying conditions are generally not asymptomatic, the notion of screening for coexisting PH arises because its presence has prognostic importance. However, the evidence for effectiveness of pulmonary arterial vasomodulating drug therapy remains limited and variable.

Early Detection

Although comprehensive rest Doppler echocardiography is accepted as the standard for initially

---

Box 1
Updated clinical classification of PH[a]

1. PAH
    1.1. Idiopathic PAH
    1.2. Heritable
        1.2.1. BMPR2
        1.2.2. ALK1, endoglin (with or without hereditary hemorrhagic telangiectasia)
        1.2.3. Unknown
    1.3. Drug- and toxin-induced
    1.4. Associated with
        1.4.1. Connective tissue diseases
        1.4.2. HIV infection
        1.4.3. Portal hypertension
        1.4.4. Congenital heart diseases
        1.4.5. Schistosomiasis
        1.4.6. Chronic hemolytic anemia
    1.5. Persistent PH of the newborn
    1.6. Pulmonary veno-occlusive disease and/or pulmonary capillary hemangiomatosis
2. PH owing to left heart disease
    2.1. Systolic dysfunction
    2.2. Diastolic dysfunction
    2.3. Valvular disease
3. PH owing to lung diseases and/or hypoxia
    3.1. Chronic obstructive pulmonary disease
    3.2. Interstitial lung disease
    3.3. Other pulmonary diseases with mixed restrictive and obstructive pattern
    3.4. Sleep-disordered breathing
    3.5. Alveolar hypoventilation disorders
    3.6. Chronic exposure to high altitude
    3.7. Developmental abnormalities
4. Chronic thromboembolic PH
5. PH with unclear multifactorial mechanisms
    5.1. Hematologic disorders: myeloproliferative disorders, splenectomy
    5.2. Systemic disorders: sarcoidosis, pulmonary Langerhans cell histiocytosis: lymphangioleiomyomatosis, neurofibromatosis, vasculitis
    5.3. Metabolic disorders: glycogen storage disease, Gaucher disease, thyroid disorders
    5.4. Others: tumoral obstruction, fibrosing mediastinitis, chronic renal failure on dialysis

[a] Presented at the 2008 4th World Symposium on Pulmonary Hypertension held in Dana Point, California.
  Adapted from Simonneau G, Robbins IM, Beghetti M, et al. Updated clinical classification of pulmonary hypertension. J Am Coll Cardiol 2009;54(Suppl 1):S43–54; with permission.

---

detecting PH, its usefulness as a screening tool is compromised by issues of expense and accuracy. Furthermore, because it requires that PH be present at rest (and accurately detected) to raise the suspicion of disease, it may fail to detect earlier stages of pulmonary vasculopathy in which no overt hemodynamic abnormalities are exhibited in a resting state.

GENETIC BACKGROUND

It is reasonable to wonder whether individuals harboring a genetic mutation associated with PAH might be at risk of having or developing phenotypic clinically relevant PAH that may merit therapy.[25–27] Although it is currently generally accepted that a genetic substrate likely requires a "second hit" (such as an environmental trigger or modifier gene) to produce the PAH phenotype, recognition that a genetic predisposition is present in a patient could lead to specific assessment to detect the early manifestation of disease and, if appropriate, the introduction of treatment.[28] Potential genetic predispositions include bone morphogenetic protein receptor 2 (BMPR2) heterozygous germline mutations, ALK1 or endoglin mutations in patients with hereditary hemorrhagic telangiectasia, HLA genotype profile, polymorphisms of serotonin transporter, or reduced expression of prostacyclin synthase, endothelial nitric oxide synthase, and endothelin-converting enzyme, to name a few.

Currently, however, the usefulness of genotyping is uncertain. Because even individuals with documented BMPR2 mutations or multiple effected family members have an approximately 1 in 10 chance of developing PAH, the initiation of potentially toxic and expensive treatment regimens in asymptomatic patients based on genotype is unfounded. Nevertheless, family counseling is warranted and careful periodic assessment for the development of PAH is recommended.

EXERCISE

The application of exercise-induced changes in pulmonary hemodynamics has been suggested as a means of detecting PH at an early stage. A high proportion of individuals (31.6%) related to patients with idiopathic or familial PAH (with or without known BMPR2 gene mutation) have a Doppler echocardiographic measurement of exercise tricuspid regurgitant velocity exceeding the 90th percentile value of normal individuals. This finding suggests that patients with a potential genetic risk of having or developing PAH could be identified through noninvasive exercise assessment. The occurrence of exercise-related PH may be further elicited by simultaneous exposure to hypoxic conditions.[29,30]

Previous observations suggest that low or decreasing carbon dioxide diffusing capacity in patients with systemic sclerosis is predictive of a higher likelihood of future development of PAH.[31] In 54 patients who had systemic sclerosis with these markers of high risk and a Doppler echocardiographically estimated right ventricular systolic pressure (RVSP) between 30 and 50 mm Hg, exercise resulted in a "positive" test (defined as an increase of RVSP by at least 20 mm Hg within 1 minute of achieving 85% of predicted maximal heart rate on a Bruce protocol treadmill test) in 44%.[32] Among these, right heart catheterization (RHC) confirmed the presence of PAH (defined as mean pulmonary artery pressure [mPAP] >30 mm Hg and pulmonary arterial opening pressure of <18 mm Hg with arm weight–resistance exercise, or as mPAP >25 mm Hg at rest) in 81% (62% exercise-defined, 19% at rest). A more recent study of asymptomatic and symptomatic patients with connective tissue disease who were assessed with both exercise Doppler-echocardiography and cardiopulmonary exercise testing identified 36 of 54 patients who had either exercise-induced estimated RVSP greater than 40 mm Hg or a peak oxygen uptake (peak Vo_2) less than 75% predicted. Of the 28 patients who had subsequent RHC, 1 had a systolic pulmonary artery pressure at rest greater than 40 mm Hg and 24 had an exercise value greater than 40 mm Hg.[33] Although these results showed a level of congruence of "risk factors" and degree of correlation between echocardiographic and/or exercise aerobic capacity and invasive exercise results, their implications in predicting clinically important PAH remains unclear.

A study of invasive hemodynamic monitoring during simultaneous cardiopulmonary exercise testing in patients with symptoms or fatigue of unclear origin examined the relationship of aerobic capacity with hemodynamics. Patients meeting the definition of exercise-induced PH with normal resting hemodynamics exhibited a pattern of exercise-related Vo_2 and pulmonary arterial pressure response intermediate between those with normal pulmonary hemodynamics and those with documented resting PH, suggesting that exercise-induced PH has functional consequences and that it is a stage in the trajectory from clinical normalcy to definitive pulmonary vasculopathy.[34] Moreover, preliminary evidence shows that treatment with endothelin antagonists or phosphodiesterase-5 inhibitors of symptomatic patients with exercise-induced PAH results in improved 6-minute walk distance.[35]

Whether the findings in these symptomatic patients also apply to asymptomatic high-risk patients for whom screening studies might be useful is unclear.[36] It is uncertain not only what the likelihood is that asymptomatic patients who exhibit exaggerated pulmonary hypertensive responses will ultimately exhibit traditionally defined PAH or symptoms, or what the duration of "latent" preclinical disease is, but also what the cut-off should be for defining a "high-risk" abnormal response. This ambiguity is amplified further by technical and interpretative difficulties of noninvasive screening and the lack of procedural uniformity in invasively monitored exercise tests.

Although the concept of screening is typically applied to a search for evidence of pulmonary vasculopathy in asymptomatic patients, it also applies to looking for evidence of PH occurring in patients who may be symptomatic because of comorbid conditions. The supervention of PH in the setting of hypoxic lung disease is prognostically important and may raise consideration of treatment (currently of unproven efficacy) of associated pulmonary vascular disease, especially if it is disproportionately severe. Methods for screening for PH in entities such as interstitial lung disease have been described (in which the diffusing capacity of carbon dioxide during routine pulmonary function testing can be used to sensitively detect the presence of a mean pulmonary arterial pressure >25 mm Hg).[37,38]

OTHER MARKERS

Other biomarkers that have been reported to suggest the presence of PAH in high-risk populations include endothelin-1, interleukin-8, tissue necrosis factor α, and endoglin levels.[39] Because these markers were correlated with echocardiographic diagnosis of PAH, whether they currently add anything to the recommendation for simply screening with Doppler echocardiography is unclear.

If Detected, Then What?

The early detection of PAH has intuitive appeal, but the actual course of action in the real-life clinical arena if screening suggests the presence of PAH remains elusive. The dilemma revolves around several inter-related issues: what is the reliability of the screening method and results, what should be done to confirm the results, what is the importance of asymptomatic PAH (especially if it is mild), and what are the implications for management?

RELIABILITY OF SCREENING METHOD

Although echocardiography is commonly used to estimate pulmonary arterial pressure through extrapolating from Doppler-measured systolic tricuspid regurgitant velocity and estimated right atrial pressure,[40,41] its accuracy has been criticized in studies comparing it with direct measurement using RHC.[42] Comparison of echocardiographically estimated right ventricular pressure and invasive measurement obtained within 1 hour showed that the former was within 10 mm Hg of the latter in only 48% of measurements among 65 patients assessed for various types of PH; the mean overestimate was 19 ± 11 mm Hg and underestimate was 30 ± 16

mm Hg.[43] The likelihood of underestimation was particularly high when the Doppler images were suboptimal.

More recent studies support these findings; Doppler echocardiographic measurements were inaccurate with respect to the RHC in more than 50% of patients when performed from 48 hours or less[44] up to 30 days apart.[45] Moreover, a high degree of discrepancy was still seen when the studies were performed simultaneously.[45] Unfortunately, other information derived from the echocardiogram, such as estimates of right atrial size or right ventricular size and function, were not reported in these studies. The authors concluded that echocardiography remains an "indispensable"[43] and "critically important"[45] tool for assessing PH. The dilemma is how results in individual patients should be considered in light of this degree of apparent inaccuracy. How should an estimated right ventricular systolic pressure of 40 mm Hg be integrated into the diagnostic framework and assessment of a patient if it has a 50% chance of being either an overestimate by an average of 19 mm Hg (in which case the patient does not have PH) or an underestimate by an average of 30 mm Hg (consistent with severe PH)? Is it reasonable or feasible to do RHC in all of these patients who are screened for PH despite lack of symptoms?

CONFIRMATION

The reliability of any screening result (resting echocardiographic estimated RVSP, exercise hemodynamics, or other markers) can be assessed through either direct evaluation with a gold standard (RHC) or through accumulation of other indirect markers that indicate the same conclusion. Thus, although isolated indicators of PH or its sequelae may lack accuracy in individual cases (such as echocardiogram-derived correlates of mean and diastolic pulmonary arterial pressure, cardiac output, or pulmonary vascular resistance; semiquantitative right ventricular size and function, right atrial size, inferior vena cava size, and respiratory variation; coronary sinus dilatation; N-terminal prohormone of brain natriuretic peptide (NT-proBNP) or BNP serum sodium concentration; uric acid level; electrocardiographic signs of right ventricular hypertrophy or right atrial enlargement; or central pulmonary enlargement on chest radiograph), a composite picture may nevertheless emerge, and should be considered in developing a tentative diagnosis to direct further management.

Although a direct threshold for raising the index of suspicion of PH cannot be specified, an equivocally elevated RVSP in the absence of other indicators of PH raises the likelihood of a false-positive screening result, whereas the presence of cumulative evidence would justify definitive confirmation with RHC. Even if the RVSP is believed to be a false-positive, a repeat assessment in the near future is appropriate, especially in a high-risk population.

WHAT IS THE IMPORTANCE OF MILD PH?

Perhaps equally perplexing is how much significance to attach to a borderline elevation of pulmonary pressure, even when it is definitively assessed using RHC. A mean pulmonary arterial pressure of 20 to 25 mm Hg is higher than the normal range but not in the range that is formally defined as clinically abnormal. The ambiguity posed by values in this range led the participants at the 4th World Symposium on Pulmonary Hypertension to formally decline making recommendations for management. Moreover, the clinical significance of truly mild PH (25–30 mm Hg mean pulmonary arterial pressure) in the asymptomatic screened patient is not clear.

MANAGEMENT WHEN SCREENING REVEALS PH

If treatment for PAH was both benign and inexpensive, then empiric treatment to prevent progression of vasculopathy in higher risk patients would be reasonable. However, most treatment modalities are potentially toxic, complex, or expensive; efficacy in this setting has not been assessed; and the natural history of progression at this stage of disease is unclear. Even when mild PH is identified in some populations and seems to have prognostic consequences (such as in patients with sickle cell anemia), treatment may be ineffective or even harmful.

Sufficient evidence can be cited from other diseases to suggest that empiric but logical treatment can be harmful enough to warrant a cautious and vigilant approach in mild PH. Although specific algorithms are difficult to create, the approach based on results of screening should incorporate these guidelines:

1. Noninvasive screening should use multiple parameters, rather than depend on a single criterion.
2. A negative (or likely negative) outcome should not necessarily lead to invasive confirmation. An exception to this may be if the estimated RVSP is very high despite no apparent other correlations, necessitating RHC to either confirm the presence of PH or allay anxiety. Otherwise, continued observation and periodic screening according to the underlying risk-status should be pursued.
3. A likely positive screening assessment warrants RHC to either confirm that treatment is

reasonable (if PAH is severe) or to establish an accurate hemodynamic baseline for follow-up comparison if ongoing surveillance is more appropriate (if borderline or mild).

EVALUATING A SYMPTOMATIC PATIENT WITH SUSPECTED PH

The approach to diagnostic assessment of a symptomatic patient differs from that of screening the high-risk asymptomatic patient. The goal is to identify the cause of symptoms so that they might be treated. The presence of symptoms implies that the disease is in an advanced stage and that life expectancy is predictably reduced. Thus, treatment is also directed toward promoting longevity. Available therapies, although not curative, have proven (but limited) benefits regarding symptoms, functional status, and survival in this context. The evaluation of symptomatic patients, as represented in **Fig. 1**, is designed to assure that these patients are correctly identified to initiate appropriate treatment.

Despite the high level of consensus regarding the diagnostic algorithms, dilemmas remain that the algorithms do not address. As PH is becoming more broadly recognized among diverse patient groups encountered in daily practice, the number of dilemmas increasingly expands. One major source of difficulty in daily practice is that PH is often seen in association with other diseases outside the spectrum of the well-studied groups of patients with group I PH (PAH). How PH impacts these patients and how it should be treated remains enigmatic and therefore controversial.

Non-PAH PH

Some pathophysiologic conditions predispose to the development of PH. Elevated pulmonary venous pressures in group II PH can lead to high pressures measured in the precapillary pulmonary vessels from passive back pressure, pulmonary vasoconstriction, and eventual vascular remodeling. Hypoxia is a stimulus for vasoconstriction and also can lead to vascular remodeling. PH associated with hypoxic lung or ventilatory disorders are classified as group II PH. PH caused by chronic thromboembolism is group IV PH.[8] Taken together, these groups have been referred to as "non–pulmonary arterial hypertension pulmonary hypertension (non-PAH PH)"[46] or "secondary (non–category 1) pulmonary hypertension."[47]

If the PH is caused by the coexisting condition, then the simplest recommendation is to treat the underlying cause. With distressingly rare exceptions (such as correction of mitral stenosis or normalization of severe systemic hypertension), treatment of the substrate is not very effective or even available. Furthermore, whether the PH was caused by the associated condition or simply represents two diseases in the same patient is not always clear, in which case sole treatment of the putative underlying cause may not adequately ameliorate the PH. The most commonly encountered scenario, however, is the presence of PH that is out of proportion to what would be expected for the underlying cause. Although the associated condition may have triggered the PH (perhaps in association with a permissive genetic profile), the hemodynamic abnormality becomes sufficiently severe to become a separate problem, such as causing symptoms, producing right heart failure, and increasing mortality, independent of and compounding the original disease.

Several dilemmas arise from this: what constitutes a degree of PH that is disproportionate to the substrate condition, how should these patients be evaluated, and should treatment be directed specifically at the PH?

Pulmonary Venous Hypertension

PH occurs in up to two-thirds of patients with chronic severe left heart disease.[48] Left-sided myocardial or valvular heart disease can be suspected based on physical examination, chest radiograph, electrocardiogram, and, of course, echocardiogram. An essential part of the evaluation of any patient with PH is the accurate determination of pulmonary venous pressure even (or perhaps especially) in patients without preexisting evidence of postcapillary PH, and this is a major impetus behind the universal recommendation that all patients with suspected PH undergo hemodynamic catheterization, including pulmonary capillary wedge pressure measurement (PCWP; with wedge position confirmed with oxygen saturation) or left atrial or left ventricular end-diastolic pressure if necessary. The results of a PCWP determination must always be put into the clinical context. Errors in measurement of PCWP are frequent, because of factors such as failure to recognize a damped PA tracing or to account for effects of respiration on the measurement. Involvement of a vigilant and thoughtful hemodynamicist is essential to optimizing usefulness of this critical aspect of PH evaluation.

The number of patients with PH associated with PVH (elevated PCWP) caused by diastolic dysfunction is increasing, likely because of the prevalence of diastolic dysfunction in an aging population,[49] PH in the setting of left heart failure with preserved ejection fraction (HFpEF) seems also to be promoted by morbid obesity, atrial arrhythmias, hypoxemia, and coexisting chronic obstructive pulmonary disease (COPD),[50] all of which are becoming more common in the population. This trend has produced a growing dilemma for physicians: how should patients with PH with an elevated PCWP be treated? The answer likely depends partly on the degree to which the PH is "proportional to" the PVH. Patients with PH and a normal transpulmonary gradient between the mean pulmonary artery pressure and mean PCWP (generally taken as 12 mm Hg)[51] have PH from "passive" back transmission of postcapillary pressure elevation. The higher the transpulmonary gradient, the more a precapillary "reactive" component of pulmonary vasoconstriction or remodeling is playing a role.

Acute assessment of hemodynamic manipulation is particularly important when PVH is suspected. When the mean PCWP is normal at baseline, volume loading or exercise may disclose a high value, suggesting PVH. Nitric oxide, a potent short-acting selective pulmonary arterial vasodilator, is normally administered primarily to assess whether the patient has a vasodilator response that would justify a trial of treatment with calcium channel blockers. In patients with a degree of PVH, pulmonary selective vasodilator assessment should be performed with caution and mainly to assess whether vasodilation is acutely tolerated at all. Symptomatic worsening, systemic hypotension, arterial desaturation, decreasing cardiac output, or pulmonary congestion indicates that the presence of PVH contraindicates long-term use of a medication with selective pulmonary vasodilator effects. Under these circumstances, precapillary vasodilation without reduction in PVH from high left-sided pressures may lead to fluid extravasation into the alveoli.[52–55] Conversely, if normal or high systemic pressure is present, the use of nitroprusside may reveal that reduction of systemic blood pressure may markedly improve PH, suggesting the best initial treatment strategy. Similarly, if the patient is volume overloaded, effective diuresis may lower both PCWP and PH.

An additional facet of the dilemma concerning PH with elevated PCWP is where the cutoff is between normal and abnormal PCWP. Patients with primary (now called *idiopathic*) PH enrolled into the National Institutes of Health (NIH) registry in the 1980s were required to have a PCWP of 12 mm Hg or less. Virtually all subsequent clinical drug trials have used a cutoff value of 15 mm Hg. Thus, for frequently encountered patients with higher PCWPs, guidelines and approval for medications are not available. To gain insight into this group, an ongoing US registry (REVEAL) permitted inclusion of patients with a mean pulmonary artery pressure greater than 25 mm Hg and PCWP up to 18 mm Hg.[56] Of 2967 patients enrolled, 239 (8.1%)

had PCWPs of 16 to 18 mm Hg. These patients were significantly older, more obese, walked less far in 6-minute walk testing, and had more co-morbid conditions (systemic hypertension, sleep apnea, renal insufficiency, and diabetes), but their treatment profile was not different from that of the group with a lower PCWP[57] suggesting that physicians are already extrapolating data from safety and efficacy studies and outcome data in traditionally defined PAH to those with higher PCWP. Whether this strategy provides comparable benefit remains uncertain, particularly because PCWP may underestimate true left ventricular end diastolic pressure in a substantial number of patients.[58] These patients may have left ventricular diastolic dysfunction or HFpEF as a comorbidity superimposed on what otherwise would have been pure PAH. A suggested algorithm for consideration of these patients is shown in **Fig. 2.** Proper patient characterization can also be enhanced by consideration of the relative severity of the PH and the diastolic abnormality. The more severe the PH, and the milder the degree of diastolic dysfunction, the more likely it is that the patient has the pathophysiology of group I PAH modified by diastolic dysfunction as a comorbidity. This calculus may be further modified by the presence or absence of group I PAH risk factors. This

concept is illustrated in **Fig. 3**, which is also relevant for patients with elements of group III PH. If a decision is made to initiate PAH therapy in patients with group II features, agents that may also lower left-sided filling pressures, such as phosphodiesterase-5 inhibitors or investigational agents such as soluble guanylate cyclase activators, may be more logical than more purely pulmonary vasodilating agents that may pose greater risk of pulmonary congestion.

Hypoxic Pulmonary or Ventilatory Disease

PH is common in hypoxic lung disease, but even severe hypoxic pulmonary diseases do not generally cause more than modest PH.[37,38,59–65] However, a minority of patients develop marked PH though its presence does not correlate with lung function.[66–69] Multiple factors likely contribute to both the PH and to right ventricular dysfunction in some patients with chronic obstructive lung disease or interstitial lung disease, some of which are common to all causes (hypoxemia, myocardial ischemia, acidemia, hypercarbia, blood vessel destruction).[47] Other subsets may have genetic predispositions or associated connective tissue disease. The clinical dilemma is whether severe PH in this setting indicates a superimposed

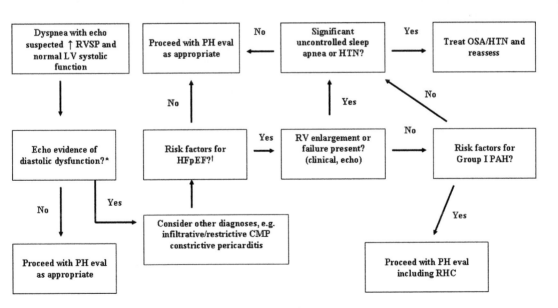

* Abnormal mitral Doppler; LA enlargement; Increased LV wall thickness

† HTN, obesity, sleep apnea, elderly, diabetes, CAD

Fig. 2. Algorithm for assessment of patients with dyspnea, preserved left ventricular systolic function, and echocardiographic findings of elevated tricuspid regurgitant velocity with diastolic filling abnormalities. CAD, coronary artery disease; CMP, cardiomyopathy; HFpEF, heart failure with preserved ejection fraction; HTN, hypertension; LA, left atrial; LV, left ventricular; OSA, obstructive sleep apnea; RHC, right heart catheterization; RVSP, right ventricular systolic pressure.

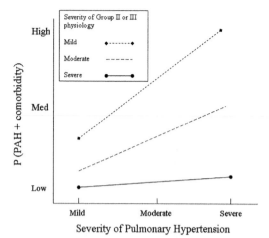

Fig. 3. Relationship among severity of group II or III pathophysiology, severity of pulmonary hypertension, and the probability of PAH-like disease with group II or III pathophysiology as a comorbidity. The probability that a patient has primarily features of group I PAH with group II or III as comorbidity can be assessed through weighing the severity of the PH against the severity of group II or III pathophysiology. If the patient also has risk factors for group I PAH, then the probability is further increased. The probability that the patient will benefit from PAH-specific treatment is suspected to be similarly related, but this is not clearly established. Group II, World Health Organization (WHO) group II (PH with left-sided heart disease); Group III, WHO group III (PH with lung diseases/hypoxia); Med, medium; P, probability.

vasculopathy or is a consequence of the pulmonary process.[70] If the former, therapy with pulmonary vascular targeted therapy may seem worth considering. However, even mild PH is associated with reduced survival in COPD.[64,71–74]

Unfortunately, several reasons exist to use caution regarding treatment directed at PH in the setting of lung disease: no systematic clinical study has provided evidence for drug efficacy or safety, pulmonary vasodilation may exacerbate hypoxemia through promoting poor gas exchange caused by ventilation-perfusion (V/Q) mismatching,[75] and symptoms from the pulmonary process will not be affected even if hemodynamics are improved. Finally, PH may partly be a marker for severe associated disease but may not be directly causal of prognosis, and pulmonary vascular treatment therefore may not alter the main source of poor outcome.[76] In view of these limitations, medications aimed at treatment of pulmonary vascular disease in these patients cannot generally be recommended.[46,69] In individual circumstances in which the severity of PH is substantially disproportionate to the severity of the group III pathophysiology, these medications may merit cautious consideration. This area is ripe for additional

investigation; when possible, these patients should be referred for consideration of participation in applicable clinical trials.

Sleep-Disordered Breathing

Although 20% to 40% of patients with sleep apnea may have associated PH,[77] sleep apnea is not likely to be an independent cause of severe pulmonary vascular disease and is seldom associated with significant right ventricular dysfunction.[78–82] When PH is present in association with obstructive sleep apnea, treatment with continuous positive airway pressure can lower pulmonary arterial pressure.[83–86] Obesity hypoventilation syndrome can cause severe cor pulmonale, and given the worldwide epidemic of obesity, clinicians must be vigilant in considering this diagnosis.[87]

CTEPH

The recognition that chronic thromboembolic disease is a potentially surgically correctable cause of severe PH makes it especially important to diagnose. This clinical responsibility raises several diagnostic dilemmas: should CTEPH be looked for in patients who have had an acute pulmonary embolic event, what is the most appropriate screening test for patients with symptomatic PH, and is there a role for nonsurgical treatment?

Screening for PH in asymptomatic patients with a history of pulmonary embolism is not warranted. However, the presence of CTEPH must be conscientiously and reliably ruled out in all patients with PH, even in the absence of a history suggestive of pulmonary embolism. Approximately 40% of patients with CTEPH lack this history.[46,88–90]

The prevalence of a chronic thromboembolic origin of PH is less well defined. Of 2924 consecutively evaluated patients in the Pulmonary Hypertension Center at Mayo Clinic, 200 (6.8%) had a main diagnosis of CTEPH. Because of the low pretest probability and the importance of avoiding false-negative results, the diagnostic strategy must emphasize high sensitivity while allowing for low specificity, which has led to a consensus that radionuclide V/Q scanning is the appropriate modality, because a normal or low-probability test virtually excludes a thromboembolic substrate, whereas an intermediate- or high-probability study mandates further evaluation. The sensitivity of V/Q scan for detection of chronic pulmonary thromboembolism confirmed by digital subtraction angiography was reported in the range of 97%, compared with 51% for multidetector chest CT angiography when performed from 2000 to 2005.[91] More recently, higher sensitivity has been reported for 64-row CT scanners (94%–98%).[92] With continuing enhancement of CT resolution, both sensitivity and specificity are likely to improve. CT angiography also provides important anatomic information about the location of thromboembolic disease, and about associated lung and cardiac structure and disease.

Does the recommendation to use V/Q scanning for CTEPH detection still apply? Although the gap in sensitivity compared with CT angiography is narrowing, V/Q scanning is still reasonable to recommend, although this may need to be reconsidered in the near future. Nonetheless, the quality of CT imaging and interpretation is variable, and cases persist in which CT imaging was interpreted as negative, whereas high-probability V/Q scans and additional evaluation confirmed CTEPH. The most immediate question is what the relative roles are of CT angiography versus invasive angiography once a positive V/Q scan is obtained. Current multidetector CT angiography with three-dimensional reconstruction techniques provides anatomic accuracy sufficient for guiding pulmonary thromboendarterectomy and avoids the risk of an additional invasive procedure.

HOW SHOULD PATIENTS BE FOLLOWED?

The evaluation of patients with PH does not end with diagnosis. The determination over time of whether treatment is producing desired effects is pivotal to management. The challenge for physicians is devising a strategy for follow-up that informs the decision to maintain or alter treatment. This determination requires a clear understanding of the factors that define treatment efficacy, establishing the baseline status of the patient in terms of those factors, and reevaluating the patient at intervals appropriate for detecting meaningful clinical changes.

The effectiveness of therapy is a function of the extent to which treatment goals are met. The goal of treatment is to improve symptoms and functional capacity and to improve prognosis. These objectives are related: measures of functional capacity and symptomatic status correlate with survival, and are largely determined by right ventricular function and cardiac output. Thus, assessment of functional capacity and other markers of right ventricular function are appropriate indices of treatment efficacy. Although improvements in pulmonary arterial pressure and resistance are implicit in these goals, clinical measurements of pulmonary hemodynamics correlate less strongly with outcome. This finding may seem to present a perplexing dilemma, but it is very important in understanding how the treatment of PH should best be monitored.

The explanation for why pulmonary pressure is a poor correlate with symptoms and survival is multifaceted. First, pulmonary pressure can fluctuate significantly and unpredictably over short periods of time and can be affected by position, activity, intravascular volume, anxiety, altitude, and other factors. Second, assessment of pulmonary pressure, whether through noninvasive echocardiographic estimation or through catheterization, occurs at isolated times with limited sampling duration under conditions that may not represent the average state of the patient. Third, measurement techniques are subject to error and may not even correlate with one another in an individual patient. Each of these factors warrants further consideration.

Spontaneous fluctuation of pulmonary hemodynamics in patients with PH has long been recognized. Rich and colleagues[93] observed in 1985 that the mean coefficient of variation for hourly mean pulmonary arterial pressure during 6 hours of monitoring in 12 supine resting patients was more than 8%, and for total pulmonary resistance was 12.9%. The fluctuation tended to be more pronounced for patients with more severe PH. They calculated that a mean change of pulmonary arterial pressure of 22% (36% for pulmonary resistance) would be necessary to attribute the change to an intervention in an individual patient. Therefore, even over a short time, the "noise" in measuring pulmonary hemodynamics may overwhelm any small (but true) effect that a drug may produce.

By extension, measurement of pulmonary hemodynamics during periodic brief RHC provides only an "ice pick" view of a patient's status. This finding has recently been vividly illustrated by the experience with long-term measurement of right ventricular systolic pressure and extrapolation of mean pulmonary arterial pressure in 24 patients with implanted ambulatory pulmonary hemodynamic monitors. In these patients, a wide variation in pressures around the daily median was consistently observed.[94,95] In some of these patients, assessment of PH (through echocardiography) frequently diverged from the median daily pressure but was nevertheless within the range of variation, occasionally leading to a failure to detect changes in the trend of daily pressures during the course of treatment (**Fig. 4**).

The unreliability of Doppler echocardiography in consistently mirroring invasive hemodynamic findings has been discussed earlier. When superimposed on spontaneous hemodynamic variations, this additional discordance would seem to make echocardiography an unreliable means to assess the hemodynamic trajectory of the patient on treatment. This observation is emphasized in a recent study of patients in the REVEAL registry, in which

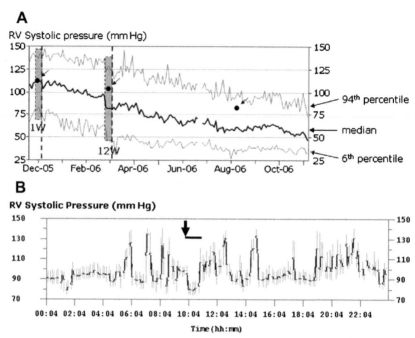

A

RV Systolic pressure (mm Hg)

94th percentile

median

6th percentile

1W and 12W

Dec-05   Feb-06   Apr-06   Jun-06   Aug-06   Oct-06

B

RV Systolic Pressure (mm Hg)

00:04 02:04 04:04 06:04 08:04 10:04 12:04 14:04 16:04 18:04 20:04 22:04

Time (hh:mm)

Fig. 4. Representative examples obtained from implanted hemodynamic monitors. (*A*) Depiction of daily median values (*dark line*) of RVSP over the course of 1 year in a patient on treatment with multiple pulmonary vasomodulating drugs. Daily 6th and 94th percentiles for values are also shown, illustrating the variation in pressures. 1W and 12 W show the first- and twelfth-week monitoring intervals. The dots and arrows show the RVSP estimated using Doppler echocardiography at three points in time. Although the echocardiographic data reflect the downward trend in pressures, they are not consistently congruent with the actual invasively monitored daily medians. Because they fall within the range of pressures measured for those days, however, the values may be accurate. RV, right ventricular. (*B*) Depiction of 6-minute median RVSP values (*dark line*) over the course of 1 day in a different patient. The vertical bars represent the range between the 6th and 94th percentile of RVSP values for each 6-minute interval. A Doppler echocardiogram obtained on this day reported an estimated RVSP of 75 mm Hg, which was "lower than the pressure 3 months ago of 102 mm Hg." The daily median RVSP at this time was consistently 98 mm Hg. The echocardiographic study began at the point marked by the arrow and lasted the duration indicated by the horizontal line, during which the monitored RVSP was usually in the range of 80 mm Hg. This finding suggested that the echocardiographic result was accurate, but nevertheless was not representative of the patient's median daily RVSP. RV, right ventricular.

the level of discrepancy between echocardiographic and catheterization data was virtually unchanged regardless of the interval that separated the two tests, from the same day up to 1 year apart.[96]

These observations suggest that pulmonary hemodynamics, and particularly measurements (and especially estimations) of pulmonary arterial pressure, may be an unreliable means to assess patient well-being or response to treatment. Unreliability of this single parameter is a function of not only measurement technique but also pathophysiology: pulmonary arterial pressure, when considered out of context, may seem to paradoxically decrease ("improve") despite clinical deterioration, because it may be a reflection of worsening right ventricular pump function.

Clearly inaccuracy, biologic fluctuation, and intermittent measurement of isolated hemodynamic parameters conspire to raise doubts that anything of more than vague clinical relevance is provided by these tests. Perhaps then the attempt to measure a precise hemodynamic parameter is misdirected, and the goal should be to take a broader and longer-term view to obtain a representation of the patient's overall clinical status and prognosis. This process would involve assessment of clinical features that correspond with symptomatic status and risk of early mortality.

Right Ventricular Function

The functional status of the right ventricle is a strong determinant of prognosis in patients with PH and left ventricular failure or COPD.[97] Historically, measurement of right ventricular function has been neglected because reliability was difficult with available imaging or functional techniques. However, methodologies for assessing the right ventricle, such as cardiac MRI[98,99] and CT imaging,[100] are undergoing increasing refinement. Right ventricular ejection fraction measured with radionuclide angiography is a function of right ventricular stroke volume, cardiac index, pulmonary vascular resistance, age, and sex in patients with PAH.[101] However, animal models suggest that pulmonary pressure alone may be insufficient to explain the development of right ventricular dysfunction and failure.[102]

Although echocardiographic images are not as volumetrically reliable as newer imaging techniques, indirect measures of right ventricular function (such as tricuspid annular plane systolic excursion) have been shown to have a strong correlation with functional status and survival.[103]

Indices of right ventricular function, when combined with indices of pulmonary vascular disease, have shown strong predictive value for outcome and association with functional status.[104] A simple measure of pulmonary artery capacitance includes stroke volume (SV) and pulmonary vascular pulse pressure (PP) in the equation SV/PP, and thus incorporates the relationship of right heart pump function and pulmonary arterial stiffness. This relationship is strongly predictive of survival.[105–107]

Functional Capacity

Functional classification according to subjective limitations of activity tolerance is a crude semiquantitative way to describe functional capacity. Despite vagaries of interpretation that lead to ambiguities of interpretation,[108] functional classification by World Health Organization or New York Heart Association criteria has repeatedly been shown to have strong predictive value for duration of survival.[109]

In an effort to more quantitatively and consistently measure functional capacity, the 6-minute walk test (6MWT) has been used in patients with PH and has been the primary end point in numerous clinical drug studies.[110] Distance walked in a 6MWT correlates with cardiac output, PVR, and peak Vo_2 (but not with mean pulmonary arterial pressure), and is predictive of survival.[111] The 6MWT, therefore, has been regarded as "an indirect test of right ventricular function."[110] A recent meta-analysis of randomized clinical drug studies showed that 6MWT distance improved with treatment, as did functional status, hemodynamics, and survival, although correlation among these outcomes was not specifically assessed.[112] Nevertheless, the 6MWT is subject to confounding influences, including effort and noncardiopulmonary (eg, musculoskeletal factors, pain) limitations.[113,114] In

addition, patients with a high (>450 m) 6MWT distance at presentation tend to be younger and have lower body mass index than comparably symptomatic patients with a shorter 6MWT distance. In these patients, improvement in functional status is not associated with change in 6MWT distance during treatment.[115]

Cardiopulmonary exercise testing provides more objective data and is useful for distinguishing cardiac, pulmonary, and other sources of exertional disability, and correlates with improvement in pulmonary hemodynamics during chronic treatment.[116] Patients with PH have lower peak oxygen consumption (Vo_2), higher ratio of minute ventilation to carbon dioxide production (expired volume per unit time/carbon dioxide consumption [VE/Vco_2]) and slope, and diminished partial pressure of end-tidal carbon dioxide ($PETco_2$), although the predictive value and usefulness in treatment monitoring of these variables remains unclear.[117] The use of a simplified submaximal cardiopulmonary exercise test using a step test and laptop-based system (SHAPE Medical Systems, St Paul, MN, USA) was recently described.[118] Data from this methodology could serve as a useful way to follow patients, and as an end point in clinical trials. It avoids some of the issues of lack of standardization/uniform interpretation that have plagued prior efforts to use cardiopulmonary exercise testing as an end point.

Outcome Goals

For reasons outlined earlier, the success of therapy is most productively defined in terms of functional response and other indices that reflect right ventricular function in the face of elevated pulmonary resistance. Systematic goal-directed follow-up is the lynchpin of optimal therapy.[119] The treat-to-target strategy for PAH was most systematically articulated first in 2005 when the availability of multiple approved drugs made combination therapy a possibility.[120] The treatment objective used was a composite of 6MWT distance greater than 380 m, peak Vo_2 greater than 10.4 mL/min/kg, and peak exercise systemic systolic blood pressure greater than 120 mm Hg based on the previously observed prognostic significance of each of these parameters.[121,122] Failure to achieve all three components of the treatment goal warranted advancement of therapy. Survival using this strategy surpassed that of a historical control group but was not specifically compared with alternative strategies, such as continuation of unchanged medication regimen, substitution (rather than addition) of medications, initiation of combination therapy at the outset, or use of different treatment goals. Nevertheless, the important concept was introduced that a composite (more global) clinical end point reflecting functional status and cardiopulmonary efficiency should be used in patient management decisions.

Innumerable reports are available on the prognostic value of various clinical or hemodynamic variables. The growing plethora of predictors has posed a dilemma for the practitioner: what should the conclusion be when different criteria point in different directions? For example, does a patient on monotherapy with a self-described poor functional capacity, a 6MWT distance of 430 m, and NT-proBNP of 1200 require an additional drug? Rather than relying on a single parameter, the principle of incorporating multiple clinical considerations into a global assessment of a patient's status to select or alter therapy has been advocated.[1,123] Although the original NIH registry of primary pulmonary hypertension incorporated three hemodynamic parameters (mean pulmonary arterial pressure, mean right atrial pressure, and cardiac index) into a predictive equation,[109] this equation seems to lack as much predictive value in the current era. The same variables have been used in a modified predictive equation based on exponential regression analysis of a single-institution population of patients with idiopathic, familial, or anorexigen-associated PAH.[124] Other variables may be more relevant in other populations of patients with PAH, such as those with scleroderma.[125]

Updating the clinician's ability to prognosticate underlies recent efforts to consolidate multiple relevant clinical factors into an accessible risk calculating model that predicts 1-year survival. Using data from the REVEAL registry, Benza and colleagues[126,127] developed a multivariable formula for clinical use. Demographic, clinical, biomarker, and hemodynamic variables are included. The attractiveness of the risk calculator for clinical use is that, although it incorporates multiple variables, the accuracy of prediction does not require that all variables be available; that is, it holds up even if missing values are present. Moreover, because the predictive equation was derived from a large patient population at different stages of disease and treatment, it is applicable at points of time other than at the baseline presentation of a treatment-naïve patient. This fact raises the possibility (as yet unproven) that altering treatment among patients shown to be at higher risk of early mortality may improve survival. Therefore, a risk score of this type may serve as an objective in a treat-to-goal strategy. Despite the potential usefulness of the current risk calculator,

incorporation of extent of change in parameters over time and/or inclusion of other variables, such as tricuspid annular plane systolic excursion, stroke volume/pulse pressure, or right ventricular volume, is likely to fine-tune it further in the future.

One dilemma confronting the clinician is how to equate the results of clinical trials (end points) with treatment objectives in practice. Does a statistically significant improvement in 6MWT distance or in delay in time to clinical worsening (TTCW) among study patients provide information about what to expect or aim for in an individual patient? This query has two components: (1) is the end point itself a clinically important or desirable variable to follow, and, if so, (2) to what extent must the end point be different from baseline to reflect a meaningful therapeutic effect?

In 19 clinical drug studies, 6MWD changed by a mean of -10 to 108 m (mean, 35.6 m).[112] However, how to predict which patient will respond to any given drug to this extent or more is unclear, as is what degree of improvement really represents an effect that is noticeable in terms of symptomatic improvement or survival benefit. Some evidence suggests that it is not the extent to which 6MWT distance improves while on treatment that impacts survival but rather whether it improves to a specific distance (ie, approximately 380 m).[121] Based on one study of patients enrolled in a randomized study of sildenafil, an improvement of 41 m in the 6MWT distance corresponded with improvement in quality-of-life measures.[128]

Appropriately adjudicated TTCW (incorporating all-cause mortality, nonelective hospitalization for PAH indications, and 15% or greater worsening of 6MWT distance) has been advocated as a potentially useful end point for clinical trials because it incorporates a broader perspective of relevant potential outcomes.[129–131] For clinical utility, however, worsening (or its absence) may be less than ideal as an end point because a patient could remain stable but severely symptomatic and limited. Under these circumstances, neglecting to advance therapeutic aggressiveness may be inappropriate.

A multiparameter index reflecting improvement seems like a desirable end point candidate that would assess drug efficacy and provide guidance for clinical practice. This index would include measures of both symptomatic/functional parameters and duration of effect. The inclusion of duration would address the issue of whether a beneficial functional effect may be only short-lived or even be associated with an augmented mortality risk, as has been seen in some heart failure–related drug studies. The simplest construct might be change in 6MWT distance over time, in which the area-

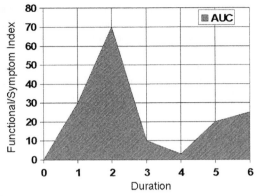

Fig. 5. Hypothetical illustration of an area-under-the-curve (AUC) graph measuring therapeutic benefit of an intervention.

under-the-curve represented degree of benefit and a target area would represent a clinical treatment goal at various intervals (**Fig. 5**). Possible alternative indices to measure over time might be functional classification, peak Vo_2, absolute 6MWT distance, standardized quality-of-life scores, quantitative measures of right ventricular function, biomarker levels, and hemodynamics. Ideally, a composite index of multiple parameters analogous to the REVEAL risk calculator could be constructed. Although theoretically appealing, no direct evidence in support of this concept currently exists. Nevertheless, this represents a useful mode of thought for physicians to bring to clinical decision making for patients with PAH.

SUMMARY

Understanding of the appropriate role for PH screening, in terms of both target population and selection of screening tools, remains limited. Diagnostic evaluation of suspected PH has benefited from published guidelines on classification and evaluation, and education regarding rigorous application of these tools. Suggested strategies for following response to therapy have been discussed and remain open to further evolution. Most patients with suspected PH fall outside group I PAH, and many patients have overlapping features. This article addresses issues in evaluating and characterizing these patients. For most of these patients, evaluation and therapy directed at the non–group I features represents the mainstay of approach. However, patients with risk factors for group I PAH who also have elements of groups II or III that formally remove them from classical group I membership are common in clinical practice, as are patients without obvious risk factors for group I PAH who have PH that seems disproportionate

to their group II or III features. At a minimum, the thoughtful clinician must fully characterize and track the particular pathophysiology of individual patients, and target the non–group I characteristics with appropriate therapy. An understanding of the potential for harm with use of pulmonary-specific vasodilators, either through aggravating hypoxemia, causing fluid retention or pulmonary congestion, or wasting health care resources on expensive therapies that may not be effective, must be clearly understood. Further investigation is needed regarding the optimal role of medications traditionally reserved for classical group I PAH.

REFERENCES

1. McLaughlin VV, McGoon MD. Pulmonary arterial hypertension. Circulation 2006;114(13):1417–31.
2. McLaughlin VV, Archer SL, Badesch DB, et al. ACCF/AHA 2009 expert consensus document on pulmonary hypertension: a report of the American College of Cardiology Foundation Task Force on Expert Consensus Documents and the American Heart Association: developed in collaboration with the American College of Chest Physicians, American Thoracic Society, Inc., and the Pulmonary Hypertension Association. Circulation 2009; 119(16):2250–94.
3. Galie N, Hoeper MM, Humbert M, et al. Guidelines for the diagnosis and treatment of pulmonary hypertension: the Task Force for the Diagnosis and Treatment of Pulmonary Hypertension of the European Society of Cardiology (ESC) and the European Respiratory Society (ERS), endorsed by the International Society of Heart and Lung Transplantation (ISHLT). Eur Heart J 2009;30(20):2493–537.
4. Rich S, Dantzker DR, Ayres SM, et al. Primary pulmonary hypertension: a national prospective study. Ann Intern Med 1987;107(2):216–23.
5. Humbert M, Sitbon O, Chaouat A, et al. Pulmonary arterial hypertension in France: results from a national registry. Am J Respir Crit Care Med 2006;173(9):1023–30.
6. Brown LM, Chen H, Halpern SD, et al. Delay in recognition of pulmonary arterial hypertension: factors identified from the REVEAL Registry. Chest 2011;140(1):19–26.
7. Galie N, Rubin LJ, Hoeper MM, et al. Treatment of patients with mildly symptomatic pulmonary arterial hypertension with bosentan (EARLY study): a double-blind, randomised controlled trial. Lancet 2008;371:2093–100.
8. Simonneau G, Robbins IM, Beghetti M, et al. Updated clinical classification of pulmonary hypertension. J Am Coll Cardiol 2009;54(Suppl 1):S43–54.
9. Hachulla E, Gressin V, Guillevin L, et al. Early detection of pulmonary arterial hypertension in

systemic sclerosis: a French nationwide prospective multicenter study. Arthritis Rheum 2005; 52(12):3792–800.

10. Bull TM. Screening and therapy of pulmonary hypertension in systemic sclerosis. Curr Opin Rheumatol 2007;19(6):598–603.

11. Hachulla E, deGroote P, Gressin V, et al. The three-year incidence of pulmonary arterial hypertension associated with systemic sclerosis in a multicenter nationwide longitudinal study in France. Arthritis Rheum 2009;60(6):1831–9.

12. Colle IO, Moreau R, Godinho E, et al. Diagnosis of portopulmonary hypertension in candidates for liver transplantation: a prospective study. Hepatology 2003;37:401–9.

13. Hadengue A, Benyahoun MK, Lebrec D, et al. Pulmonary hypertension complicating portal hypertension: prevalence and relation to splanchnic hemodynamics. Gastroenterology 1991;100:520–8.

14. Kawut SM, Krowka MJ, Trotter JF, et al. Clinical risk factors for portopulmonary hypertension. Hepatology 2008;48(1):196–203.

15. Krowka MJ, Swanson KL, Frantz RP, et al. Portopulmonary hypertension: results from a 10-year screening algorithm. Hepatology 2006;44:1502–10.

16. Condliffe R, Kiely DG, Peacock AJ, et al. Connective tissue disease-associated pulmonary arterial hypertension in the modern treatment era. Am J Respir Crit Care Med 2009;179(2):151–7.

17. Sitbon O, Lascoux-Combe C, Delfraissy JF, et al. Prevalence of HIV-related pulmonary arterial hypertension in the current antiretroviral therapy era. Am J Respir Crit Care Med 2008;177(1):108–13.

18. Almodovar S, Cicalini S, Petrosillo N, et al. Pulmonary hypertension associated with HIV infection. Chest 2010;137(Suppl 6):6S–12S.

19. Abenhaim L, Moride Y, Brenot F, et al. Appetite-suppressant drugs and the risk of primary pulmonary hypertension. International primary pulmonary hypertension study group. N Engl J Med 1996; 335(9):609–16.

20. Klok F, van Kralingen K, van Dijk A, et al. Prospective cardiopulmonary screening program to detect chronic thromboembolic pulmonary hypertension in patients after acute pulmonary embolism. Haematologica 2010;95(6):970–5.

21. Pengo V, Lensing A, Prins M, et al. Incidence of chronic thromboembolic pulmonary hypertension after pulmonary embolism. N Engl J Med 2004; 350(22):2257–64.

22. Dentali F, Donadini M, Gianni M, et al. Incidence of chronic pulmonary hypertension in patients with previous pulmonary embolism. Thromb Res 2009; 124(3):256–8.

23. Adatia I, Kothari SS, Feinstein JA. Pulmonary hypertension associated with congenital heart disease. Chest 2010;137(Suppl 6):52S–61S.

24. Beghetti M, Galiè N. Eisenmenger syndrome: a clinical perspective in a new therapeutic era of pulmonary arterial hypertension. J Am Coll Cardiol 2009; 53(9):733–40.

25. Bull TM, Coldren CD, Geraci MW, et al. Gene expression profiling in pulmonary hypertension. Proc Am Thorac Soc 2007;4(1):117–20.

26. Rubin LJ. BMPR2 mutation and outcome in pulmonary arterial hypertension: clinical relevance to physicians and patients. Am J Respir Crit Care Med 2008;177(12):1300–1.

27. Machado RD, Eickelberg O, Elliott CG, et al. Genetics and genomics of pulmonary arterial hypertension. J Am Coll Cardiol 2009;54(Suppl 1):S32–42.

28. Geraci MW, Bull TM, Tuder RM. Genomics of pulmonary arterial hypertension: implications for therapy. Heart Fail Clin 2010;6(1):101–14.

29. Grunig E, Weissmann S, Ehlken N, et al. Stress Doppler echocardiography in relatives of patients with idiopathic and familial pulmonary arterial hypertension: results of a multicenter European analysis of pulmonary artery pressure response to exercise and hypoxia. Circulation 2009;119(13):1747–57.

30. Kiencke S, Bernheim A, Maggiorini M, et al. Exercise-induced pulmonary artery hypertension: a rare finding? J Am Coll Cardiol 2008;51(4): 513–4.

31. Steen V, Medsger T. Predictors of isolated pulmonary hypertension in patients with systemic sclerosis and limited cutaneous involvement. Arthritis Rheum 2003;48(2):516–22.

32. Steen V, Chou M, Shanmugam V, et al. Exercise-induced pulmonary arterial hypertension in patients with systemic sclerosis. Chest 2008;134(1):146–51.

33. Kovacs G, Maier R, Aberer E, et al. Assessment of pulmonary arterial pressure during exercise in collagen vascular disease. Chest 2010;138(2):270–8.

34. Tolle JJ, Waxman AB, Van Horn TL, et al. Exercise-induced pulmonary arterial hypertension. Circulation 2008;118(21):2183–9.

35. Park MH, Ramani GV, Kop WJ, et al. Exercise-uncovered pulmonary arterial hypertension and pharmacologic therapy: clinical benefits. J Heart Lung Transplant 2010;29(2):228–9.

36. Oudiz RJ, Rubin LJ. Exercise-induced pulmonary arterial hypertension: a new addition to the spectrum of pulmonary vascular diseases. Circulation 2008;118(21):2120–1.

37. Zisman DA, Karlamangla AS, Kawut SM, et al. Validation of a method to screen for pulmonary hypertension in advanced idiopathic pulmonary fibrosis. Chest 2008;133(3):640–5. DOI:10.1378/chest.07-2488.

38. Zisman DA, Ross DJ, Belperio JA, et al. Prediction of pulmonary hypertension in idiopathic pulmonary fibrosis. Respir Med 2007;101(10):2153–9.

39. Coral-Alvarado P, Quintana G, Garces M, et al. Potential biomarkers for detecting pulmonary

arterial hypertension in patients with systemic sclerosis. Rheumatol Int 2009;29(9):1017–24.

40. Berger M, Haimowitz A, Van Tosh A, et al. Quantitative assessment of pulmonary hypertension in patients with tricuspid regurgitation using continuous wave Doppler ultrasound. J Am Coll Cardiol 1985;6:359–65.

41. Currie PJ, Seward JB, Chan KL, et al. Continuous wave Doppler determination of right ventricular pressure: a simultaneous Doppler-catheterization study in 127 patients. J Am Coll Cardiol 1985; 6(4):750–6.

42. Arcasoy SM, Christie JD, Ferrari VA, et al. Echocardiographic assessment of pulmonary hypertension in patients with advanced lung disease. Am J Respir Crit Care Med 2003;167(5):735–40.

43. Fisher MR, Forfia PR, Chamera E, et al. Accuracy of Doppler echocardiography in the hemodynamic assessment of pulmonary hypertension. Am J Respir Crit Care Med 2009;179:615–21.

44. Testani JM, St. John Sutton MG, Wiegers SE, et al. Accuracy of noninvasively determined pulmonary artery systolic pressure. Am J Cardiol 2010;105(8):1192–7.

45. Rich JD, Shah SJ, Swamy R, et al. The inaccuracy of Doppler echocardiographic estimates of pulmonary artery pressures in patients with pulmonary hypertension: implications for clinical practice. Chest 2011;139(5):988–93.

46. Hoeper MM, Barberà JA, Channick RN, et al. Diagnosis, assessment, and treatment of non-pulmonary arterial hypertension pulmonary hypertension. J Am Coll Cardiol 2009;54(Suppl 1):S85–96.

47. Rich S, Rabinovitch M. Diagnosis and treatment of secondary (non-category 1) pulmonary hypertension. Circulation 2008;118(21):2190–9.

48. O'Callaghan DS, McNeil K. Pulmonary hypertension and left heart disease: emerging concepts and treatment strategies. Int J Clin Pract 2008; 62(s160):29–31.

49. Shapiro BP, McGoon MD, Redfield MM. Unexplained pulmonary hypertension in elderly patients. Chest 2007;131(1):94–100.

50. Leung CC, Moondra V, Catherwood E, et al. Prevalence and risk factors of pulmonary hypertension in patients with elevated pulmonary venous pressure and preserved ejection fraction. Am J Cardiol 2010;106(2):284–6.

51. Oudiz RJ. Pulmonary hypertension associated with left-sided heart disease. Clin Chest Med 2007; 28(1):233–41.

52. Palmer SM, Robinson LJ, Wang A, et al. Massive pulmonary edema and death after prostacyclin infusion in a patient with pulmonary veno-occlusive disease. Chest 1998;113:237–40.

53. Preston IR, Klinger JR, Houtchens J, et al. Pulmonary edema caused by inhaled nitric oxide therapy in two patients with pulmonary hypertension

associated with the CREST syndrome. Chest 2002;121:656–9.

54. Farber HW, Graven KK, Kokolski G, et al. Pulmonary edema during acute infusion of epoprostenol in a patient with pulmonary hypertension and limited scleroderma. J Rheumatol 1999;26(5):1195–6.

55. Humbert M, Maitre S, Capron F, et al. Pulmonary edema complicating continuous intravenous prostacyclin in pulmonary capillary hemangiomatosis. Am J Respir Crit Care Med 1998;157: 1681–5.

56. McGoon MD, Krichman A, Farber H, et al. Design of the REVEAL registry for US patients with pulmonary arterial hypertension. Mayo Clin Proc 2008; 83(8):923–31.

57. Badesch DB, Raskob GE, Elliott CG, et al. Pulmonary arterial hypertension: baseline characteristics from the REVEAL registry. Chest 2009;137(2):376–87.

58. Halpern SD, Taichman DB. Misclassification of pulmonary hypertension due to reliance on pulmonary capillary wedge pressure rather than left-ventricular end-diastolic pressure. Chest 2009; 136(1):37–43.

59. Scharf SM, Iqbal M, Keller C, et al. Hemodynamic characterization of patients with severe emphysema. Am J Respir Crit Care Med 2002;166(3):314–22.

60. Nadrous H, Pellikka PA, Krowka M, et al. The impact of pulmonary hypertension on survival in patients with idiopathic pulmonary fibrosis. Chest 2005;128:616–7.

61. Grubstein A, Bendeyan D, Schactman I, et al. Concomitant upper-lobe bullous emphysema, lower-lobe interstitial fibrosis and pulmonary hypertension in heavy smokers: report of eight cases and review of the literature. Respir Med 2005;99:948–54.

62. Lettieri C, Nathan S, Barnett S, et al. Prevalence and outcomes of pulmonary arterial hypertension in advanced idiopathic pulmonary fibrosis. Chest 2006;129(3):746–52.

63. Shorr A, Wainright J, Cors C, et al. Pulmonary hypertension in patients with pulmonary fibrosis awaiting lung transplantation. Eur Respir J 2007; 30(4):715–21.

64. Hamada K, Nagai S, Tanaka S, et al. Significance of pulmonary arterial pressure and diffusion capacity of the lung as prognosticator in patients with idiopathic pulmonary fibrosis. Chest 2007; 131(3):650–6.

65. Weitzenblum E, Chaouat A, Canuet M, et al. Pulmonary hypertension in chronic obstructive pulmonary disease and interstitial lung diseases. Semin Respir Crit Care Med 2009;30(4):458–70.

66. Chaouat A, Naeije R, Weitzenblum E. Pulmonary hypertension in COPD. Eur Respir J 2008;32(5): 1371–85.

67. Thabut G, Dauriat G, Stern JB, et al. Pulmonary hemodynamics in advanced COPD candidates

for lung volume reduction surgery or lung transplantation. Chest 2005;127:1531–6.

68. Nathan SD, Shlobin OA, Ahmad S, et al. Pulmonary hypertension and pulmonary function testing in idiopathic pulmonary fibrosis. Chest 2007;131(3): 657–63.

69. Burger CD. Pulmonary hypertension in COPD: a review and consideration of the role of arterial vasodilators. COPD 2009;6(2):137–44.

70. Weitzenblum E. Severe pulmonary hypertension in COPD: is it a distinct disease? [editorial]. Chest 2005;127(5):1480–2.

71. Burrows B, Kettel LJ, Niden AH, et al. Patterns of cardiovascular dysfunction in chronic obstructive lung disease. N Engl J Med 1972;286:912–8.

72. Traver GA, Cline MG, Burrows B. Predictors of mortality in chronic obstructive pulmonary disease. A 15-year follow-up study. Am Rev Respir Dis 1970;119:895–902.

73. Weitzenblum E, Hirth C, Ducolone A, et al. Prognostic value of pulmonary artery pressure in chronic obstructive pulmonary disease. Thorax 1981;36:752–8.

74. Patel NM, Lederer DJ, Borczuk AC, et al. Pulmonary hypertension in idiopathic pulmonary fibrosis. Chest 2007;132(3):998–1006.

75. Stolz D, Rasch H, Linka A, et al. A randomised, controlled trial of bosentan in severe COPD. Eur Respir J 2008;32(3):619–28.

76. Girgis RE, Mathai SC. Pulmonary hypertension associated with chronic respiratory disease. Clin Chest Med 2007;28(1):219–32.

77. Sajkov D, McEvoy RD. Obstructive sleep apnea and pulmonary hypertension. Prog Cardiovasc Dis 2009;51(5):363–70.

78. Somers VK, White DP, Amin R, et al. Sleep apnea and cardiovascular disease: an American Heart Association/American College of Cardiology Foundation Scientific Statement From the American Heart Association Council for High Blood Pressure Research Professional Education Committee, Council on Clinical Cardiology, Stroke Council, and Council on Cardiovascular Nursing In Collaboration With the National Heart, Lung, and Blood Institute National Center on Sleep Disorders Research (National Institutes of Health). J Am Coll Cardiol 2008;52(8): 686–717.

79. Chaouat A, Weitzenblum E, Krieger J, et al. Pulmonary hemodynamics in the obstructive sleep apnea syndrome: results in 220 consecutive patients. Chest 1996;109(2):380–6.

80. Laks L, Lehrhaft B, Grunstein RR, et al. Pulmonary hypertension in obstructive sleep apnoea. Eur Respir J 1995;8:537–41.

81. Sanner BM, Doberauer C, Konermann M, et al. Pulmonary hypertension in patients with obstructive sleep apnea syndrome. Arch Intern Med 1997;157: 2483–7.

82. Yamakawa H, Shiomi T, Sasanabe R, et al. Pulmonary hypertension in patients with severe obstructive sleep apnea. Psychiatry Clin Neurosci 2002; 56:311–2.

83. Sajkov D, Wang T, Saunders NA, et al. Continuous positive airway pressure treatment improves pulmonary hemodynamics in patients with obstructive sleep apnea. Am J Respir Crit Care Med 2002; 165:152–8.

84. Kessler R, Chaouat A, Weitzenblum E, et al. Pulmonary hypertension in the obstructive sleep apnoea syndrome: prevalence, causes and therapeutic consequences. Eur Respir J 1996;9:787–94.

85. Alchanatis M, Tourkohorti G, Kakouros S, et al. Daytime pulmonary hypertension in patients with obstructive sleep apnea: the effect of continuous positive airway pressure on pulmonary hemodynamics. Respiration 2001;68(6):566–72.

86. Arias M, Garcia-Rio F, Alonso-Fernandez A, et al. Pulmonary hypertension in obstructive sleep apnea: effects of continuous positive airway pressure. Eur Heart J 2006;27(9):1106–13.

87. Piper A. Obesity hypoventilation syndrome: therapeutic implications for treatment. Expert Review of Respir Med 2010;4(1):57–70.

88. Bonderman D, Skoro-Sajer N, Jakowitsch J, et al. Predictors of outcome in chronic thromboembolic pulmonary hypertension. Circulation 2007; 115(16):2153–8.

89. Bonderman D, Wilkens H, Wakounig S, et al. Risk factors for chronic thromboembolic pulmonary hypertension. Eur Respir J 2009;33:325–31.

90. Condliffe R, Kiely DG, Gibbs JSR, et al. Prognostic and aetiological factors in chronic thromboembolic pulmonary hypertension. Eur Respir J 2009;33: 332–8.

91. Tunariu N, Gibbs SJR, Win Z, et al. Ventilation-perfusion scintigraphy is more sensitive than multidetector CTPA in detecting chronic thromboembolic pulmonary disease as a treatable cause of pulmonary hypertension. J Nucl Med 2007;48(5):680–4.

92. Reichelt A, Hoeper MM, Galanski M, et al. Chronic thromboembolic pulmonary hypertension: evaluation with 64-detector row CT versus digital substraction angiography. Eur J Radiol 2009;71(1): 49–54.

93. Rich S, D'Alonzo GE, Dantzker DR, et al. Magnitude and implications of spontaneous hemodynamic variability in primary pulmonary hypertension. Am J Cardiol 1985;55(1):159–63.

94. Frantz R, Kjellstrom B, McGoon M. Ambulatory hemodynamic monitoring in pulmonary arterial hypertension. Adv Pulm Hypertens 2008;7(4):405–10.

95. Frantz RP, Benza RL, Kjellstrom B, et al. Continuous hemodynamic monitoring in patients with pulmonary arterial hypertension. J Heart Lung Transplant 2008;27(7):780–8.

96. Farber HW, Foreman AJ, Miller DP, et al. REVEAL registry: correlation of right heart catheterization and echocardiography in patients with pulmonary arterial hypertension. Congest Heart Fail 2011;17:56–64.

97. McLure LER, Peacock AJ. Cardiac magnetic resonance imaging for the assessment of the heart and pulmonary circulation in pulmonary hypertension. Eur Respir J 2009;33(6):1454–66.

98. Biederman RW. Cardiovascular magnetic resonance imaging as applied to patients with pulmonary arterial hypertension. Int J Clin Pract 2009; 63(Suppl 162):20–35.

99. van Wolferen SA, Marcus JT, Boonstra A, et al. Prognostic value of right ventricular mass, volume, and function in idiopathic pulmonary arterial hypertension. Eur Heart J 2007;28(10):1250–7.

100. Ley S, Grünig E, Kiely DG, et al. Computed tomography and magnetic resonance imaging of pulmonary hypertension: pulmonary vessels and right ventricle. J Magn Reson Imaging 2010;32(6):1313–24.

101. Kawut SM, Al-Naamani N, Agerstrand C, et al. Determinants of right ventricular ejection fraction in pulmonary arterial hypertension. Chest 2009;135(3):752–9.

102. Bogaard HJ, Natarajan R, Henderson SC, et al. Chronic pulmonary artery pressure elevation is insufficient to explain right heart failure. Circulation 2009;120(20):1951–60.

103. Forfia PR, Fisher MR, Mathai SC, et al. Tricuspid annular displacement predicts survival in pulmonary hypertension. Am J Respir Crit Care Med 2006;174:1034–41.

104. Champion HC, Michelakis ED, Hassoun PM. Comprehensive invasive and noninvasive approach to the right ventricle-pulmonary circulation unit: state of the art and clinical and research implications. Circulation 2009;120(11):992–1007.

105. Mahapatra S, Nishimura RA, Oh JK, et al. The prognostic value of pulmonary vascular capacitance determined by Doppler echocardiography in patients with pulmonary arterial hypertension. J Am Soc Echocardiogr 2006;19(8):1045–50.

106. Mahapatra S, Nishimura RA, Sorajja P, et al. Relationship of pulmonary arterial capacitance and mortality in idiopathic pulmonary arterial hypertension. J Am Coll Cardiol 2006;47(4):799–803.

107. Campo A, Mathai SC, Le Pavec J, et al. Hemodynamic predictors of survival in scleroderma-related pulmonary arterial hypertension. Am J Respir Crit Care Med 2010;182(2):252–60.

108. Taichman DB, McGoon MD, Harhay MO, et al. Wide variation in clinicians' assessment of New York Heart Association/World Health Organization functional class in patients with pulmonary arterial hypertension. Mayo Clin Proc 2009;84(7): 586–92.

109. D'Alonzo GE, Barst RJ, Ayres SM, et al. Survival in patients with primary pulmonary hypertension: results from a national prospective registry. Ann Intern Med 1991;115:343–9.

110. Naeije R. The 6-min walk distance in pulmonary arterial hypertension. Chest 2010;137(6):1258–60.

111. Miyamoto S, Nagaya N, Satoh T, et al. Clinical correlates and prognostic significance of six-minute walk test in patients with primary pulmonary hypertension: comparison with cardiopulmonary exercise testing. Am J Respir Crit Care Med 2000;161:487–92.

112. Galie N, Manes A, Negro L, et al. A meta-analysis of randomized controlled trials in pulmonary arterial hypertension. Eur Heart J 2009;30(4):394–403.

113. Garin MC, Highland KB, Silver RM, et al. Limitations to the 6-minute walk test in interstitial lung disease and pulmonary hypertension in scleroderma. J Rheumatol 2009;36(2):330–6.

114. Pamidi S, Mehta S. Six-minute walk test in scleroderma-associated pulmonary arterial hypertension: are we counting what counts? J Rheumatol 2009;36(2):216–8.

115. Degano B, Sitbon O, Savale L, et al. Characterization of pulmonary arterial hypertension patients walking more than 450 m in 6 min at diagnosis. Chest 2010;137(6):1297–303.

116. Provencher S, Herve P, Sitbon O, et al. Changes in exercise haemodynamics during treatment in pulmonary arterial hypertension. Eur Respir J 2008;32(2):393–8.

117. Arena R, Lavie CJ, Milani RV, et al. Cardiopulmonary exercise testing in patients with pulmonary arterial hypertension: an evidence-based review. J Heart Lung Transplant 2010;29(2):159–73.

118. Sitbon O, Hoeper MM, Simonneau G. Assessing effectiveness of pulmonary arterial hypertension therapies in daily practice. Curr Opin Pulm Med 2010;16:S21–6.

119. Woods PR, Frantz RP, Johnson BD. The usefulness of submaximal exercise gas exchange in pulmonary arterial hypertension: a case series. Clin Med Insights Circ Respir Pulm Med 2010;4(1):35–40.

120. Hoeper MM, Markevych I, Spiekerkoetter E, et al. Goal-oriented treatment and combination therapy for pulmonary arterial hypertension. Eur Respir J 2005;26(5):858–63.

121. Sitbon O, Humbert M, Nunes H, et al. Long-term intravenous epoprostenol infusion in primary pulmonary hypertension: prognostic factors and survival. J Am Coll Cardiol 2002;40(4):780–8.

122. Wensel R, Opitz CF, Anker SD, et al. Assessment of survival in patients with primary pulmonary hypertension: importance of cardiopulmonary exercise testing. Circulation 2002;106:319–24.

123. Sitbon O, Galie N. Treat-to-target strategies in pulmonary arterial hypertension: the importance of using multiple goals. Eur Respir Rev 2010;19(118):272–8.

124. Thenappan T, Shah SJ, Rich S, et al. Survival in pulmonary arterial hypertension: a reappraisal of

the NIH risk stratification equation. Eur Respir J 2010;35(5):1079–87.

125. Johnson SR, Swinton JR, Granton JT. Prognostic factors for survival in scleroderma associated pulmonary arterial hypertension. J Rheumatol 2008; 35:1584–90.

126. Benza RL, Miller DP, Gomberg-Maitland M, et al. Predicting survival in pulmonary arterial hypertension. insights from the registry to evaluate early and long-term pulmonary arterial hypertension disease management (REVEAL). Circulation 2010; 2010(122):164–72.

127. Benza RL, Gomberg-Maitland M, Miller DP, et al. The REVEAL registry risk score calculator in patients newly diagnosed with pulmonary arterial hypertension. Chest 2012;141:354–62.

128. Gilbert C, Brown MCJ, Cappelleri JC, et al. Estimating a minimally important difference in pulmonary arterial hypertension following treatment with sildenafil. Chest 2009;135(1):137–42.

129. McLaughlin VV, Badesch DB, Delcroix M, et al. End points and clinical trial design in pulmonary arterial hypertension. J Am Coll Cardiol 2009;54(Suppl 1): S97–107.

130. Haworth SG, Beghetti M. Assessment of endpoints in the pediatric population: congenital heart disease and idiopathic pulmonary arterial hypertension. Curr Opin Pulm Med 2010;16:S35–41.

131. Peacock AJ, Naeije R, Galie N, et al. End-points and clinical trial design in pulmonary arterial hypertension: have we made progress? Eur Respir J 2009;34(1):231–42.

Imaging in the Evaluation of Pulmonary Artery Hemodynamics and Right Ventricular Structure and Function

Asghar A. Fakhri, MD, Rachel A. Hughes-Doichev, MD*,
Robert W.W. Biederman, MD, Srinivas Murali, MD

KEYWORDS

• Pulmonary hypertension • Echocardiography • Cardiac magnetic resonance • Cardiac imaging

KEY POINTS

- Imaging is an important adjunct to heart catheterization for diagnosing pulmonary hypertension (PH) and discerning the etiology of elevated pulmonary artery pressures.
- Echocardiography is useful for screening patients for PH and to obtain a baseline assessment of right ventricular function.
- Doppler echocardiography provides useful hemodynamic information and assesses left ventricular diastolic dysfunction and valvular disease and can also be used to screen for intracardiac shunts.
- Cardiac magnetic resonance imaging (CMR) has gained importance in patients with PH and is the gold standard for assessing 3-dimensional right ventricular structure and function.
- CMR plays a crucial role in quantifying and locating intracardiac shunts, identifying myocardial fibrosis due to right ventricular strain, and also provides highly reproducible measurements that can be used to track response to PH therapy.
- Cardiac computed tomography (CT) is important for diagnosing thromboembolic disease and pathologies of the lung parenchyma.
- Ventilation/perfusion nuclear scans have greater sensitivity than CT for diagnosing chronic thromboembolic disease.

INTRODUCTION

The term pulmonary hypertension (PH) encompasses several disorders that manifest with elevated pressures in the pulmonary arterial (PA) circulation and subsequent dysfunction of the right ventricle (RV).[1] These disorders are grouped by the World Health Organization (WHO) into 5 distinct subsets: PA hypertension (PAH), PH from left-sided heart disease, PH from lung disease or hypoxemia, PH from chronic thrombotic and/or embolic disease (CTEPH), and miscellaneous (extrinsic compression of pulmonary vessels and so forth).[1] Along with clinical and laboratory evaluation, several imaging modalities play a crucial role in establishing the etiology, severity, prognosis, and response to

Echocardiography Laboratory, Cardiovascular Magnetic Resonance Imaging Laboratory, and Section of Heart Failure and Pulmonary Hypertension, Division of Cardiology, Department of Medicine, Gerald McGinnis Cardiovascular Institute, Allegheny General Hospital, 320 East North Avenue, Pittsburgh, PA 15212, USA
* Corresponding author. Claude Joyner Echocardiography Laboratory, Gerald McGinnis Cardiovascular Institute, Allegheny General Hospital, 320 East North Avenue, Pittsburgh, PA 15212.
E-mail address: rhughesd@wpahs.org

Heart Failure Clin 8 (2012) 353–372
doi:10.1016/j.hfc.2012.04.004
1551-7136/12/$ – see front matter © 2012 Elsevier Inc. All rights reserved.

therapy in the patient population with PH.[1] Imaging is used to assess physical characteristics of the PA, hemodynamic parameters, and pathologic changes in the right atrium (RA) and RV. The most commonly used modalities in current clinical practice for non-invasive hemodynamic and RV assessment are echocardiography (transthoracic, transesophageal) and cardiac magnetic resonance imaging (CMR).[1]

Pathophysiology of PH and RV Dysfunction

A full review of the pathophysiology of PH is beyond the scope of this discussion. However, an overview of the causes of PH and the effects of PH on RV function is pertinent to this review of imaging in PH. A lesion leading to elevated pulmonary pressure, currently defined as mean PA pressure (MPAP) greater than 25 mm Hg, can lie anywhere along a path from the PAs, pulmonary capillaries, pulmonary veins, up to the left heart. PH can also result from destruction or extrinsic compression of these structures by other intrathoracic abnormalities. The gamut of imaging techniques is used to evaluate all the earlier-mentioned structures.

The major focus of imaging in PH remains the evaluation of the RV because RV function is closely linked to symptoms and mortality.[2] Normally, the RV is the most anterior chamber of the heart and can be subdivided using an embryologic approach (inlet, trabeculated apex, and infundibulum/outflow tract) or using anatomic localization (anterior, lateral, and inferior walls).[3] The normal RV has a complex shape, appearing crescent shaped in cross section, with the septum being concave toward the left ventricle (LV).[3] A simplified

schematic of the RV is depicted in **Fig. 1**. Although the volume of the RV is greater than that of the LV in the normal adult, RV mass is significantly less than the LV mass.[3] These characteristics render the RV a much more compliant structure.[2] The muscular wall of the RV is composed of a network of myofibers with a circumferential orientation in the superficial layers and a longitudinal (base to apex) orientation in the deep layers.[3] Thus, RV contractile function consists of both longitudinal shortening and circumferential contraction, both of which can be assessed using imaging techniques. Under normal conditions, the primary functions of the RV are to (1) maintain low filling pressures to facilitate rapid systemic venous return and (2) generate adequate systolic pressure to permit blood flow through a normally low-impedance and low-resistance pulmonary vascular circuit.[3] Although the RV is well suited for these functions given the normally low afterload, it is much less tolerant of increases in afterload compared with the LV. When PA pressure increases acutely to more than 40 mm Hg, RV dilatation and dysfunction usually ensue due to greater distensibility and vulnerability to afterload.[2–4] One important mechanism for reduced cardiac output (CO) is the worsening of ventricular interdependence from an enlarging RV. Because the pericardial space constrains the RV and LV within a fixed volume, expansion of the RV can impinge on the LV, impairing the filling of the latter.[2] With chronically elevated PA pressures, the RV has time to hypertrophy to generate progressively greater systolic pressures. This remodeling also leads to flattening of the normally concave right side of the interventricular septum,

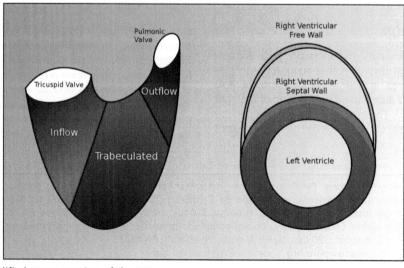

Fig. 1. A simplified representation of the RV.

which in turn affects LV diastolic performance.[2] RV dilatation and exacerbation of ventricular interdependence occur in the later stages of chronic PH. The combination of RV hypertrophy, increased RV wall stress, and reduced CO can produce RV ischemia, resulting in a cascade of progressive RV dysfunction and dilatation.[2]

Role of Imaging in PH

In current clinical practice, echocardiography and CMR are the major modalities used to evaluate noninvasive hemodynamics and cardiac structure and function. In addition, computed tomography (CT) of the chest can be used to evaluate for pulmonary parenchymal disease, intravascular thromboembolism, and other important intrathoracic pathologies. Although first-pass radionuclide angiography had been used in the past to assess RV ejection fraction (RVEF), this application for nuclear imaging has largely been replaced by echocardiography and CMR. However, radionuclide imaging still retains an essential role for evaluating the pulmonary vasculature in patients with PH. Although CT angiography is accurate for identifying acute thromboembolism in the proximal PAs, CTEPH often involves the smaller branch vessels that are less well resolved by CT angiography. In contrast, ventilation/perfusion scintigraphy or ventilation/perfusion

scanning has demonstrated superior sensitivity to CT angiography for detecting CTEPH and is therefore the test of choice to screen for this disease.[5] Each modality offers complementary information for establishing the etiology and severity of PH. Echocardiography is often the first-line imaging technique in patients with PH, because it is easily available, is inexpensive, lacks ionizing radiation, and provides well-validated hemodynamic information along with structural and functional assessment with excellent spatial and temporal resolution. CMR, with its high-resolution 3-dimensional (3D) capabilities, ability to assess tissue characteristics, increasingly better validated hemodynamic assessments, and high degree of reproducibility, has become the mainstay for initial and follow-up imaging of patients with PH in referral centers. There is growing advocacy for using CMR-derived end points to improve clinical trial design.[6] A summary of available imaging modalities and their uses is provided in **Table 1**.

NONINVASIVE HEMODYNAMICS ASSESSMENT

The first step in the diagnostic pathway of PH is performing a hemodynamic assessment. In the past, this was exclusively performed using invasive right-sided heart catheterization (RHC) to

Table 1
Imaging modalities available for evaluation of PA hemodynamics and RV structure and function

Desired Diagnostic Information	Preferred Imaging Modality
Screening for PH	Transthoracic echocardiography to measure the SPAP
Screening for intracardiac shunt	Transthoracic echocardiography • Color Doppler flow • Shunt calculation • Impact of shunt on RV function
Preliminary assessment of RV function	2D echocardiography
RV mass	Cardiac MRI
Confirmatory assessment and quantification of RV function	Cardiac MRI 3D echocardiography
Significant valvular disease	Transesophageal echocardiography Cardiac MRI
Quantification of shunt	Cardiac MRI
Locating shunt and preoperative assessment of shunt	Transesophageal echocardiography or cardiac MRI
Myocardial fibrosis or infiltrative disease (sarcoidosis, amyloidosis)	Cardiac MRI
Chronic thromboembolism	Ventilation perfusion scintigraphy (V/Q Scan) CT with contrast Cardiac MRI Pulmonary angiography
Interstitial lung disease	CT

evaluate pressures, CO, shunt physiology, and vascular resistance. Increasingly, echocardiography and CMR are used to establish the presence of PH, although RHC remains the gold standard for confirming the diagnosis and monitoring response to therapy. In addition, although noninvasive evaluations are extremely safe, RHC is associated with a very low but nonnegligible rate of morbidity and mortality.[7]

Echocardiography for Noninvasive Hemodynamics

Doppler echocardiography has grown to become a useful noninvasive tool for hemodynamic measurements. This modality is used to measure pressure gradients between chambers of the heart and also to quantify blood flow through various chambers. Yock and Popp first described the method to estimate RV systolic pressure and thus systolic PA pressure (SPAP) by measuring the velocity of tricuspid regurgitation (TR).[8,9] The peak velocity of TR (TRv) depends on the pressure difference between the RV and the RA during systole. This velocity is then used to calculate the pressure difference with a simplified form of the Bernoulli equation:

$$P_{RV} - P_{RA} = 4 \times (TRv)^2$$

RA pressure is determined using a standardized approach and then added to the pressure gradient, providing an estimate of RV systolic pressure (**Fig. 2**). The American Society of Echocardiography (ASE) currently recommends performing this measure routinely in adults undergoing echocardiographic evaluation.[8] In one general population study, each 10 mm Hg increase in SPAP by echocardiography had an adjusted hazard ratio of 1.46 for mortality.[10] In another study of patients with systolic and diastolic heart failure, this measurement had a specificity of 96% in diagnosing heart failure, compared with diagnosis by history taking, LV ejection fraction, and N-terminal probrain natriuretic peptide (NT-proBNP).[11] In addition, study patients in the highest quartile of SPAP (>45 mm Hg) had a markedly increased mortality compared with those in the lower 3 quartiles.[11] Although this measure may be helpful toward diagnosis and prognosis, it has also been studied as a marker for monitoring response to therapy. One study of patients with idiopathic PAH (IPAH) demonstrated improvement in SPAP by echocardiography after administration of sildenafil and epoprostenol.[12,13] Strengths of this measure include ease of performance and reproducibility. However, there is potential for underestimating SPAP because of variation in the angle of Doppler interrogation and or because of the presence of severe TR.[8,14] In general, use of TRv to estimate SPAP often leads to underestimation compared with SPAP as determined by RHC.[13,15,16] Thus, it must be emphasized that the role of the earlier-mentioned method remains in screening and that it should not be used to confirm a diagnosis. It is recommended that a patient with an SPAP of 40 mm Hg by Doppler echocardiography undergo further evaluation.[1,8] There may be

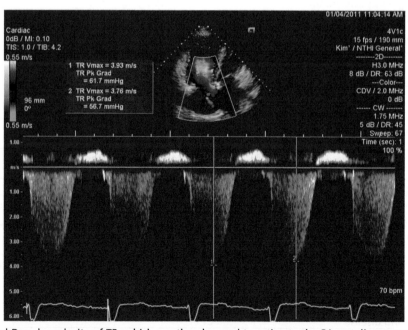

Fig. 2. Spectral Doppler velocity of TR, which can then be used to estimate the PA systolic pressure.

a role for serial measurements in monitoring response to therapy as described earlier, although this is not currently recommended.[12,13]

In addition to SPAP, Doppler echocardiography can be used to estimate diastolic PA pressure (DPAP) and MPAP.[8] Like SPAP, DPAP is also estimated using the simplified Bernoulli equation, except it is done using the velocity of pulmonic regurgitation at end diastole. This measurement is the PA-RV pressure gradient at end diastole and can be added to RA pressure to derive DPAP (r = 0.93, as compared with invasive measurement).[17] The Doppler profile through the PA can be used to obtain acceleration time (PAAT), which correlates with MPAP and, more recently, has been shown to correlate very well with the technique described earlier for measuring SPAP.[8,18] The PA Doppler profile is obtained by placing the pulsed wave (PW) Doppler cursor in the PA in the parasternal or subcostal short-axis views. Using a validated regression equation, PAAT estimates MPAP as follows:

$$MPAP = 79 - (0.45 \times PAAT)$$

The advantage of using PAAT is that adequate images to measure PAAT can be obtained in 99.6% of patients, whereas the correlation between PAAT and SPAP by TR velocity is very strong (r = −0.96).[18] This has an advantage over using TRv, because up to 25% of patients may not have sufficient TR to allow for accurate measurement of velocity.[18] Like SPAP measured by Doppler echocardiography, PAAT has been shown to improve within hours after the administration of sildenafil in patients with IPAH.[12] In addition to pressure measurements, echocardiography can be used to calculate pulmonary vascular resistance (PVR) by using the TRv and the PA Doppler profile together. The PVR is calculated as follows:

$$PVR = \frac{Vmax_{TR}}{TVI_{RVOT}} \times 10 + 0.16$$

where PVR is in Woods units, $Vmax_{TR}$ is the TRv jet (m/s), and TVI_{RVOT} is the pulsed Doppler time-velocity integral (cm) in the RV outflow tract (RVOT).[19] Measuring PVR may be important to distinguish patients with elevated PA pressures due to high flow states from those with pathologic changes in the pulmonary vasculature.[8] However, because of lack of sufficient validation and imprecise estimates for values of PVR greater than 8 Woods units, this method is currently not recommended for routine clinical use.[8]

In patients being evaluated for dyspnea who have normal resting measures of pulmonary hemodynamics and without any evidence of coronary disease, the ASE has established a framework to perform exercise stress echocardiography to evaluate for exercise-induced PH. The current recommendation is to perform the resting and supine bicycle exercise measurement of SPAP at a nonextreme workload.[8] In this setting, abnormal SPAP has been defined as a pressure of 43 mm Hg or greater in patients without valvular heart disease.[8] However, because exercise is a condition that increases flow, elevation in SPAP may simply be due to an increased flow state rather than true PH. This can be seen in subjects older than 55 years or in well-trained athletes.[8,20] To differentiate pathologic exercise-induced PH from an increased flow, it may be necessary to simultaneously measure stress PVR as described earlier. Although exercise echocardiography is recommended only for investigational uses, it has recently demonstrated promise as a potential screening tool in certain patient groups.[1] For example, in family members of patients with IPAH or familial PAH, 32% of relatives were shown to have exercise-induced PH by echocardiography in comparison with only 10% of controls, and, of these subjects, the relatives with mutations in the BMPR2 gene had the greatest likelihood of exercise-induced PH.[21] Other studies have shown that in patients with systemic sclerosis who do not have previously diagnosed PAH, there is a high prevalence of exercise-induced PH.[20]

Given that the most common cause of RV dysfunction is left-sided heart failure, echocardiography is also an important tool for determining elevated left-sided filling pressures as an etiology of PH. Such elevations can be due to LV dysfunction or valvular disease. The most reproducible parameter to estimate pulmonary capillary wedge pressure (PCWP) by echocardiography is the ratio between early diastolic mitral inflow velocity (E) and early diastolic mitral annulus velocity (E'), or E/E'.[22] This measure has been validated in several cardiac conditions.[22] In the past, this ratio was used to directly calculate an estimate of the PCWP.[23]

However, subsequent studies have demonstrated that direct calculation of PCWP is not as robust as simply using the ratio to categorize patients as normal versus having elevated LV filling pressures.[24] Thus, current approaches recommend using this measure in a qualitative rather than quantitative manner.[22] An E/E' of 8 or less reflects normal filling pressures, E/E' of 15 or more reflects elevated filling pressure, and the intermediate range is indeterminate.[22] A recent study of patients with normal LV ejection fraction has shown that when E/E' is combined with measurement of left atrial size, an E/E' between

8 and 13 with an enlarged left atrium or an E/E′ greater than 13 has a sensitivity of 87% and a specificity of 88% in comparison with LV filling pressure directly measured by heart catheterization.[25] Thus, this is potentially a very useful marker for patients who may have PH due to diastolic heart failure.

In addition to estimating pressures, pulsed Doppler echocardiography can be used to estimate volumetric flow such as RV stroke volume (SV), CO, and pulmonary to systemic shunt ratio (Qp:Qs).[26] The Qp:Qs is determined by obtaining the SVs of the LV and RV. The main measurements needed for this are the PW Doppler velocity profile at the LV outflow tract (LVOT) and RVOT and the diameter of each of these outflow tracts. The PW Doppler profile for the RVOT is traced to obtain the velocity time integral (VTI). The cross-sectional area of the RVOT is calculated using the measured diameter of the RVOT. The RV SV (or Qp) is determined by multiplying the VTI by the cross-sectional area. The same procedure is repeated in the LVOT for Qs component, which finally provides the Qp:Qs estimate. This measurement assumes the absence of significant valvular regurgitation. If significant aortic or pulmonic regurgitation is present, then the measurements must instead be performed at the mitral and tricuspid annuli, respectively, although this approach is much less reproducible. Although echocardiographic estimation of shunt has limitations, it can serve as a useful screening tool in patients with known intracardiac shunts. The results must be interpreted with caution and should be confirmed with other testing when appropriate because the amount of error, driven principally by estimation of the cross-sectional area, can be as much as 20%.[26]

Although Doppler echocardiography offers a variety of approaches for assessing PA hemodynamics, particularly PA pressures and resistance, the earlier discussion was mostly limited to methods with standardized approaches outlined by the ASE.[8] There are many additional approaches that are currently investigational but that may gain importance as more validation studies are performed.[27]

CM for Noninvasive Hemodynamics

The principle advantage of phase contrast CMR (PC-CMR) over any other modalities of hemodynamic assessment is its ability to accurately and reproducibly quantify volumetric flow to assess SV, CO, and regurgitant fractions (RFs).[28–31] With Doppler echocardiography, volumetric flow is estimated by measuring peak velocity and then multiplying this by an assumed cross-sectional area of interest. This approach has several assumptions that can lead to significant variability in the estimate of volumetric flow. First, many of the calculations for cross-sectional areas assume a circular geometry, which may not be applicable. Second, this approach does not account for changes in the cross-sectional area during the cardiac cycle. Third, it assumes laminar flow and therefore that the velocity measured at one point is exactly the same at all other points in a given cross-sectional area. Last, velocity measurements by Doppler can be underestimated with a nonparallel angle of interrogation. In contrast, with PC-CMR, the cross-sectional area of the region of interest is measured directly by planimetry at many time points throughout the cardiac cycle. Further, the velocity of blood flow is measured not just at a single point but numerous points with high resolution in a given cross-sectional area, thus accounting for differences in blood flow velocities where flow is nonlaminar. Moreover, any plane of imaging can be selected, so obtaining the correct angle of interrogation is not an issue. There are several applications of PC-CMR in the assessment of RV hemodynamics. First, RV SV can be obtained at the level of the PA by integrating the systolic portion of the flow curve. Similarly, LV SV can be obtained at the level of the aorta and Qp:Qs computed with the 2 measurements (**Fig. 3**). When compared with shunt quantification by RHC in patients with congenital heart disease, shunt determination by PC-CMR has been shown to correlate very well ($r = 0.91$).[31] Similarly, PC-CMR can generate volumetric flow curves for a given valve during systole and diastole, which can then be used to quantitatively estimate the severity of valvular regurgitation.[29,30] A framework for categorizing the RF in terms of severity has been proposed as follows: mild for an RF of 15% or less, moderate for an RF of 16% to 25%, moderate to severe for an RF of 25% to 48%, and severe for an RF greater than 48%.[30] PC-CMR can be used visually to help localize a shunt that may be difficult to find using other modalities (**Fig. 4**).

Although the determination of volumetric flow by PC-CMR is relatively accurate and reproducible, the literature on PA pressure assessment by CMR is still conflicting. Direct estimation of PA pressures by CMR has proved challenging. A method described by Laffon and colleagues[32] computes MPAP using PC-CMR to determine mean blood flow velocity across the cross-sectional area of the main PA (MPA) at peak systole and the maximal cross-sectional area of the MPA. This technique initially showed excellent

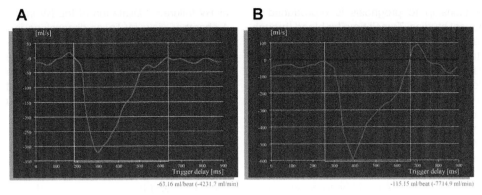

Fig. 3. The SVs for the LV (*A*) and RV (*B*) are obtained by performing phase-contrast CMR through the aorta and PA, respectively. This patient with an atrial septal defect was found to have a Qp:Qs ratio of 1.8.

correlation (r = 0.92) in control subjects with MPAP measured by RHC,[32] but the correlation did not exist when patients with PH were selectively evaluated (r = 0.21).[33] Other approaches using acceleration time and acceleration/ejection time ratio have also yielded poor correlations.[33] One indirect approach for estimating PA pressures is by determining the ratio of ventricular mass of the RV to that of the LV or ventricular mass index (VMI). The VMI has demonstrated reasonable correlation with MPAP while also being shown to be reasonably reproducible.[33–35] Nevertheless,

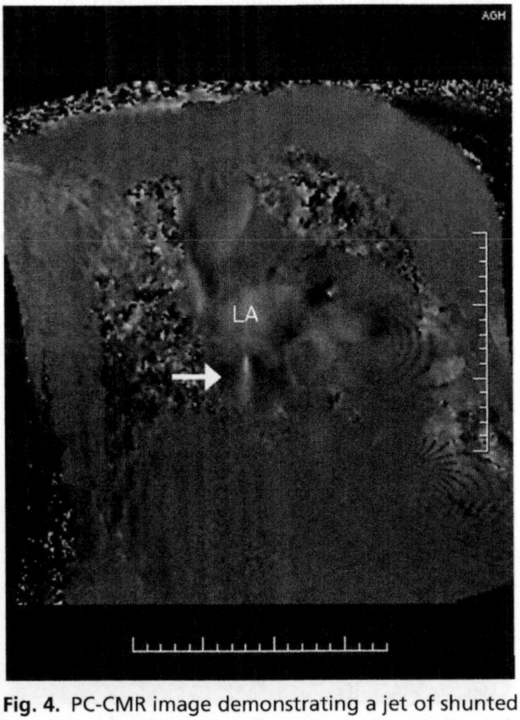

![Fig. 4 PC-CMR image]

Fig. 4. PC-CMR image demonstrating a jet of shunted blood flowing from the left atrium to the RA (*arrow*).

the automation of current CMR methodologies to estimate PA pressures is limited at present, resulting in an approach that can be time and labor intensive without a significant incremental yield in information.

Although direct estimation of PA pressures by CMR has proved challenging, the modality has emerged as uniquely suitable for measuring PA stiffness. Dynamic imaging with high temporal and spatial resolution in any plane makes CMR highly suitable for quantifying PA stiffness. Decreased PA elasticity seen in patients with PH may result from a combination of increased distending pressures and pathologic changes in the vascular wall.[36] Such changes may have a role in the pathogenesis of PH progression and appear to be linked to prognosis.[36] One of these measures, relative area change (RAC), determines the change in cross-sectional area during the cardiac cycle in a proximal portion of the PA.[37] This measure is computed as follows:

$$RAC = \frac{(CSA_{Max} - CSA_{Min})}{CSA_{Min}}$$

where *CSA* is cross-sectional area of a proximal segment of the PA, both maximal and minimal. The mean *RAC* was lower in patients with PAH than in controls (20 ± 10% vs 58 ± 21%, P<.05).[37] Moreover, in patients with PAH, RAC was significantly lower in nonsurvivors than in survivors, and patients with an RAC of 16% or less had a significantly lower survival rate than those with an RAC greater than 16%. Moreover, RAC was a better marker for death than other known prognostic indicators, including 6-minute walk distance (6MWD), systemic venous oxygen saturation, invasively measured RA pressure, and invasively measured PVR. This marker of PA stiffness holds much promise and may become central to the evaluation of patients with PH if this relationship to prognosis is reproduced in subsequent studies. Transit time for blood through the pulmonary circulation has emerged as an important CMR marker in patients with PAH. Using time-resolved magnetic resonance angiography, PA blood volume (PaBV) and PA transit time (PaTT) are directly determined.[38] In one small study of 12 patients with WHO Group I PH and 10 controls, PaTT of 2 seconds had a sensitivity of 92% and a specificity of 90% for predicting PAH as confirmed by RHC. If validated in larger studies, certain hemodynamic markers such as PaTT and RAC of the PA could become an essential component of noninvasive hemodynamic assessment.

EVALUATION OF RA AND RV STRUCTURE AND FUNCTION

Because the RV is subject to many of the pathologic consequences of PH, reliable imaging of this structure is essential for establishing the severity of PH and prognosis. Thus, echocardiography and CMR play essential roles in the evaluation of patients with PH. These modalities provide information on the size and morphology of RA and RV, RV systolic function, and RV diastolic function.

Echocardiography in the Quantification of Size and Morphology of RA and RV

The apical 4-chamber view focused on the RV is the view of choice for measuring dimensions of the RA and RV.[8] In this view, the size of the RA can be quantified by length (major dimension), diameter (minor dimension), and area obtained by planimetry. A length greater than 53 mm, a diameter greater than 44 mm, or an area greater than 18 cm^2 has been classified as RA enlargement, which is an indirect marker of RV diastolic dysfunction.[8] In validation studies with primary PAH, an RA area greater than 27 cm^2 or an RA area index greater than 5 cm^2/m^2 has been shown to be a strong echocardiographic predictor of death or transplantation.[39,40] More recently, Grapsa and colleagues[41] showed that RA sphericity index by 3D echocardiography was an extremely strong predictor of clinical deterioration (96% sensitivity, 90% specificity, and area under the curve of 0.97). In this prospective study, this 3D marker was a clinical predictor stronger than parameters assessing change in RV geometry and even change in 3D RVEF (sensitivity, 91.1%; specificity, 35.3%; and area under the curve, 0.479).[41]

Whereas RA enlargement reflects RV diastolic dysfunction and TR severity, RV enlargement results from chronic pressure or volume overload

or RV failure.[2–4] Dilatation of the RV in the apical 4-chamber view by linear dimensions is defined as a basal diameter greater than 42 mm, a midlevel diameter greater than 35 mm, or a longitudinal dimension greater than 86 mm.[8] In patients with chronic pulmonary disease, RV enlargement based on indexed linear dimension has been shown to predict survival (hazard ratio, 1.27; 95% confidence interval [CI], 1.08–1.48).[42] An assessment of the size of RV can also be performed qualitatively. In a normal-sized RV, the midlevel RV diameter is smaller than the diameter of the LV at the same level and the apex is occupied primarily by the LV.[43] With moderate enlargement, the RV and LV cavity areas are of similar size and the apex is shared equally by the LV and RV.[43] With severe enlargement, RV cavity area is greater than that of the LV and the apex is formed primarily by the RV (**Fig. 5**).[43]

In addition to RV size, several assessments of RV morphology can be performed by echocardiography. An assessment of RV wall thickness is important because this indicates RV hypertrophy in response to chronic pressure overload.[4] An RV wall thickness greater than 5 mm at end diastole in the subcostal view indicates RV hypertrophy. However, this finding can also be due to other causes, such as infiltrative or hypertrophic cardiomyopathies.[8] In addition, with pressure or volume overload, flattening of the normally concave interventricular septum toward the LV cavity occurs at various stages in the cardiac cycle (**Fig. 6**). This flattening can be assessed best in the parasternal short-axis view at midcavity level, where it appears qualitatively as a D-shaped LV cavity. Quantitatively, flattening of the septum is measured by an eccentricity index, which is defined as the ratio of the anteroposterior dimension to the septolateral dimension of the LV.[8] An eccentricity index greater than 1.0 suggests RV pressure or volume overload.[8] With isolated volume overload, septal

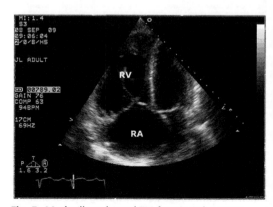

Fig. 5. Markedly enlarged RV forming the apex.

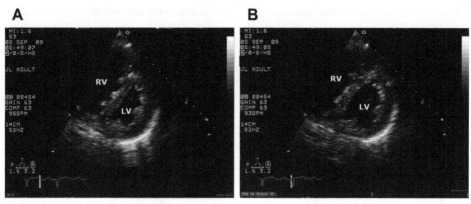

Fig. 6. Flattening of the interventricular septum during systole (A) and diastole (B).

flattening occurs primarily in end diastole, whereas with isolated RV pressure overload, flattening occurs both at end systole and end diastole.[8] In patients with primary PAH, each 0.5-unit increase in diastolic eccentricity index has been shown to correlate with a hazard ratio of 1.45 (95% CI, 1.12–1.86) for transplantation or mortality.[40,44] Measurement of the eccentricity index can be confounded by the presence of concomitant conduction system disease such as a left bundle branch block.[8] In addition to 2D assessment, one recent study has demonstrated variation in 3D RV remodeling based on several etiologies of PH, including PAH, CTEPH, and PH secondary to mitral regurgitation.[45] Remodeling of the RV by 3D imaging was affected most adversely in patients with PAH.[45] The presence of a pericardial effusion can provide important prognostic information and has been shown to be an independent predictor of mortality.[40,46] In a large prospective registry of patients with PAH using a multivariable model incorporating clinical, laboratory, catheterization, and echocardiographic data, the presence of any pericardial effusion on echocardiography conferred a hazard ratio of 1.35 (P = .014) for mortality.[46]

CMR for Evaluating RV Size and Morphology

Perhaps the most established use for CMR in PAH is for the evaluation of the structure and function of RV. Although many other technologies can reasonably approach the accuracy of CMR for the estimation of the size and function of RV, all are ill suited for interrogating the irregular geometry and free wall myocardium. Thus, no other imaging technique, noninvasive or invasive, approaches the inherent accuracy of CMR for the RV. It naturally follows that one of the major strengths of CMR relative to other modalities is the ability to obtain RV volumes and mass in an

accurate and extremely reproducible manner.[47,48] Typically, images are acquired using steady state free precession (SSFP) technique and can be obtained in either short-axis planes from base to apex or transverse axial planes from the pulmonic valve level to the diaphragmatic level. For quantifying the volume and mass of RV, the short-axis view may be preferable because using the transverse axial plane may result in inaccurate assessment of endocardial and epicardial borders at the level of the diaphragmatic (inferior) wall.[49] However, the transverse axial approach has advantages for evaluating RV systolic function as described later. After image acquisition is complete, epicardial and endocardial contours are delineated using semiautomated computer algorithms and then manually edited (**Fig. 7**). The papillary muscles and RV trabeculations are excluded from the RV mass. After the borders are defined, the area of myocardium and the RV cavity in each slice is multiplied by the slice thickness to yield a volume of myocardium and volume of RV cavity per slice. These volumes are then summated to yield a total RV myocardial volume and RV cavity volume. The RV myocardial volume, multiplied by the density of muscle 1.055 g/cm,[3] provides a measure of RV mass.

In one study of patients with PAH, the ratio of RV mass to LV mass or VMI showed a stronger correlation with MPAP by RHC than with echocardiographically estimated MPAP.[34] The sensitivity and specificity for VMI were 84% and 71%, respectively, for predicting PAH. However, a subsequent study of 44 patients with PAH found the correlation to be less robust for VMI, with a relatively high false-negative rate of 20%.[33] At present, a mass cutoff for right ventricular hypertrophy is not formally specified, but age-based normative data are available to help guide assessments.[50,51] Another study by van Wolferen and colleagues[52] evaluated the volumes and mass of

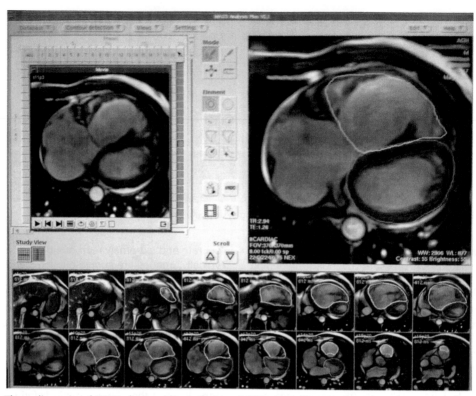

Fig. 7. Three-dimensional RVEF obtained by outlining of RV volume at several levels.

RV in the PAH population using CMR and compared these measures with other conventional assessments such as New York Heart Association functional class, 6MWD, and RHC hemodynamic parameters. In the multivariate analysis of all variables, only CMR-derived volumes both at baseline and during follow-up predicted mortality. Among the other variables, 6MWD predicted mortality only at baseline and invasively measured PVR-predicted mortality only during follow-up. An RV end-diastolic volume (EDV) index greater than the median (84 mL/m^2) conferred a hazard ratio of 1.61 for mortality ($P<.001$).[52] With further validation studies, the reproducibility, precision, and accuracy of CMR-derived volume and mass could prove to be uniquely suitable traits for monitoring response to therapy in the PAH population.

Another distinct aspect of CMR assessment of the RV is the ability to assess tissue characteristics using gadolinium contrast (**Fig. 8**). A growing body of literature has emerged regarding the significance of myocardial contrast enhancement in the PH population.[53–56] Gadolinium chelates allow for water visualization in the extravascular tissue space.[57] In necrotic or fibrotic myocardium, the kinetics of gadolinium uptake are altered such that there is a higher concentration of gadolinium in the diseased myocardium than in the viable

myocardium at 10 minutes after contrast administration. The late gadolinium-enhanced (LGE) areas can be visualized and quantified to assess the impact of certain disease states on the myocardium. Irrespective of the etiology of PAH, patients often demonstrate myocardial LGE at the insertion point of the RV free wall into the interventricular septum.[54–56] It has been hypothesized that this finding is related to chronic RV pressure overload. Although the mass of LGE tissue correlates with RVEF, RV EDV, RV mass, and invasively measured MPAP, the prognostic significance of this finding remains to be determined by future validation studies.[53,55,56] The use of gadolinium should be avoided in patients with end-stage renal disease because of the rare risk of developing nephrogenic systemic fibrosis.[57]

Assessing RV Function by Echocardiography

An assessment of RV systolic and diastolic function is essentially an assessment of the functional impact of PH on cardiac performance. Compared with the LV, the geometry of the RV is complex, making an assessment of its function similarly complex. Moreover, the relative anterior position of the RV in the chest wall has made echocardiographic imaging of the RV especially challenging, particularly in the

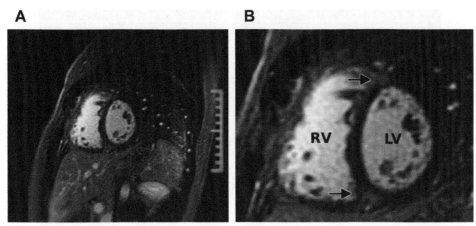

Fig. 8. Late gadolinium enhancement at the insertion of the RV into the interventricular septum (*A*), with an inset (*B*) in a patient with PH (*arrows*).

setting of significant RV enlargement or coexisting pulmonary disease. Given these difficulties, several approaches for echocardiographic assessment of RV function have been proposed and studied. It must be understood that these approaches are complementary, and a multifaceted assessment is recommended.

M-Mode and 2-Dimensional Echocardiography

Given the complex geometry of the RV, extrapolation of chamber volume from 2-dimensional (2D) views using geometric assumptions has proved less reliable for the RV than for the LV. Consequently, some of the research on RV function assessment has used simpler measures as surrogates for RV systolic function such as tricuspid annular plane systolic excursion (TAPSE) and RV fractional area change (FAC). TAPSE is a linear measurement that can be performed either using M-mode through the lateral tricuspid annulus or by 2D imaging. This measure is premised on the physiologic finding that longitudinal contraction is a significant component of RV systolic function[3] and that measurement of TAPSE serves as a useful approximation of global RV systolic function. TAPSE is determined by subtracting the apex to lateral tricuspid annular distance during systole from the distance during diastole (**Fig. 9**).[14] A TAPSE value less than 16 mm has been defined as impaired RV systolic function.[8] This is a reliable measure because it is simple to perform, is easily reproduced, does not require outlining of the entire endocardial border, and does not use geometric assumptions. Given these strengths, TAPSE has been well studied in many patient populations and has been shown to predict mortality in the PAH

population. In a study of patients with IPAH by Ghio and colleagues,[44] a TAPSE less than 16 mm conferred a hazard ratio of 2.74 (95% CI, 1.11–6.67) for mortality. In another cohort study of patients with PAH, those with reduced TAPSE had reduced cardiac index on RHC as well as a hazard ratio of 5.7 (*P* = .02) for mortality.[58] However, TAPSE is less valid in several of the following situations: when regional RV dysfunction is present, when RV visualization is incomplete, when severe TR is present, in the patient after cardiac surgery, or when RV dysfunction is severe.[59–61] RV dysfunction causes a paradoxic increase in TAPSE because of rocking motion of the heart. Despite these limitations, TAPSE is quantitative and is performed quickly, and so it is currently recommended to perform this measure as a standard component of RV assessment.[8]

In addition to linear measures, area measures can also be used to assess RV function. Measurement of RV cavity area is performed using planimetry of the cavity circumscribed by the endocardial borders, which are traced in an apical 4-chamber view focused on the RV. The RV cavity area is measured at end systole and end diastole, and RV FAC is computed as follows:

$$FAC = \frac{Area_{Diastole} - Area_{Systole}}{Area_{Diastole}} \times 100$$

This 2D variable has correlated reasonably well with CMR-derived RVEF[62,63] and has been shown to predict mortality.[44] However, reproducibility of the measure has proved challenging[64] because RV visualization may be incomplete with severe RV enlargement, endocardial border definition may be difficult, and the angle-imaging plane may vary from one study to the next.

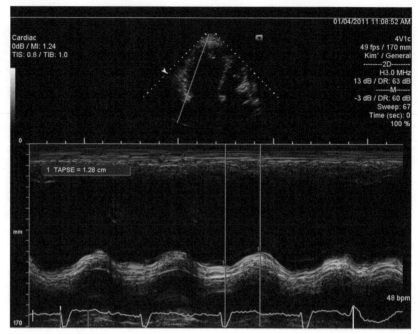

Fig. 9. Measurement of TAPSE in M-mode.

Some of the test-retest variability that occurs with 2D techniques because of complex RV geometry may be overcome by using a 3D approach. Current ultrasound transducer and processing equipment permits acquisition of real-time 3D volumetric data at a sufficient temporal resolution (20 volumes per second) to estimate RV systolic function. The 3D volumetric data are obtained using a matrix array transducer placed at the apical position. Endocardial borders are then outlined in the short-axis view at several levels using automated detection algorithms, excluding trabeculations and papillary muscles. These automated borders must then be confirmed by manual editing. The EDV and end-systolic volume (ESV) are then estimated using a summation disks method (**Fig. 10**). RVEF is calculated as follows:

$$RVEF = \frac{EDV - ESV}{EDV} \times 100$$

At present, a lower reference limit for RVEF has been set at 44% based on available data, although large-scale normative data are still lacking.[8] Although reasonable agreement between CMR and 3D echocardiography has been demonstrated in patients with PAH for EDV and ESV ($r = 0.74$ and $r = 0.75$, respectively), the agreement for ejection fraction was shown to be less robust ($r = 0.66$).[65] However, 3D echocardiography is faced with some limitations. The larger size of matrix array

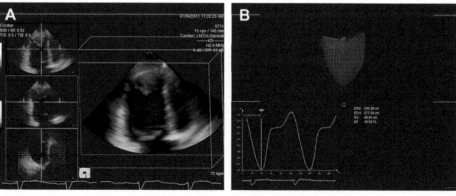

Fig. 10. Three-dimensional echocardiography used for determining RVEF (A & B).

transducers can occasionally limit adequate acoustic windows. As with 2D echocardiography, inclusion of the entire RV can be difficult in patients with severe RV enlargement. Nevertheless, volumetric assessment by 3D echocardiography is reproducible and may prove to be a useful method to monitor response to therapy in patients with PAH.[65] At present, a multicenter prospective observational trial of patients with PAH is underway to assess whether this measure adds useful prognostic information and whether it has utility in assessing efficacy of therapy.[66]

Doppler Techniques for Assessing RV Function

There are several important markers of RV function derived from Doppler echocardiography. These include change in RV pressures over change in time (RV dP/dT), myocardial performance index (MPI), tricuspid annular velocities, tricuspid inflow for diastolic function, and strain imaging.

RV dP/dT was first described as an invasive measure of contractile performance that reflected the ability of a normal ventricle to rapidly generate pressure.[67] Echocardiographically, this is measured using the velocity profile of the tricuspid regurgitant jet using continuous wave Doppler of the TR jet; dP/dT is the time interval for the TR velocity to rise from 1 to 2 m/s.[8] Although relatively easy to measure, RV dP/dT can be dependent on loading conditions and may be less accurate in the setting of severe TR. Because of lack of normative data, this measure is not recommended for routine

use and should only be used in patients who have suspected RV dysfunction.[8]

Another important Doppler measure is the RV myocardial performance index or Tei index. This marker measures both global systolic and diastolic function, and it has been validated in CTEPH, PH in the setting of congenital heart disease, IPAH, and PAH from connective tissue disease.[68–71] RV MPI is the ratio of nonejection work to ejection work of the RV:

$$MPI_{RV} = \frac{IVCT + IVRT}{ET}$$

where $IVCT$ = isovolumic contraction time, $IVRT$ = isovolumic relaxation time, and ET = ejection time.[8] The measurement of these time intervals can be performed by separate PW Doppler evaluation of the tricuspid inflow and RVOT. An alternative approach is to perform a single-tissue Doppler interrogation of the lateral tricuspid annulus (**Fig. 11**).[8] These velocities are then used to measure the respective time intervals. RV MPI by the single-tissue Doppler method been shown to have a better correlation to RVEF and RV FAC in comparison with the method using separate PW Doppler of tricuspid inflow and RVOT.[72] Compared with other Doppler techniques, this measurement is less dependent on the angle of interrogation because the magnitude of the velocity is not as important as the time intervals. Original data in the congenital heart disease population suggested that another strength of the MPI was its relative independence from loading conditions, although subsequent studies have

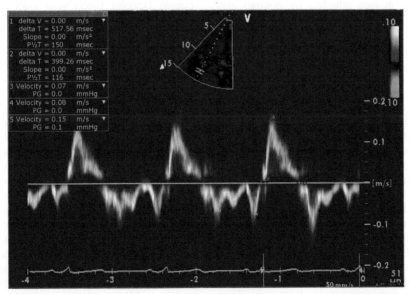

Fig. 11. Tissue Doppler echocardiography can be used to measure the velocity of RV systolic contraction and also the Tei index.

called this finding into question.[69,73] Nevertheless, RV MPI is an important adjunct to the visual estimation of RV function that has been validated in many clinical settings and integrates evaluation of both systolic and diastolic function. The threshold for abnormal MPI by PW Doppler has been defined as greater than 0.40, whereas for tissue Doppler MPI, the threshold is greater than 0.55.

Another important marker of global RV systolic function, the tricuspid annular velocity or S', is a tissue Doppler corollary of TAPSE. S' can be measured online using pulsed tissue Doppler or offline by performing color-coded tissue Doppler and selecting the tricuspid annulus as the region of interest during postprocessing. The highest velocity in the systolic velocity profile is measured (see **Fig. 11**). In contrast to many other echocardiographic parameters, this measure has a substantial amount of normative data to support its use.[74] Its strengths and limitations are similar to those described earlier for TAPSE. In addition, as with many Doppler measurements, accurate S' depends on a parallel angle of interrogation to avoid underestimation of velocities. With these considerations in mind, it is recommended to perform this measurement when possible.[8] The lower limit of normal is 10 cm/s by pulsed tissue Doppler and 6 cm/s by color-coded tissue Doppler.[8] In addition to the peak velocity, the tissue Doppler profile can be used to measure isovolumic acceleration (IVA). The tissue Doppler velocity waveform usually has 2 distinct components: an isovolumic contraction phase and an ejection phase. The IVA, which is the slope of the first component, has been validated in many disorders and is less affected by preload and afterload conditions.[8] However, this measure is not recommended for routine clinical use because normal cutoff values have not yet been established.[8]

CMR for Evaluating RV Systolic Function

Given its 3D capabilities and excellent spatial resolution, CMR has become the standard for evaluating the accuracy of other modalities to assess RV systolic function (see **Fig. 7**). Its primary role has become that of a confirmatory test to quantify RV function when dysfunction is suspected based on other modalities. Functional RV assessment, such as assessment of RV volumes, is usually performed using bright blood sequences such as SSFP that are used to generate dynamic (cine) images during a 5- to 18-second breath-hold to limit respiratory motion artifact.[75,76]

Distinct from RV volume and mass assessments, RVEF is better assessed in the transverse

axial plane rather than the short-axis plane. This is because inclusion of basal short-axis segment contributes to a significant proportion of RV volume, and variability in measuring this segment can result in substantial variation in RVEF assessment. In contrast, using the transverse axial approach, there is clear delineation of the valve planes and thus elimination of the error in RVEF assessment at the base of the RV. Conversely, there is somewhat increased variability in the measurement of the diaphragmatic portion of the RV using the transverse axial approach, although this may be counterbalanced by the reduction in error at the basal portion of the RV. Thus, although short-axis images are excellent for volume and mass measurements, it may be more reliable to use transverse axial assessments for RVEF.[49,77,78] Compared with CMR, volumes are underestimated by 3D echocardiography and often overestimated using cardiac CT.[48] Thus, CMR-derived RVEF seems to have the greatest accuracy among the various imaging modalities. This was demonstrated recently by the authors' laboratory, where they showed a strong correlation ($r = 0.96$) between CMR-derived RV mass and actual RV mass measured in explanted hearts from transplant recipients.[79]

Echocardiographic Evaluation of RV Diastolic Function

A growing area of interest is the study of RV diastolic function. Many components of the assessment of RV diastolic function are similar to those of the LV. The major components include transtricuspid Doppler blood flow velocities, tricuspid annular tissue Doppler velocities, hepatic vein Doppler flow, inferior vena cava size and collapsibility, and RA size. The latter indicators of diastolic dysfunction, inferior vena cava distention/loss of collapsibility and RA enlargement, have been discussed earlier. Transtricuspid flow is measured using PW Doppler in a medially angulated apical 4-chamber view with the sample volume placed at the tips of the tricuspid leaflets.[80] As with the LV, there are 2 distinct peak diastolic flow velocities, the early (E) and late diastolic (A) peak velocities, which are used to compute the ratio between the two (E/A). These velocities can be significantly affected by breathing and, for the purpose of standardization, should be performed at an end-expiratory breath-hold.[81] Transtricuspid flow velocities are also affected by loading conditions, so it is important to obtain diastolic tissue Doppler velocities (early diastolic or E', late diastolic or A') of the lateral tricuspid annulus as well. These velocities are less susceptible to changes in loading conditions and are important in differentiating normal filling from pseudonormal filling. Along with transtricuspid and tricuspid annular velocities, it is important to obtain PW Doppler flow in the hepatic veins (subcostal view) and PA (parasternal or subcostal view).

In noncardiac surgical patients, a ratio of tricuspid E/E' greater than 4 predicts RA pressure greater than 10 mm Hg in noncardiac surgical patients with a sensitivity and specificity of 88% and 85%, respectively[82]; whereas in cardiac transplant recipients, an E/E' greater than 8 has a sensitivity and specificity of 78% and 85%, respectively.[83] An E/A less than 0.8 suggests impaired relaxation, whereas an E/A of 0.8 or greater and 2.1 or lesser is pseudonormal if the E/E' is greater than 6 or there is a diastolic flow predominance in the hepatic veins.[8] An E/A greater than 2.1 with an E wave deceleration time less than 120 milliseconds or late diastolic forward flow in the PA indicates restrictive filling of the RV.[8]

CMR for Evaluating RV Diastolic Function

CMR has emerged as an important tool in the evaluation of RV diastolic function.[75,84] The ability of CMR to simultaneously visualize the motion of the entire pulmonic and tricuspid valves with excellent spatial and temporal resolution offers a unique window into RV diastolic function that is unavailable with other modalities. Using SSFP imaging, Gan and colleagues[85] were able to obtain 2-chamber RV views for simultaneously visualizing pulmonic valve closure and tricuspid valve opening to determine isovolumic relaxation time (IVRT) in 25 patients with PH and 11 controls. This method seems to be promising in that IVRT strongly correlated with other clinically used markers including NT-proBNP ($r = 0.70$; $P<.001$), cardiac index on RHC ($r = -0.70$; $P<.001$), and RVEF ($r = -0.69$; $P<.001$). In addition, sildenafil therapy was shown to decrease IVRT in this patient population.[85]

Along with IVRT, CMR can be used to generate diastolic RV filling profiles similar to echocardiography. There are 2 methods for obtaining these volume curves, either using PC-CMR through the tricuspid annulus or tracing RV volumes at each frame taken in the diastolic portion of the cardiac cycle. The latter technique was used by Gan and colleagues, who showed that patients with PH have reduced early diastolic filling rate (similar to echocardiographic E velocity), reduced E/A filling ratio, and an increased A filling rate. However, this approach of tracing multiple RV volumes is relatively more labor intensive than tracing the contour of the tricuspid valve orifice during

diastole for PC-CMR. The latter approach was compared with Doppler echocardiographic evaluation of RV diastolic function and found to have excellent correlation for early (E) filling, atrial-systolic (A) filling, and E/A ratio ($r>0.89$) in normal subjects.[86] In addition, this approach can be used to assess superior vena cava flow profiles, similar to the echocardiographic assessment of pulmonary vein flows.[86] Although there is early evidence that RV diastolic function may have prognostic significance, validation in larger studies and therapeutic trials will be important to understand the clinical significance.

Strain Imaging

Strain echocardiography for evaluation of RV function

Strain imaging is a quantitative tool for assessing regional myocardial deformation (shortening or lengthening of the myocardium), which serves as a measure of myocardial contractility. It is expressed as a percentage of change in myocardial length between end diastole and end systole relative to the original length in end diastole or

$$\varepsilon = \frac{\Delta L}{L_O}$$

where ε is strain, ΔL is change in length of a specified region of myocardium from end diastole to end systole, and L_O is the original length at end diastole. This was originally performed using tissue Doppler techniques. However, this approach has now largely been replaced by the use of speckle-tracking technology on 2D B-mode echocardiography. The latter technique does not rely on Doppler techniques but rather uses echocardiographic tissue speckle signatures that are unique to the region of interest and can be tracked over time through the cardiac cycle using a software algorithm. These techniques, because they do not require Doppler, are not angle dependent, in contrast to tissue Doppler strain. Although there are multiple components of strain that can be measured when evaluating the LV, strain measurements in the RV are most reproducible in the apical 4-chamber view and are thus limited to measures of longitudinal strain.[8] Normative data for RV strain are limited, therefore this technology is still experimental. However, patients with PH have clearly been shown to have reduced longitudinal strain in comparison with normal controls.[87] Moreover, based on preliminary data, it seems that PAH can also adversely affect LV mechanics as assessed by strain.[87]

Strain by CMR for evaluation of RV function

Tissue tagging can be performed during CMR to track the motion of ventricular tissue during the cardiac cycle.[88] Given that the RV is a thin-walled structure, use of such magnetic tags is more difficult because they are spaced far apart. An alternative approach is through the use of strain-encoded (SENC) CMR. This approach generates 2 sets of images, with bright areas designating static tissue in the first image set and contracting tissue in the second image set.[89] The 2 sets of images are then combined to generate a strain image. RV strain measurement by CMR has some advantages over echocardiography, principally that there is no angle dependence as there is with Doppler echocardiography. Also, some of the limitations of measuring strain in a 2D imaging plane are overcome with the use of SENC. This approach has been demonstrated to accurately assess regional RV systolic function.[89] Along with assessing systolic function, strain imaging by CMR has been used to study LV diastolic mechanics such as LV diastolic torsion recovery rate (also known as untwisting).[90] Such measures correlate extremely well with the relaxation constant tau, with little influence from variations in loading conditions such as elevated left atrial pressure or elevated aortic pressures.[90] Such techniques may have important applications for assessing RV diastolic function but have not yet been studied for this purpose. If validated in clinical trials, strain by CMR may become an important and highly reproducible quantitative marker of RV systolic and diastolic function.

SUMMARY

Evaluating hemodynamics and determining RV function are cornerstones in the assessment and management of patients with PH. For this purpose, echocardiography and CMR are indispensable tools in the patient population with PH. Echocardiography provides a well-validated, widely available, inexpensive, and reliable method to screen and follow pulmonary pressures and RV function without exposure to ionizing radiation. CMR techniques are highly accurate, are highly reproducible, have excellent 3D capabilities, and allow for complete visualization of any structure in any imaging plain. These technologies offer complementary information and, as more data become available, will be used increasingly to track the severity of PH in patients as well as the response of patients with PH to specific therapies.

REFERENCES

1. McLaughlin VV, Archer SL, Badesch DB, et al. ACCF/AHA 2009 expert consensus document on pulmonary hypertension: a report of the American College of Cardiology Foundation Task Force on Expert Consensus Documents and the American Heart Association: developed in collaboration with the American College of Chest Physicians, American Thoracic Society, Inc., and the Pulmonary Hypertension Association. Circulation 2009;119(16):2250–94.
2. Chin KM, Kim NH, Rubin LJ. The right ventricle in pulmonary hypertension. Coron Artery Dis 2005; 16(1):13–8.
3. Haddad F, Hunt SA, Rosenthal DN, et al. Right ventricular function in cardiovascular disease, part I: anatomy, physiology, aging, and functional assessment of the right ventricle. Circulation 2008;117(11): 1436–48.
4. Haddad F, Doyle R, Murphy DJ, et al. Right ventricular function in cardiovascular disease, part II: pathophysiology, clinical importance, and management of right ventricular failure. Circulation 2008;117(13): 1717–31.
5. Tunariu N, Gibbs SJ, Win Z, et al. Ventilation-perfusion scintigraphy is more sensitive than multidetector CTPA in detecting chronic thromboembolic pulmonary disease as a treatable cause of pulmonary hypertension. J Nucl Med 2007;48(5):680–4.
6. Freed BH, Patel AR, Lang RM. Redefining the role of cardiovascular imaging in patients with pulmonary arterial hypertension. Curr Cardiol Rep 2012. [Epub ahead of print]. DOI: 10.1007/s11886-012-0253-2.
7. Hoeper MM, Lee SH, Voswinckel R, et al. Complications of right heart catheterization procedures in patients with pulmonary hypertension in experienced centers. J Am Coll Cardiol 2006;48(12):2546–52.
8. Rudski LG, Lai WW, Afilalo J, et al. Guidelines for the echocardiographic assessment of the right heart in adults: a report from the American Society of Echocardiography: endorsed by the European Association of Echocardiography, a registered branch of the European Society of Cardiology, and the Canadian Society of Echocardiography. J Am Soc Echocardiogr 2010;23(7):685–713.
9. Yock PG, Popp RL. Noninvasive estimation of right ventricular systolic pressure by Doppler ultrasound in patients with tricuspid regurgitation. Circulation 1984;70(4):657–62.
10. Lam CS, Borlaug BA, Kane GC, et al. Age-associated increases in pulmonary artery systolic pressure in the general population. Circulation 2009;119(20): 2663–70.
11. Damy T, Goode KM, Kallvikbacka-Bennett A, et al. Determinants and prognostic value of pulmonary arterial pressure in patients with chronic heart failure. Eur Heart J 2010;31(18):2280–90.
12. Behzadnia N, Najafizadeh K, Sharif-Kashani B, et al. Noninvasive assessment of acute cardiopulmonary effects of an oral single dose of sildenafil in patients with idiopathic pulmonary hypertension. Heart Vessels 2010;25(4):313–8.

13. Hinderliter AL, Willis PW 4th, Barst RJ, et al. Effects of long-term infusion of prostacyclin (epoprostenol) on echocardiographic measures of right ventricular structure and function in primary pulmonary hypertension. Primary Pulmonary Hypertension Study Group. Circulation 1997;95(6):1479–86.

14. Horton KD, Meece RW, Hill JC. Assessment of the right ventricle by echocardiography: a primer for cardiac sonographers. J Am Soc Echocardiogr 2009;22(7):776–92 [quiz: 861–2].

15. Fisher MR, Forfia PR, Chamera E, et al. Accuracy of Doppler echocardiography in the hemodynamic assessment of pulmonary hypertension. Am J Respir Crit Care Med 2009;179(7):615–21.

16. McGoon M, Gutterman D, Steen V, et al. Screening, early detection, and diagnosis of pulmonary arterial hypertension: ACCP evidence-based clinical practice guidelines. Chest 2004;126(Suppl 1):14S–34S.

17. Tanabe K, Asanuma T, Yoshitomi H, et al. Doppler estimation of pulmonary artery end-diastolic pressure using contrast enhancement of pulmonary regurgitant signals. Am J Cardiol 1996;78(10):1145–8.

18. Yared K, Noseworthy P, Weyman AE, et al. Pulmonary artery acceleration time provides an accurate estimate of systolic pulmonary arterial pressure during transthoracic echocardiography. J Am Soc Echocardiogr 2011;24(6):687–92.

19. Abbas AE, Fortuin FD, Schiller NB, et al. A simple method for noninvasive estimation of pulmonary vascular resistance. J Am Coll Cardiol 2003;41(6):1021–7.

20. Lau EM, Manes A, Celermajer DS, et al. Early detection of pulmonary vascular disease in pulmonary arterial hypertension: time to move forward. Eur Heart J 2011;32(20):2489–98.

21. Grunig E, Weissmann S, Ehlken N, et al. Stress Doppler echocardiography in relatives of patients with idiopathic and familial pulmonary arterial hypertension: results of a multicenter European analysis of pulmonary artery pressure response to exercise and hypoxia. Circulation 2009;119(13):1747–57.

22. Nagueh SF, Appleton CP, Gillebert TC, et al. Recommendations for the evaluation of left ventricular diastolic function by echocardiography. J Am Soc Echocardiogr 2009;22(2):107–33.

23. Nagueh SF, Middleton KJ, Kopelen HA, et al. Doppler tissue imaging: a noninvasive technique for evaluation of left ventricular relaxation and estimation of filling pressures. J Am Coll Cardiol 1997;30(6):1527–33.

24. Ommen SR, Nishimura RA, Appleton CP, et al. Clinical utility of Doppler echocardiography and tissue Doppler imaging in the estimation of left ventricular filling pressures: a comparative simultaneous Doppler-catheterization study. Circulation 2000;102(15):1788–94.

25. Dokainish H, Nguyen JS, Sengupta R, et al. Do additional echocardiographic variables increase the accuracy of E/e' for predicting left ventricular filling pressure in normal ejection fraction? An echocardiographic and invasive hemodynamic study. J Am Soc Echocardiogr 2010;23(2):156–61.

26. Quinones MA, Otto CM, Stoddard M, et al. Recommendations for quantification of Doppler echocardiography: a report from the Doppler Quantification Task Force of the Nomenclature and Standards Committee of the American Society of Echocardiography. J Am Soc Echocardiogr 2002;15(2):167–84.

27. Milan A, Magnino C, Veglio F. Echocardiographic indexes for the non-invasive evaluation of pulmonary hemodynamics. J Am Soc Echocardiogr 2010;23(3):225–39 [quiz: 332–4].

28. Colletti PM. Evaluation of intracardiac shunts with cardiac magnetic resonance. Curr Cardiol Rep 2005;7(1):52–8.

29. Fujita N, Chazouilleres AF, Hartiala JJ, et al. Quantification of mitral regurgitation by velocity-encoded cine nuclear magnetic resonance imaging. J Am Coll Cardiol 1994;23(4):951–8.

30. Gelfand EV, Hughes S, Hauser TH, et al. Severity of mitral and aortic regurgitation as assessed by cardiovascular magnetic resonance: optimizing correlation with Doppler echocardiography. J Cardiovasc Magn Reson 2006;8(3):503–7.

31. Petersen SE, Voigtlander T, Kreitner KF, et al. Quantification of shunt volumes in congenital heart diseases using a breath-hold MR phase contrast technique—comparison with oximetry. Int J Cardiovasc Imaging 2002;18(1):53–60.

32. Laffon E, Vallet C, Bernard V, et al. A computed method for noninvasive MRI assessment of pulmonary arterial hypertension. J Appl Phys 2004;96(2):463–8.

33. Roeleveld RJ, Marcus JT, Boonstra A, et al. A comparison of noninvasive MRI-based methods of estimating pulmonary artery pressure in pulmonary hypertension. J Magn Reson Imaging 2005;22(1):67–72.

34. Saba TS, Foster J, Cockburn M, et al. Ventricular mass index using magnetic resonance imaging accurately estimates pulmonary artery pressure. Eur Respir J 2002;20(6):1519–24.

35. Biederman RW. Cardiovascular magnetic resonance imaging as applied to patients with pulmonary arterial hypertension. Int J Clin Pract Suppl 2009;(162):20–35.

36. Sanz J, Kariisa M, Dellegrottaglie S, et al. Evaluation of pulmonary artery stiffness in pulmonary hypertension with cardiac magnetic resonance. JACC Cardiovasc Imaging 2009;2(3):286–95.

37. Gan CT, Lankhaar JW, Westerhof N, et al. Noninvasively assessed pulmonary artery stiffness predicts mortality in pulmonary arterial hypertension. Chest 2007;132(6):1906–12.

38. Jeong HJ, Vakil P, Sheehan JJ, et al. Time-resolved magnetic resonance angiography: evaluation of intrapulmonary circulation parameters in pulmonary arterial hypertension. J Magn Reson Imaging 2011; 33(1):225–31.

39. Bustamante-Labarta M, Perrone S, De La Fuente RL, et al. Right atrial size and tricuspid regurgitation severity predict mortality or transplantation in primary pulmonary hypertension. J Am Soc Echocardiogr 2002;15(10 Pt 2):1160–4.

40. Raymond RJ, Hinderliter AL, Willis PW, et al. Echocardiographic predictors of adverse outcomes in primary pulmonary hypertension. J Am Coll Cardiol 2002;39(7):1214–9.

41. Grapsa J, Gibbs JS, Cabrita IZ, et al. The association of clinical outcome with right atrial and ventricular remodelling in patients with pulmonary arterial hypertension: study with real-time three-dimensional echocardiography. Eur Heart J Cardiovasc Imaging 2012. [Epub ahead of print]. DOI: 10.1093/ehjci/jes003.

42. Burgess MI, Mogulkoc N, Bright-Thomas RJ, et al. Comparison of echocardiographic markers of right ventricular function in determining prognosis in chronic pulmonary disease. J Am Soc Echocardiogr 2002;15(6):633–9.

43. Lang RM, Bierig M, Devereux RB, et al. Recommendations for chamber quantification: a report from the American Society of Echocardiography's Guidelines and Standards Committee and the Chamber Quantification Writing Group, developed in conjunction with the European Association of Echocardiography, a branch of the European Society of Cardiology. J Am Soc Echocardiogr 2005;18(12):1440–63.

44. Ghio S, Klersy C, Magrini G, et al. Prognostic relevance of the echocardiographic assessment of right ventricular function in patients with idiopathic pulmonary arterial hypertension. Int J Cardiol 2010;140(3): 272–8.

45. Grapsa J, Gibbs JS, Dawson D, et al. Morphologic and functional remodeling of the right ventricle in pulmonary hypertension by real time three dimensional echocardiography. Am J Cardiol 2012; 109(6):906–13.

46. Benza RL, Miller DP, Gomberg-Maitland M, et al. Predicting survival in pulmonary arterial hypertension: insights from the Registry to Evaluate Early and Long-Term Pulmonary Arterial Hypertension Disease Management (REVEAL). Circulation 2010; 122(2):164–72.

47. Grothues F, Moon JC, Bellenger NG, et al. Interstudy reproducibility of right ventricular volumes, function, and mass with cardiovascular magnetic resonance. Am Heart J 2004;147(2):218–23.

48. Sugeng L, Mor-Avi V, Weinert L, et al. Multimodality comparison of quantitative volumetric analysis of the right ventricle. JACC Cardiovasc Imaging 2010;3(1):10–8.

49. Mooij CF, de Wit CJ, Graham DA, et al. Reproducibility of MRI measurements of right ventricular size and function in patients with normal and dilated ventricles. J Magn Reson Imaging 2008;28(1): 67–73.

50. Hudsmith LE, Petersen SE, Francis JM, et al. Normal human left and right ventricular and left atrial dimensions using steady state free precession magnetic resonance imaging. J Cardiovasc Magn Reson 2005;7(5):775–82.

51. Maceira AM, Prasad SK, Khan M, et al. Reference right ventricular systolic and diastolic function normalized to age, gender and body surface area from steady-state free precession cardiovascular magnetic resonance. Eur Heart J 2006;27(23): 2879–88.

52. van Wolferen SA, Marcus JT, Boonstra A, et al. Prognostic value of right ventricular mass, volume, and function in idiopathic pulmonary arterial hypertension. Eur Heart J 2007;28(10):1250–7.

53. Blyth KG, Groenning BA, Martin TN, et al. Contrast enhanced-cardiovascular magnetic resonance imaging in patients with pulmonary hypertension. Eur Heart J 2005;26(19):1993–9.

54. McCann GP, Beek AM, Vonk-Noordegraaf A, et al. Delayed contrast-enhanced magnetic resonance imaging in pulmonary arterial hypertension. Circulation 2005;112(16):e268.

55. McCann GP, Gan CT, Beek AM, et al. Extent of MRI delayed enhancement of myocardial mass is related to right ventricular dysfunction in pulmonary artery hypertension. AJR Am J Roentgenol 2007;188(2): 349–55.

56. Sanz J, Dellegrottaglie S, Kariisa M, et al. Prevalence and correlates of septal delayed contrast enhancement in patients with pulmonary hypertension. Am J Cardiol 2007;100(4):731–5.

57. Hundley WG, Bluemke DA, Finn JP, et al. ACCF/ACR/AHA/NASCI/SCMR 2010 expert consensus document on cardiovascular magnetic resonance: a report of the American College of Cardiology Foundation Task Force on Expert Consensus Documents. J Am Coll Cardiol 2010;55(23):2614–62.

58. Forfia PR, Fisher MR, Mathai SC, et al. Tricuspid annular displacement predicts survival in pulmonary hypertension. Am J Respir Crit Care Med 2006; 174(9):1034–41.

59. Giusca S, Dambrauskaite V, Scheurwegs C, et al. Deformation imaging describes right ventricular function better than longitudinal displacement of the tricuspid ring. Heart 2010;96(4):281–8.

60. Hsiao SH, Lin SK, Wang WC, et al. Severe tricuspid regurgitation shows significant impact in the relationship among peak systolic tricuspid annular velocity, tricuspid annular plane systolic excursion, and right ventricular ejection fraction. J Am Soc Echocardiogr 2006;19(7):902–10.

61. Tamborini G, Muratori M, Brusoni D, et al. Is right ventricular systolic function reduced after cardiac surgery? A two- and three-dimensional echocardiographic study. Eur J Echocardiogr 2009; 10(5):630–4.

62. Anavekar NS, Gerson D, Skali H, et al. Two-dimensional assessment of right ventricular function: an echocardiographic-MRI correlative study. Echocardiography 2007;24(5):452–6.

63. Schenk P, Globits S, Koller J, et al. Accuracy of echocardiographic right ventricular parameters in patients with different end-stage lung diseases prior to lung transplantation. J Heart Lung Transplant 2000;19(2):145–54.

64. Wang J, Prakasa K, Bomma C, et al. Comparison of novel echocardiographic parameters of right ventricular function with ejection fraction by cardiac magnetic resonance. J Am Soc Echocardiogr 2007; 20(9):1058–64.

65. Grapsa J, O'Regan DP, Pavlopoulos H, et al. Right ventricular remodelling in pulmonary arterial hypertension with three-dimensional echocardiography: comparison with cardiac magnetic resonance imaging. Eur J Echocardiogr 2010;11(1): 64–73.

66. Badano LP, Ginghina C, Easaw J, et al. Right ventricle in pulmonary arterial hypertension: haemodynamics, structural changes, imaging, and proposal of a study protocol aimed to assess remodelling and treatment effects. Eur J Echocardiogr 2010;11(1):27–37.

67. Gleason WL, Braunwald E. Studies on the first derivative of the ventricular pressure pulse in man. J Clin Invest 1962;41:80–91.

68. Blanchard DG, Malouf PJ, Gurudevan SV, et al. Utility of right ventricular Tei index in the noninvasive evaluation of chronic thromboembolic pulmonary hypertension before and after pulmonary thromboendarterectomy. JACC Cardiovasc Imaging 2009;2(2):143–9.

69. Eidem BW, O'Leary PW, Tei C, et al. Usefulness of the myocardial performance index for assessing right ventricular function in congenital heart disease. Am J Cardiol 2000;86(6):654–8.

70. Tei C, Dujardin KS, Hodge DO, et al. Doppler echocardiographic index for assessment of global right ventricular function. J Am Soc Echocardiogr 1996; 9(6):838–47.

71. Vonk MC, Sander MH, van den Hoogen FH, et al. Right ventricle Tei-index: a tool to increase the accuracy of non-invasive detection of pulmonary arterial hypertension in connective tissue diseases. Eur J Echocardiogr 2007;8(5):317–21.

72. Zimbarra Cabrita I, Ruisanchez C, Dawson D, et al. Right ventricular function in patients with pulmonary hypertension; the value of myocardial performance index measured by tissue Doppler imaging. Eur J Echocardiogr 2010;11(8):719–24.

73. Cheung MM, Smallhorn JF, Redington AN, et al. The effects of changes in loading conditions and modulation of inotropic state on the myocardial performance index: comparison with conductance catheter measurements. Eur Heart J 2004;25(24): 2238–42.

74. Lindqvist P, Waldenstrom A, Henein M, et al. Regional and global right ventricular function in healthy individuals aged 20-90 years: a pulsed Doppler tissue imaging study: Umeå General Population Heart Study. Echocardiography 2005;22(4): 305–14.

75. Biederman RW, Doyle M, Yamrozik J. Cardiovascular MRI tutorial: lectures and learning. 1st edition. Philadelphia: Lippincott Williams & Wilkins; 2008.

76. Benza R, Biederman R, Murali S, et al. Role of cardiac magnetic resonance imaging in the management of patients with pulmonary arterial hypertension. J Am Coll Cardiol 2008;52(21):1683–92.

77. Alfakih K, Plein S, Bloomer T, et al. Comparison of right ventricular volume measurements between axial and short axis orientation using steady-state free precession magnetic resonance imaging. J Magn Reson Imaging 2003;18(1):25–32.

78. Fratz S, Schuhbaeck A, Buchner C, et al. Comparison of accuracy of axial slices versus short-axis slices for measuring ventricular volumes by cardiac magnetic resonance in patients with corrected tetralogy of Fallot. Am J Cardiol 2009;103(12): 1764–9.

79. Farber N, Doyle M, Williams RB, et al. The evaluation of right and left ventricular morphology by CMR with comparison to recipient heart after heart transplant: a surgical perspective. J Cardiovasc Magn Reson 2011;13(Suppl 1):O16.

80. Berman GO, Reichek N, Brownson D, et al. Effects of sample volume location, imaging view, heart rate and age on tricuspid velocimetry in normal subjects. Am J Cardiol 1990;65(15):1026–30.

81. Klein AL, Leung DY, Murray RD, et al. Effects of age and physiologic variables on right ventricular filling dynamics in normal subjects. Am J Cardiol 1999; 84(4):440–8.

82. Sade LE, Gulmez O, Eroglu S, et al. Noninvasive estimation of right ventricular filling pressure by ratio of early tricuspid inflow to annular diastolic velocity in patients with and without recent cardiac surgery. J Am Soc Echocardiogr 2007; 20(8):982–8.

83. Sundereswaran L, Nagueh SF, Vardan S, et al. Estimation of left and right ventricular filling pressures after heart transplantation by tissue Doppler imaging. Am J Cardiol 1998;82(3):352–7.

84. Rathi VK, Biederman RW. Expanding role of cardiovascular magnetic resonance in left and right ventricular diastolic function. Heart Fail Clin 2009; 5(3):421–35, vii.

85. Gan CT, Holverda S, Marcus JT, et al. Right ventricular diastolic dysfunction and the acute effects of sildenafil in pulmonary hypertension patients. Chest 2007;132(1):11–7.

86. Mostbeck GH, Hartiala JJ, Foster E, et al. Right ventricular diastolic filling: evaluation with velocity-encoded cine MRI. J Comput Assist Tomogr 1993; 17(2):245–52.

87. Puwanant S, Park M, Popovic ZB, et al. Ventricular geometry, strain, and rotational mechanics in pulmonary hypertension. Circulation 2010;121(2):259–66.

88. Biederman RW, Doyle M, Yamrozik J, et al. Physiologic compensation is supranormal in compensated aortic stenosis: does it return to normal after aortic valve replacement or is it blunted by coexistent coronary artery disease? An intramyocardial magnetic resonance imaging study. Circulation 2005; 112(Suppl 9):I429–36.

89. Youssef A, Ibrahim el SH, Korosoglou G, et al. Strain-encoding cardiovascular magnetic resonance for assessment of right-ventricular regional function. J Cardiovasc Magn Reson 2008;10:33.

90. Dong SJ, Hees PS, Siu CO, et al. MRI assessment of LV relaxation by untwisting rate: a new isovolumic phase measure of tau. Am J Physiol Heart Circ Physiol 2001;281(5):H2002–9.

Prognostication in Pulmonary Arterial Hypertension

Richa Agarwal, MD[a,b],
Mardi Gomberg-Maitland, MD, MSc[b,*]

KEYWORDS

- Pulmonary arterial hypertension • Survival • Prognostic factors • Risk prediction

KEY POINTS

- Despite the advances in diagnostic and treatment strategies, and contemporary survival estimates suggesting improved outcomes, the prognosis of pulmonary arterial hypertension (PAH) patients remains poor.
- Many predictors of adverse prognosis have been identified and used as important outcome measures in clinical trials. To date, there is no consensus on which prognostic variables or risk prediction strategies best predict survival, at baseline and at different time points in the disease course.
- Hemodynamic evaluation is still required both for understanding prognosis and to monitor disease.
- Measures of functional capacity and right ventricular function are important components in risk assessment.
- Risk prediction strategies that integrate hemodynamic, clinical, imaging-based variables, biomarker data, and treatment targets are important and may be useful tools to improve clinical outcomes.

Pulmonary arterial hypertension (PAH) is a fatal orphan disease, characterized by abnormal remodeling of the pulmonary vasculature, increased pulmonary vascular resistance (PVR), and right ventricular (RV) failure. PAH may be idiopathic, heritable, or associated with other diseases such as connective tissue disease (CTD). This disease is hemodynamically defined as a resting mean pulmonary artery pressure (mPAP) of 25 mm Hg or more, a pulmonary capillary wedge pressure of less than 15 mm Hg, and an elevated PVR of greater than 3 Wood units.[1] Present therapies for PAH have improved the long-term outcomes and quality of life of these patients although mortality remains high, but accurate prognosticators and strategies for timely institution and escalation of advanced pharmacologic interventions are still needed.

Even as a highly specialized field, PAH does not lack clinical trial and registry data that proffer insights into the natural history and prognosis of this rare disease. Small observational clinical trials have identified clinical and hemodynamic variables having prognostic importance meriting their further study and validation as risk prediction tools. Prognostic markers of functional capacity as assessed by functional class (FC) or exercise testing and the hemodynamic variables of right atrial pressure and

Disclosures: Richa Agarwal has no disclosures. Actelion, Gilead, Medtronic, Novartis, and United Therapeutics have provided funding to the University of Chicago to support Dr Gomberg-Maitland's conduct of clinical trials. She has served as a consultant/participant on data safety monitoring board/steering committee for clinical trials for Actelion, Gilead, Medtronic, and Pfizer.

[a] New York Presbyterian Hospital, Section of Cardiology, Columbia University New York, NY, USA; [b] Section of Cardiology, Department of Medicine, University of Chicago, Chicago, IL, USA
* Corresponding author. Pulmonary Hypertension Center, University of Chicago Medicine, 5841 South, Maryland Avenue, Room L-08, MC 5403, Chicago, IL 60637.
E-mail address: mgomberg@medicine.bsd.uchicago.edu

Heart Failure Clin 8 (2012) 373–383
doi:10.1016/j.hfc.2012.04.011
1551-7136/12/$ – see front matter © 2012 Elsevier Inc. All rights reserved.

cardiac index (CI) reflecting RV performance are powerful and predict the outcomes in the studies on pulmonary hypertension (PH), as seen in 2 contemporary clinical registries.[2,3]

The measurement of most prognostic factors often occurs at the time of initial PAH diagnosis, when referral and treatment delays may have substantially affected disease progression, or at the time of enrollment in clinical trials with inherent population and prevalence biases of the cohorts studied. Such limitations affect the interpretation and application of the available data on prognosticators to individual patients at different time points in their disease course. The changes in prognostic factors over time or with therapeutic interventions and their impact on survival prediction have not been adequately addressed. Plus, at present some factors are more studied than others not neccssarily based on their quality but on cost or investigator bias. With expanding trial data on prognostic variables in PAH, clinicians continue to encounter newer surrogates and complex prediction algorithms that although valuable, may lack consensus and clinical usefulness and limit practical risk assessment. This article discusses the current prognostication in PAH, with comprehensive and critical review of the many prognostic factors predicting this disease (**Fig. 1**).

PROGNOSIS ACCORDING TO UNDERLYING CAUSE

As seen in patients with various cardiomyopathies in left ventricular (LV) failure, survival in PAH depends on the underlying cause. Scleroderma-associated PAH carries a worse prognosis, and these patients often have a less robust response to intravenous (IV) epoprostenol than patients with idiopathic PAH (IPAH).[4–7] There is evidence, however, that contemporary survival in patients with scleroderma-associated PAH has improved compared with historical controls.[8,9] Hereditary PAH with mutations in the bone morphogenetic protein receptor type 2 (BMPR2) gene has been associated with more rapid disease progression, greater hemodynamic compromise at diagnosis, and earlier disease presentation, up to 10 years in advance of noncarriers.[10–12] In patients with a family history of PAH, BMPR2 mutations can be detected in 50% to 80% of patients[10–12]; however, genetic screening is not traditionally performed because of multiple genetic variants and incomplete penetrance. HIV-associated PAH and IPAH are shown to have similar survival and histopathology of disease, despite younger age at diagnosis in the HIV subgroup.[13] Prognosis in PAH associated with congenital heart disease is more favorable although younger age and greater RV adaptation may account for this observation.

Because of the numbers of patients in clinical PAH trials are often small owing to the rarity of this disease, multiple subgroups with associated forms of PAH in World Health Organization (WHO) category I are frequently combined with IPAH, and long-term controlled data for distinct PAH subpopulations are lacking. Not all PAH subgroups are adequately represented (eg, portoPH), and prespecified subgroup analyses are not routinely part of PAH trial design. Associated forms of PAH and IPAH likely have biological differences with varying therapeutic response, and the available trial data make it difficult to appreciate the differential influence of the cause of PAH on survival.[14] Furthermore, the less well-studied prognosticators that emerge from noncontrolled clinical trials may not be appropriate targets or offer the same utility in guiding management decisions in associated forms of PAH as in IPAH.

THE VALUE OF FUNCTIONAL ASSESSMENT AND EXERCISE CAPACITY

Functional assessment, whether objectively determined by exercise testing or subjectively by New York Heart Association (NYHA)/WHO FC, assumes central importance for determining clinical severity and for predicting outcomes in both untreated and treated patients with cardiorespiratory illnesses. Determination of FC is a low cost but subjective measure on behalf of both the patient and physician. Patients who are NYHA/WHO FC III, and especially FC IV, have a clear survival disadvantage compared with NYHA/WHO FC I or II patients. Long-term survival discrimination between patients in FC III and IV is also striking and is apparent early from the time of diagnostic right heart catheterization (RHC).[15] Although the landmark National Institutes of Health (NIH) registry data showed worse survival estimates than in recent studies, with a median survival time of 6 years among FC I or II patients compared with 2.5 years for FC III and 6 months for FC IV,[16] these survival trends according to FC prevail nonetheless. Both at presentation and after 1 year of therapy with epoprostenol, exercise tolerance and improvements in FC were significant predictors of survival and instructive for delaying or proceeding to lung transplantation.[15,17] The persistence of late FC III or IV with therapy should prompt aggressive medication titration and/or the addition of combination pharmacologic therapy in conjunction with transplantation evaluation.[15,17]

Essentially all PAH trials have relied on objective measures of functional capacity as primary end points for assessing drug efficacy and prognosis.

Prognostic Surrogates in PAH

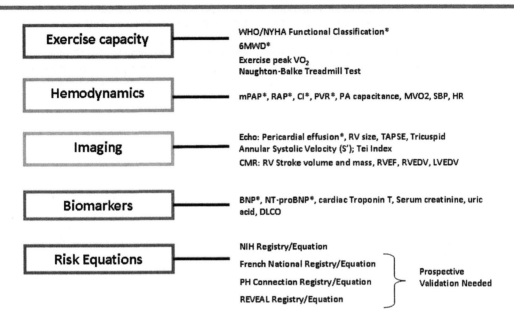

Fig. 1. Main categories of prognostic surrogates in PAH. WHO, World Health Organization; NYHA, New York Heart Association; 6MWD, 6-minute walk distance; peak VO$_2$, maximal oxygen consumption; mPAP, mean pulmonary artery pressure; RAP, right atrial pressure; CI, cardiac index; PVR, pulmonary vascular resistance; MVO$_2$, mixed venous oxygen; SBP, systolic blood pressure; HR, heart rate; TAPSE, tricuspid annular plane systolic excursion; CMR, cardiac magnetic resonance; RV, right ventricular; LV, left ventricular; EF, ejection fraction; EDV, end-diastolic volume; BNP, brain natriuretic peptide; NT-proBNP, N = terminal pro-brain natriuretic peptide; D$_{LCO}$, diffusing capacity of lung for carbon monoxide; NIH, National Institutes of Health. *Prognostic tools with the greatest evidence (multiple studies) for use or consensus among experts.

The 6 minute walk distance (6MWD) is the most commonly used end point in PAH trials, after it was found to correlate with survival in the pivotal prospective, randomized epoprostenol IPAH trial.[18] Although reproducible, inexpensive, and simple to perform, the 6MWD has several limitations in that it is effort-dependent and susceptible to motivational factors, especially in FC I and II patients. 6MWD may be less sensitive for detecting clinically meaningful change in less sick patients with PH or those who are in the early stages of the disease course. Because the average 12- or 16-week improvement in 6MWD on drug therapy-ranged from 30 to 60 m to a final walk distance still notably less than 400 m, this measure may not accurately reflect drug benefit or associated changes in survival, and such modest changes in 6MWD have defined success of the clinical trials and have led to many drug approvals. Only structured exercise training in PAH resulted in an impressive change in the 6MWD, with a mean difference of 111 m, more than that seen from any of the approved therapies.[19] The REVEAL registry (the Registry to Evaluate Early and Long-Term PAH Disease Management) discovered that 6MWD thresholds of greater than 440 m are associated with longer survival and greater than 165 m with increased mortality.[2] Recently, however, the value of 6MWD as a surrogate of survival has been questioned after a recent meta-analysis of PAH clinical trials[20] found no association between change in 6MWD and survival, leading some to conclude that 6MWD may not be an adequate end point in PH.[21]

To address the limitations of 6MWD, exercise treadmill testing (ETT) has been proposed as an alternative functional measure capable of better risk stratification. Reduced exercise capacity measured in metabolic equivalents on treadmill testing is associated with worse hemodynamic profile and increased mortality, even in FC I and II PH patients.[22] Because one of the challenges in managing PH is to identify at-risk patients early in the disease course, ETT may be a more useful method of prognostication than 6MWD, especially in patients who are less sick. The Naughton–Balke treadmill test is safe, correlates well with 6MWD, and is more widely available than cardiopulmonary exercise testing (CPET), and has been validated as a predictor of oxygen consumption during exercise in the cardiac catheterization laboratory.[22,23] Future clinical trials in PAH should include the ETT as a more objective end point and prospectively validate its use for prognostication.[22]

CPET is considered as the reference standard for functional assessment and maximal oxygen consumption (peak VO_2) with proven value in heart failure (HF)[24]; however, it is the least used exercise test in PAH clinical trials. When compared with 6MWD, CPET is also a more sensitive measure in less sick patients.[25] One study reported CPET to be an important predictor of survival in patients with PAH, and found that patients with a peak VO_2 greater than 10.4 mL/kg/min had a significantly better prognosis than those with lower peak VO_2.[26] CPET has been used as a primary end point in 2 clinical trials to date,[27,28] in contrast to the more pervasive 6MWD, presumably because of greater cost and the technical difficulties of consistently performing and interpreting CPET results in multicenter trials.

Despite limitations inherent to each exercise test, the assessment of exercise capacity continues to be important for prognostication in PAH. An individual patient's 6MWD should be carefully interpreted with respect to other clinical risk factors, the relative sensitivity of the test depending on severity of illness, and whether the change in walk distance translates to real clinical improvement. Future risk models should incorporate additional exercise measures for further validation and account for serial changes in exercise capacity to enhance risk prediction.

INVASIVE AND NONINVASIVE HEMODYNAMIC VARIABLES INFORMING PROGNOSIS

The hemodynamic evaluation in PAH is critical for understanding prognosis, both at initial RHC and at repeat invasive assessments to monitor disease progression or stabilization with therapy. The NIH registry study identified 3 hemodynamic variables associated with poor survival in both univariate and multivariate analysis: increased mPAP, increased mean right atrial pressure (mRAP), and decreased CI.[16] Although hemodynamic variables are frequently reported as valid predictors[2,3,15–17] and have the greatest number of studies supporting their association with mortality,[29] hemodynamic measures have not been used as primary end points in clinical trials and when included, they often represent secondary end points.

Given the available data, there is general consensus in using mRAP, CI, and mPAP together for predicting survival. Because RV function is an emerging focus for new therapeutic targets and

treatment algorithms, hemodynamic indices of RV performance, specifically mRAP and CI, continue to be powerful prognosticators and of interest in future studies. Cutoffs of RAP less than 10 mm Hg with a CI of greater than 2.5 L/min/m^2 or RAP of greater than 20 mm Hg with CI of less than 2.0 L/min/m^2 have been proposed as determinants of good or poor prognosis, respectively, and are meant to provide guidance to determine the nature of medical therapy.[30] An inverse association between mPAP and mortality has been reported[17] and likely signifies worsening RV function that leads to eventual decrease in the level of mPAP. A recent systematic review found that out of all the hemodynamic variables studied, mRAP had the greatest evidence for mortality prediction and identified PVR, which indicates the extent of precapillary pulmonary vascular disease and incorporates cardiac output, as a useful prognosticator.[29]

Additional hemodynamic variables with prognostic significance include decrease in stroke volume and stroke volume index,[31–35] reduced PA capacitance,[31] and decreased mixed venous oxygen.[34–36] The noninvasive hemodynamic assessment is instructive as well. A systolic blood pressure of up to 120 mm Hg with peak exercise was shown to be associated with poor outcomes at 1 year[26] In the REVEAL registry, a resting systolic blood pressure of less than 110 mm Hg and resting heart rate of greater than 92 beats/min were independently associated with increased mortality, in addition to other invasive baseline hemodynamic variables, such as elevated PVR of greater than 32 Wood units and mRAP of greater than 20 mm Hg.[2]

Approved drug therapies, with the exception of calcium channel blockers (CCB) in vasodilator responders, are not known to significantly improve pulmonary vascular disease or normalize PAP. Less than 10% of patients are responders to vasodilators (defined by reduction in mPAP of at least $\geq$10 mm Hg to an absolute mPAP <35–40 mm Hg without a decrease in cardiac output) and derive survival benefits from long-term CCBs, with up to 95% survival at 5 years.[37,38] Rarely, initial nonresponders treated with other PAH therapies will later demonstrate vasoreactivity on follow-up RHC (personal experience by the authors). This interesting phenomenon questions the mechanisms of change in the pulmonary vasculature and whether these patients follow a different disease trajectory with prognosis comparable to that of CCB responders.

THE ROLE OF IMAGING
Echocardiography

With increasing recognition of the right ventricle's importance in PH and in cardiopulmonary diseases in general, efforts have been directed toward understanding RV remodeling and mechanisms of RV adaptation using improved imaging techniques. Experienced clinicians will often make little of the estimated PA pressures on echocardiography, for instance, in favor of closely assessing RV structural and functional changes, with its effect on LV diastolic filling and cardiac output. Previous guidelines for evaluating the LV have been extensively published,[39] with little attention given to studying the RV until recently. Lack of systematic assessment of the right heart can be explained by the limited familiarity of ultrasound techniques for optimizing imaging of the RV, the complex geometry of the RV compared with the LV, difficulty in volumetric quantification for function, and insufficient data on normal values for chamber sizes. Hence, subjective assessments of the RV have been common practice.

There is now emphasis on standardizing the quantification of RV dimensions and function using newly established reference values.[40] This consensus document advocates that echocardiographic assessment includes a measure of RV size, right atrium (RA) size, estimated PAP with RA pressure estimates based on the size and collapsibility of inferior vena cava, and RV systolic function using at least 1 of the following: fractional area change, tissue Doppler-derived tricuspid lateral annular systolic velocity (S′), tricuspid annular plane systolic excursion (TAPSE), and/or RV myocardial performance index (MPI). Some of these echocardiographic parameters have known prognostic value although supporting evidence comes from small patient cohort studies.[41] With a more uniform and focused guideline-based approach to assess the RV, echocardiographic measurements may be considered as end points in future clinical trials, which along with the identification and validation of newer RV morphologic features as predictors of risk promises to make imaging ever more valuable as a tool for clinical care.

TAPSE, which reflects RV longitudinal motion, is an important index of RV systolic function. Values for TAPSE less than 1.8 cm correlate with greater RV dysfunction, RA chamber enlargement, and distortion of the RV to LV diastolic relationship. This TAPSE cutoff value was associated with significantly worse survival at 1 and 2 years in patients with PAH.[42] More recently, a lower reference value for impaired RV systolic function of 1.6 cm has been suggested by the American Society of Echocardiography.[40] S′ is easy to measure and correlates well with TAPSE and RV fractional area change.[43] An S′ of greater than 10.5 cm/s indicated normal RV function and could identify patients without significant PH in a study of

52 patients with variable disease severity.[43] As suggested by the guidelines, the cutoff of S′ less than 10 cm/s should predict abnormal RV function.[40] The Tei index, also referred to as the RV MPI, is defined as the sum of isovolumetric contraction and relaxation times divided by ejection time, and represents both RV systolic and diastolic function. The Tei index is another echocardiographic predictor of adverse outcomes in patients with PH.[44–46]

The finding of any degree of pericardial effusion on echocardiography has consistently demonstrated prognostic importance in PAH.[47] Larger effusions in patients with IPAH signify greater RA dilation, more impaired exercise tolerance, and correlate with risk of death or lung transplantation at 1 year.[48] Pericardial effusion along with RA enlargement and septal shift in diastole were shown to be significant predictors of a composite end point of death or transplantation on longer follow-up.[36]

Cardiac Magnetic Resonance Imaging

Cardiac magnetic resonance imaging (CMR) is an established imaging technique for the study of RV. Because of its high accuracy, safety, and ability to provide complete structural and functional assessment, CMR is increasingly preferred as the primary imaging modality for patients with PAH. Compared with echocardiography, CMR has low interobserver variability, making it a better tool for assessing changes in RV volumes, size, and function over time and with institution of therapies.[49] Other important information about stroke volume, cardiac output, pulmonary artery distensibility and stiffness, alterations in RV morphology, and patterns of fibrosis with disease progression can also be ascertained with CMR.[50–53] Noninvasive estimates of hemodynamic parameters such as mPAP or PVR using CMR have not yet been validated although there seems to be reasonable correlation between invasive catheterization data and CMR-derived data.[14]

In the SERAPH (Sildenafil vs Endothelin Receptor Antagonist for Pulmonary Hypertension) trial of patients with IPAH, CMR was used to assess whether there was any drug effect on RV mass, a primary end point.[54] van Wolferen and colleagues[35] found that CMR measurements of RV stroke volume of up to 25 mL/m^2, RV end-diastolic volume of 84 mL/m^2 or more, and impaired LV filling measured by reduced LV end-diastolic volume of up to 40 mL/m^2 at baseline independently predicted mortality. Worsening in these variables of RV and LV function continued to be predictive of poor outcomes at 1-year follow-up.[35]

There is interest in studying dynamic changes in RV function and size during exercise stress echocardiography or stress CMR, however, these modalities have not been thoroughly evaluated in patients with PAH. Furthermore, although three-dimensional (3D) echocardiography is more accurate for quantifying RV volumes compared with two-dimensional echocardiography (although less accurate compared with CMR), there is limited reported data demonstrating the value of 3D echocardiography in patients with PAH presently.

Biomarkers

Despite the challenges of identifying novel noninvasive markers of disease, the study of specific biomarkers for diagnosis, detection of disease progression, and treatment guidance in PAH and RV failure continues to be an active area of investigation. Plasma levels of brain natriuretic peptide (BNP) or the inactive and more stable NT-proBNP are well-established predictors of HF morbidity and mortality,[55,56] however, use of these biomarkers to tailor HF therapy is a much debated topic. In patients with PAH and RV failure, these 2 biomarkers are regularly used, both at baseline and with medical therapy, and predict survival.[57,58] Studies have shown that elevation of NT-proBNP and BNP levels correlate well with other valuable prognosticators reflecting advanced disease, including RAP, PVR, CI, 6MWD, and RV enlargement.[59–61] A study of 20 patients with PAH illustrated the usefulness of BNP for predicting the response to epoprostenol; patients with more than 50% decrease in BNP levels with treatment experienced greater event-free survival.[62]

In addition to BNP and NT-proBNP, cardiac troponin T can be a marker of acute RV failure and specifically, RV ischemia.[63] Usually found in patients with more advanced PAH also with frank hemodynamic decompensation, troponin T positivity confers a higher mortality and can urge intensified treatment aimed at alleviating RV stress. In the study by Torbicki and colleagues[63] in patients with PAH and patients with inoperable chronic thromboembolic PH, detectable troponin T levels were associated with significantly higher heart rates, reduced 6MWD, higher NT-proBNP values, and lower mixed venous oxygen saturation.

Serum uric acid levels independently predict survival in patients with IPAH, and levels proportionally increase with greater severity of disease and functional impairment.[64] Because uric acid levels are affected by multiple disease conditions, including renal failure or other hypoxemic states, this biomarker has the disadvantage of being less specific for PAH. A study by Shah and colleagues[65] demonstrated the power of using serum creatinine (SCr), an already appreciated

predictor of HF mortality, for risk assessment in patients with PAH. This study revealed that even slight elevations in the level of SCr, that is, SCr 1.0 to 1.4 mg/dL or greater than 1.4 mg/dL, were associated with higher RAP and lower CI and portended a worse prognosis.

Abnormal diffusing capacity of lung for carbon monoxide (DLco) on pulmonary function testing, when less than 43% of predicted, independently predicted death in a cohort of WHO category I patients with PAH after adjusting for associated conditions such as parenchymal lung disease on chest computed tomography, CTD etiology, and hemoglobin levels.[66] DLco testing is a readily available noninvasive test, the value of which was also attested to in the REVEAL registry.[2] Additional biomarkers reported to have prognostic utility in patients with PAH include C-reactive protein,[67] von Willebrand factor,[68] and circulating angiopoeitins.[69]

The study of biomarkers can advance the understanding of the many disease pathways involved in PAH. Many studies promoting specific biomarkers, however, are small, investigational or hypothesis generating, lack rigorous validation, and may not adequately discriminate between high- and low-risk patients. The proliferating data from ongoing biomarker studies must therefore be critically interpreted before biomarkers are accepted as novel prognostic markers with the potential for affecting treatment strategies in patients with PAH.

WHAT IS THE BEST PROGNOSTIC MARKER OR MARKERS, IF ANY?

The pharmacologic management of patients with PAH is rapidly evolving, as newer therapeutic targets that stabilize or reverse pulmonary vascular disease and target RV function are being sought and clinical practice patterns shift in favor of earlier diagnosis and aggressive treatment. Still, PAH remains a devastating disease with unacceptably poor survival. The questions remain: What is the best approach for calculating an individual patient's risk, not only at time of diagnosis but also throughout the disease trajectory? As there is not a single superior marker, how many diagnostic methods or prognostic markers should we incorporate for accurate and complete risk assessment? Importantly, what will determining a patient's risk accomplish in terms of clarifying treatment goals or follow-up, 2 critical aspects of PAH management that have not been standardized? Since the time of the NIH registry of the 1980s[16] to the current period, many new noninvasive markers of disease have been put forth, but not surprisingly, there has never been a clear guideline-supported strategy for determining prognosis.

Most centers specializing in PAH commonly obtain FC, some measure of exercise capacity, RHC data, and echocardiography for RV evaluation at baseline and at interval periods of 3 or 6 months, depending on the clinical stability of the patient and physician experience.[41] The data from these tests are indisputably important and already validated for risk stratification, but algorithms combining these and newer disease markers in multivariate models may have incremental value and be more desirable. Furthermore, for an algorithm to be truly effective, it must account for delays in diagnosis and treatment as well as changes in risk markers over the long-term.

SURVIVAL EQUATIONS: DATA FROM RECENT REGISTRIES

Estimated median survival of patients with IPAH, familial PAH, and anorexigen-associated PAH was 2.8 years after diagnosis, with 1-, 3-, and 5-year survival rates of 68%, 48%, and 34%, respectively, from the NIH registry study.[16] This registry, initiated during a time when there were no US Food and Drug Administration-approved PAH therapies, described the clinical characteristics and natural history of 194 patients. From a retrospective analysis of the risk predictors, a regression equation was derived to estimate survival using 3 baseline hemodynamic parameters (mRAP, mPAP, and CI).[16] This equation was

subsequently validated in a small cohort of 60 patients with PH[34] and became the current standard to assess therapeutic benefit. Many clinical trials without a placebo-control arm have used the NIH equation to show a survival advantage by comparing observed survival rates on study drug with the NIH-predicted survival rates. Because observed survival estimates with modern therapies seem significantly better,[3,70] the predictive accuracy and validity of the NIH equation has been recently challenged. The Pulmonary Hypertension Connection (PHC) registry analyzed 576 patients with idiopathic, familial, and anorexigen-associated PAH referred to a single US center during 1991 to 2007, compared their observed survival with the predicted survival by the NIH equation, and found that the NIH equation underestimated survival in the current era (**Fig. 2**). From the PHC, a new regression survival equation was developed that uses the same 3 hemodynamic variables as the NIH equation, albeit with different coefficients.[70] This equation performed well when compared with actual observed survival rates in other published PAH cohorts,[71,72] however, it will need prospective validation before it can be used in clinical or research settings.

Other large, modern day registries in PAH have offered insights into the determinants of survival and provide the basis for future validation of risk equations. The French National Registry described by Humbert and colleagues[3] analyzed

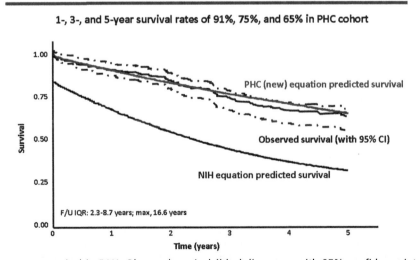

Fig. 2. Contemporary survival in PAH. Observed survival (*black lines*———; with 95% confidence interval) versus predicted survival using the Pulmonary hypertension connection (*red line*———) and National Institutes of Health (*blue line*) equations in patients with idiopathic, familial and anorexigen-associated pulmonary arterial hypertension. (*Adapted from* Thenappan T, Shah SJ, Rich S, et al. Survival in pulmonary arterial hypertension: a reappraisal of the NIH risk stratification equation. Eur Respir J 2010;35:1085.)

prognostic factors in 354 consecutive patients with idiopathic PAH, familial PAH, and anorexigen-associated PAH. A simple risk prediction equation, based on a 3-year survival rate of 58.2%, was formed from 3 significant factors on multivariate analysis: sex, 6MWD, and cardiac output at initial diagnosis.[73] The REVEAL registry[2] is a multicenter longitudinal study of 2716 patients with newly and previously diagnosed category I PAH that aimed to create a cohesive and multivariable, weighted risk formula for use at any time in the disease course. On multivariable analysis, several risk factors were independently associated with increased mortality: elevated PVR, etiology of PAH, FC, family history of PAH, renal insufficiency, RAP, resting SBP and HR, 6MWD, BNP, presence of pericardial effusion on echocardiography, and percent predicted of DLco. A prognostic equation using all of these factors was derived, and an individual could be assigned a risk category based on predicted 1-year survival. REVEAL measured prognostic factors at time of enrollment into the registry, and 1-year survival using this date was 91%, drawing some criticism that the mortality estimate may be too optimistic because of inherent prevalence and survivor bias.[74] However, the statistical method of left truncation used during model development addressed this potential bias.[2] REVEAL is additionally evaluating whether the trajectory of variables matters and what degree of change, that is, a decline 15% in 6MWD, elevates risk to possibly warrant therapeutic intervention.[75] The REVEAL equation has been modified into an uncomplicated risk calculator that is practical for clinician use.

Both the French National Registry and REVEAL registry equations maintain the importance of FC, 6MWD, and hemodynamic surrogates of RV function on multivariate analysis for risk prediction. Although such risk equations have their limitations and require broader validation, at present they offer a stronger framework for risk prediction than prior studies of single predictors.

SUMMARY

Accurate and timely prognostication in PAH is essential given the incurable nature of this disease and the high rate of death in patients who present with advanced disease. Because the disease is complex, implicates the traditionally understudied RV, and is associated with many different disease states, making sense of available prognostic tools can be understandably challenging. Risk prediction strategies, which integrate hemodynamic, clinical, imaging-based variables, biomarker data, and treatment targets are appropriate. Such strategies require proper validation, refinement, and finally consensus before determining if their use can improve the patient outcomes.

REFERENCES

1. McGoon M, Gutterman D, Steen V, et al. Screening, early detection, and diagnosis of pulmonary arterial hypertension: ACCP evidence-based clinical practice guidelines. Chest 2004;126(Suppl 1): 14S–34S.
2. Benza RL, Miller DP, Gomberg-Maitland M, et al. Predicting survival in pulmonary arterial hypertension: insights from the Registry to Evaluate Early and Long-Term Pulmonary Arterial Hypertension Disease Management (REVEAL). Circulation 2010; 122(2):164–72.
3. Humbert M, Sitbon O, Chaouat A, et al. Survival in patients with idiopathic, familial, and anorexigen-associated pulmonary arterial hypertension in the modern management era. Circulation 2010;122(2): 156–63.
4. Kawut SM, Taichman DB, Archer-Chicko CL, et al. Hemodynamics and survival in patients with pulmonary arterial hypertension related to systemic sclerosis. Chest 2003;123(2):344–50.
5. Kuhn K, Byrne D, Arbogast PG, et al. Outcome in 91 consecutive patients with pulmonary arterial hypertension receiving epoprostenol. Am J Respir Crit Care Med 2003;167(4):580–6.
6. McLaughlin VV, Presberg KW, Doyle RL, et al. Prognosis of pulmonary arterial hypertension: ACCP evidence-based clinical practice guidelines. Chest 2004;126(Suppl 1):78S–92S.
7. Stupi AM, Steen VD, Owens GR, et al. Pulmonary hypertension in the CREST syndrome variant of systemic sclerosis. Arthritis Rheum 1986;29(4): 515–24.
8. Badesch DB, McGoon MD, Barst RJ, et al. Longterm survival among patients with scleroderma-associated pulmonary arterial hypertension treated with intravenous epoprostenol. J Rheumatol 2009; 36(10):2244–9.
9. Williams MH, Das C, Handler CE, et al. Systemic sclerosis associated pulmonary hypertension: improved survival in the current era. Heart 2006; 92(7):926–32.
10. Girerd B, Montani D, Coulet F, et al. Clinical outcomes of pulmonary arterial hypertension in patients carrying an ACVRL1 (ALK1) Mutation. Am J Respir Crit Care Med 2010;181(8):851–61.
11. Rosenzweig EB, Morse JH, Knowles JA, et al. Clinical implications of determining BMPR2 mutation status in a large cohort of children and adults with pulmonary arterial hypertension. J Heart Lung Transplant 2008;27(6):668–74.
12. Sztrymf B, Coulet F, Girerd B, et al. Clinical outcomes of pulmonary arterial hypertension in

carriers of BMPR2 mutation. Am J Respir Crit Care Med 2008;177(12):1377–83.

13. Pettipretz P, Brenot F, Azarian R, et al. Pulmonary hypertension in patients with human immunodeficiency virus infection. Circulation 1994;89:2772.

14. McLaughlin VV, Badesch DB, Delcroix M, et al. End points and clinical trial design in pulmonary arterial hypertension. J Am Coll Cardiol 2009;54(Suppl 1): S97–107.

15. McLaughlin VV, Shillington A, Rich S. Survival in primary pulmonary hypertension: the impact of epoprostenol therapy. Circulation 2002;106(12):1477–82.

16. D'Alonzo GE, Barst RJ, Ayres SM, et al. Survival in patients with primary pulmonary hypertension: results from a national prospective registry. Ann Intern Med 1991;115(5):343–9.

17. Sitbon O, Humbert M, Nunes H, et al. Long-term intravenous epoprostenol infusion in primary pulmonary hypertension: prognostic factors and survival. J Am Coll Cardiol 2002;40(4):780–8.

18. Barst R, Rubin L, Long W, et al. A comparison of continuous intravenous epoprostenol (prostacyclin) with conventional therapy for primary pulmonary hypertension. N Engl J Med 1996;334: 296–301.

19. Mereles D, Ehlken N, Kreuscher S, et al. Exercise and respiratory training improve exercise capacity and quality of life in patients with severe chronic pulmonary hypertension. Circulation 2006;114(14): 1482–9.

20. Macchia A, Marchioli R, Marfisi R, et al. A meta-analysis of trials of pulmonary hypertension: a clinical condition looking for drugs and research methodology. Am Heart J 2007;153(6):1037–47.

21. Farber HW. The status of pulmonary arterial hypertension in 2008. Circulation 2008;117(23):2966–8.

22. Shah SJ, Thenappan T, Rich S, et al. Value of exercise treadmill testing in the risk stratification of patients with pulmonary hypertension. Circ Heart Fail 2009;2(4):278–86.

23. Gomberg-Maitland M, Huo D, Benza RL, et al. Creation of a model comparing 6-minute walk test to metabolic equivalent in evaluating treatment effects in pulmonary arterial hypertension. J Heart Lung Transplant 2007;26(7):732–8.

24. Mancini DM, Eisen H, Kussmaul W, et al. Value of peak exercise oxygen consumption for optimal timing of cardiac transplantation in ambulatory patients with heart failure. Circulation 1991;83(3):778–86.

25. Raeside D, Smith A, Brown A, et al. Pulmonary artery pressure measurement during exercise testing in patients with suspected pulmonary hypertension. Eur Respir J 2000;16:282–7.

26. Wensel R, Opitz C, Anker S, et al. Assessment of survival in patients with primary pulmonary hypertension: importance of cardiopulmonary exercise testing. Circulation 2002;106:319–24.

27. Barst R, McGoon M, McLaughlin V, et al. Beraprost therapy for pulmonary arterial hypertension. J Am Coll Cardiol 2003;41(12):2119–25.

28. Barst RJ, Langleben D, Frost A, et al. Sitaxsentan therapy for pulmonary arterial hypertension. Am J Respir Crit Care Med 2004;169(4):441–7.

29. Swiston JR, Johnson SR, Granton JT. Factors that prognosticate mortality in idiopathic pulmonary arterial hypertension: a systematic review of the literature. Respir Med 2010;104(11):1588–607.

30. McLaughlin VV, McGoon MD. Pulmonary arterial hypertension. Circulation 2006;114(13):1417–31.

31. Mahapatra S, Nishimura RA, Sorajja P, et al. Relationship of pulmonary arterial capacitance and mortality in idiopathic pulmonary arterial hypertension. J Am Coll Cardiol 2006;47(4):799–803.

32. Okada O, Tanabe N, Yasuda J, et al. Prediction of life expectancy in patients with primary pulmonary hypertension. A retrospective nationwide survey from 1980–1990. Intern Med 1999;38(1):12–6.

33. Rich S, Levy PS. Characteristics of surviving and nonsurviving patients with primary pulmonary hypertension. Am J Med 1984;76(4):573–8.

34. Sandoval J, Bauerle O, Palomar A, et al. Survival in primary pulmonary hypertension. Validation of a prognostic equation. Circulation 1994;89:1733–44.

35. van Wolferen SA, Marcus JT, Boonstra A, et al. Prognostic value of right ventricular mass, volume, and function in idiopathic pulmonary arterial hypertension. Eur Heart J 2007;28(10):1250–7.

36. Raymond R, Hinderliter A, Willis P, et al. Echocardiographic predictors of adverse outcomes in primary pulmonary hypertension. J Am Coll Cardiol 2002; 39(7):1214–9.

37. Rich S, Kaufman E, Levy P. The effect of high doses of calcium-channel blockers on survival in primary pulmonary hypertension. N Engl J Med 1992;327:76.

38. Sitbon O, Humbert M, Jais X, et al. Long-term response to calcium channel blockers in idiopathic pulmonary arterial hypertension. Circulation 2005; 111(23):3105–11.

39. Lang RM, Bierig M, Devereux RB, et al. Recommendations for chamber quantification: a report from the American Society of Echocardiography's Guidelines and Standards Committee and the Chamber Quantification Writing Group, developed in conjunction with the European Association of Echocardiography, a branch of the European Society of Cardiology. J Am Soc Echocardiogr 2005;18(12):1440–63.

40. Rudski LG, Lai WW, Afilalo J, et al. Guidelines for the echocardiographic assessment of the right heart in adults: a report from the American Society of Echocardiography endorsed by the European Association of Echocardiography, a registered branch of the European Society of Cardiology, and the Canadian Society of Echocardiography. J Am Soc Echocardiogr 2010;23(7):685–713 [quiz: 786–8].

41. McLaughlin VV, Archer SL, Badesch DB, et al. ACCF/AHA 2009 expert consensus document on pulmonary hypertension: a report of the American College of Cardiology Foundation Task Force on Expert Consensus Documents and the American Heart Association: developed in collaboration with the American College of Chest Physicians, American Thoracic Society, Inc., and the Pulmonary Hypertension Association. Circulation 2009;119(16):2250–94.

42. Forfia PR, Fisher MR, Mathai SC, et al. Tricuspid annular displacement predicts survival in pulmonary hypertension. Am J Respir Crit Care Med 2006;174(9):1034–41.

43. Saxena N, Rajagopalan N, Edelman K, et al. Tricuspid annular systolic velocity: a useful measurement in determining right ventricular systolic function regardless of pulmonary artery pressures. Echocardiography 2006;23(9):750–5.

44. Sebbag I, Rudski L, Therrien J, et al. Effect of chronic infusion of epoprostenol on echocardiographic right ventricular myocardial performance index and its relation to clinical outcome in patients with primary pulmonary hypertension. Am J Cardiol 2001;88:1060–3.

45. Tei C, Dujardin KS, Hodge DO, et al. Doppler echocardiographic index for assessment of global right ventricular function. J Am Soc Echocardiogr 1996;9(6):838–47.

46. Yeo T, Dujardn K, Tei C, et al. Value of a doppler-derived index combining systolic and diastolic time intervals in predicting outcome in primary pulmonary hypertension. Am J Cardiol 1998;81:1157–61.

47. Eysmann SB, Palevsky HI, Reichek N, et al. Two-dimensional and Doppler-echocardiographic and cardiac catheterization correlates of survival in primary pulmonary hypertension. Circulation 1989;80(2):353–60.

48. Hinderliter A, Willis PW 4th, Long W, et al. Frequency and prognostic significance of pericardial effusion in primary pulmonary hypertension. Am J Cardiol 1999;84:481–4.

49. Di Guglielmo L, Dore R, Vespro V. Pulmonary hypertension: role of computed tomography and magnetic resonance imaging. Ital Heart J 2005;6(10):846–51.

50. Bradlow WM, Assomull R, Kilner PJ, et al. Understanding late gadolinium enhancement in pulmonary hypertension. Circ Cardiovasc Imaging 2010;3(4):501–3.

51. Marcus J, Noordegraaf A, Roeleveld R, et al. Impaired left ventricular filling due to right ventricular pressure overload in primary pulmonary hypertension. Noninvasive monitoring using MRI. Chest 2001;119(6):1761–5.

52. Paz R, Mohiaddin RH, Longmore DB. Magnetic resonance assessment of the pulmonary arterial trunk anatomy, flow, pulsatility and distensibility. Eur Heart J 1993;14(11):1524–30.

53. Tardivon AA, Mousseaux E, Brenot F, et al. Quantification of hemodynamics in primary pulmonary hypertension with magnetic resonance imaging. Am J Respir Crit Care Med 1994;150(4):1075–80.

54. Wilkins MR, Paul GA, Strange JW, et al. Sildenafil versus Endothelin Receptor Antagonist for Pulmonary Hypertension (SERAPH) Study. Am J Respir Crit Care Med 2005;171(11):1292–7.

55. Doust JA, Pietrzak E, Dobson A, et al. How well does B-type natriuretic peptide predict death and cardiac events in patients with heart failure: systematic review. BMJ 2005;330(7492):625.

56. Hartmann F, Packer M, Coats AJ, et al. Prognostic impact of plasma N-terminal pro-brain natriuretic peptide in severe chronic congestive heart failure: a substudy of the Carvedilol Prospective Randomized Cumulative Survival (COPERNICUS) trial. Circulation 2004;110(13):1780–6.

57. Blyth KG, Groenning BA, Mark PB, et al. NT-proBNP can be used to detect right ventricular systolic dysfunction in pulmonary hypertension. Eur Respir J 2007;29(4):737–44.

58. Nagaya N, Nishikimi T, Uematsu M, et al. Plasma brain natriuretic peptide as a prognostic indicator in patients with primary pulmonary hypertension. Circulation 2000;102:865–70.

59. Andreassen AK, Wergeland R, Simonsen S, et al. N-terminal pro-B-type natriuretic peptide as an indicator of disease severity in a heterogeneous group of patients with chronic precapillary pulmonary hypertension. Am J Cardiol 2006;98(4):525–9.

60. Fijalkowska A, Kurzyna M, Torbicki A, et al. Serum N-terminal brain natriuretic peptide as a prognostic parameter in patients with pulmonary hypertension. Chest 2006;129(5):1313–21.

61. Williams MH, Handler CE, Akram R, et al. Role of N-terminal brain natriuretic peptide (N-TproBNP) in scleroderma-associated pulmonary arterial hypertension. Eur Heart J 2006;27(12):1485–94.

62. Park MH, Scott RL, Uber PA, et al. Usefulness of B-type natriuretic peptide as a predictor of treatment outcome in pulmonary arterial hypertension. Congest Heart Fail 2004;10(5):221–5.

63. Torbicki A, Kurzyna M, Kuca P, et al. Detectable serum cardiac troponin T as a marker of poor prognosis among patients with chronic precapillary pulmonary hypertension. Circulation 2003;108(7):844–8.

64. Nagaya N, Uematsu M, Satoh T, et al. Serum uric acid levels correlate with the severity and the mortality of primary pulmonary hypertension. Am J Respir Crit Care Med 1999;160:487–92.

65. Shah SJ, Thenappan T, Rich S, et al. Association of serum creatinine with abnormal hemodynamics and mortality in pulmonary arterial hypertension. Circulation 2008;117(19):2475–83.

66. Chandra S, Shah SJ, Thenappan T, et al. Carbon monoxide diffusing capacity and mortality in pulmonary arterial hypertension. J Heart Lung Transplant 2010;29(2):181–7.

67. Quarck R, Nawrot T, Meyns B, et al. C-reactive protein: a new predictor of adverse outcome in pulmonary arterial hypertension. J Am Coll Cardiol 2009;53(14):1211–8.

68. Kawut SM, Horn EM, Berekashvili KK, et al. von Willebrand factor independently predicts long-term survival in patients with pulmonary arterial hypertension. Chest 2005;128(4):2355–62.

69. Kumpers P, Nickel N, Lukasz A, et al. Circulating angiopoietins in idiopathic pulmonary arterial hypertension. Eur Heart J 2010;31(18):2291–300.

70. Thenappan T, Shah SJ, Rich S, et al. Survival in pulmonary arterial hypertension: a reappraisal of the NIH risk stratification equation. Eur Respir J 2010;35(5):1079–87.

71. McLaughlin VV, Sitbon O, Badesch DB, et al. Survival with first-line bosentan in patients with primary pulmonary hypertension. Eur Respir J 2005;25(2):244–9.

72. Sitbon O, McLaughlin VV, Badesch DB, et al. Survival in patients with class III idiopathic pulmonary arterial hypertension treated with first line oral bosentan compared with an historical cohort of patients started on intravenous epoprostenol. Thorax 2005;60(12):1025–30.

73. Humbert M, Sitbon O, Yaici A, et al. Survival in incident and prevalent cohorts of patients with pulmonary arterial hypertension. Eur Respir J 2010;36(3): 549–55.

74. McLaughlin VV, Suissa S. Prognosis of pulmonary arterial hypertension: the power of clinical registries of rare diseases. Circulation 2010;122(2):106–8.

75. Benza RL, Miller DP, Frantz RP, et al. Association between Serial 6-Minute Walk Distance (6MWD) Assessments and the REVEAL Pulmonary Arterial Hypertension (PAH) Risk Score Calculator. Presented at: The International Society for Heart and Lung Transplantation Annual Meeting. Chicago (IL), April 22, 2010.

Pharmacotherapy for Pulmonary Arterial Hypertension

Gautam V. Ramani, MD[a],*, Myung H. Park, MD[b]

KEYWORDS

- Pulmonary arterial hypertension • Pulmonary hypertension • Pharmacotherapy • Prostacyclins

KEY POINTS

- There are currently 9 disease-specific therapies for pulmonary arterial hypertension approved by the Food and Drug Administration, each with relative strengths and weaknesses and varying side-effect profiles.
- Long-term compliance and treatment success depend on selection of effective, tolerable therapy that patients can incorporate into their lifestyle.
- All disease-specific pharmacotherapies have been shown to improve exercise tolerance. Additional benefits of therapy vary based on specific study criteria for each drug, but comprehensive PAH disease-specific therapy has been shown to reduce clinical worsening and improve quality of life.
- Frequent assessment of a patient's risk profile is essential in ensuring adequate pharmacotherapy. Patients who continue to progress symptomatically or exhibit high-risk clinical features should be assessed for combination pharmacotherapy, continuous-infusion prostacyclins, and consideration for lung transplant referral.
- Despite therapeutic advances, PAH-associated morbidity and mortality remain unacceptably high.

BACKGROUND

Pulmonary arterial hypertension (PAH) is a disabling, progressive disease characterized by vasoconstriction, smooth muscle proliferation, remodeling, and thrombosis of the pulmonary vasculature. Although described and characterized as early as 1950, median survival in the absence of disease-specific therapy was less than 3 years as recently as 1991.[1,2] Progressive increases in pulmonary vascular resistance over time lead to right ventricular failure, subsequent organ hypoperfusion, and death. For many years pharmacotherapy was largely supportive, and focused on optimization of volume status with diuretics and correction of hypoxemia with supplemental oxygen.

In the 1980s it was recognized that thrombosis played a role in the pathobiology of pulmonary hypertension, and anticoagulation was recommended. The importance of vasoconstriction in the pathogenesis was highlighted in the early 1990s, and calcium-channel blockers were introduced as a treatment for pulmonary hypertension (PH).[3] Additional studies demonstrated that vasoconstriction was only one component of the pathophysiology of PAH, and novel disease-specific therapies targeting cellular physiology and endothelial dysfunction, resulting in vascular remodeling, have dramatically altered the prognosis of this rapidly progressive disease.

The past decade has seen an explosion in the available therapies for the management of PAH. Therapies now target 3 distinct molecular pathways (**Fig. 1**), and involve a variety of delivery approaches including continuous infusion (either

[a] University of Maryland School of Medicine, Baltimore VAMC, 110 South Paca Street, 7th Floor, Baltimore, MD 21201-1559, USA; [b] Cardiology Care Unit, Pulmonary Vascular Disease Program, University of Maryland School of Medicine, 110 South Paca Street, 7th Floor, Baltimore, MD 21201-1559, USA
* Corresponding author.
E-mail address: gramani@medicine.umaryland.edu

Heart Failure Clin 8 (2012) 385–402
doi:10.1016/j.hfc.2012.04.012
1551-7136/12/$ – see front matter © 2012 Elsevier Inc. All rights reserved.

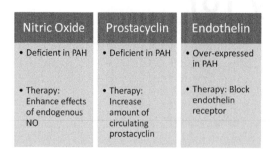

Nitric Oxide	Prostacyclin	Endothelin
• Deficient in PAH	• Deficient in PAH	• Over-expressed in PAH
• Therapy: Enhance effects of endogenous NO	• Therapy: Increase amount of circulating prostacyclin	• Therapy: Block endothelin receptor

Fig. 1. Mechanisms of therapies approved by the Food and Drug Administration. NO, nitric oxide; PAH, pulmonary arterial hypertension.

subcutaneous or intravenous), and inhaled and oral agents. Each mode of delivery and targeted mechanism of action possesses a unique side-effect profile with respective strengths and weaknesses. Choosing appropriate pharmacotherapy can be a daunting task for the practitioner, as no head-to-head comparisons between drugs have been published. Furthermore, the range of inclusion criteria, specifically with regard to allowing for background therapy for pivotal clinical trials, has evolved over time, further complicating the translation of these studies into the medical decision-making process.

This article aims to assist the practitioner in developing an evidence-based, rational pharmacologic treatment algorithm for the management of patients with PAH. Currently approved pharmacotherapy and the pivotal trials that led to approval for the respective agents are reviewed. The article concludes with a discussion of common dilemmas in the treatment of PAH for which strong evidence is lacking. Distinctions are made between recommendations supported by randomized clinical trials, consensus expert opinions, and the opinions of the authors.

DIAGNOSTIC EVALUATION OF PAH

The diagnostic evaluation of PAH is reviewed in detail elsewhere in this issue. It is of paramount importance to establish and confirm the diagnosis of PAH via right heart catheterization (RHC), and to exclude more common causes of elevated pulmonary artery pressures including pulmonary venous hypertension related to left-sided heart disease, chronic thromboembolic pulmonary hypertension (CTEPH), and chronic obstructive or interstitial lung disease. Initiation of pulmonary arterial vasodilators may worsen oxygenation and lead to hemodynamic deterioration if prescribed in these conditions. If underlying medical conditions are discovered that may predispose patients to development of associated pulmonary arterial hypertension (APAH), including intracardiac

shunts, connective tissue diseases, liver disease, or human immunodeficiency virus (HIV) infection, appropriate subspecialty consultations and targeted disease-specific therapy should be initiated. Given the potential for significant drug-drug interactions, a multidisciplinary approach to the management of these patients is advised.

SUPPORTIVE THERAPIES IN PAH

These therapies are not unique to the treatment of PAH, but play a critical role in comprehensive disease management. The benefit of an integrated exercise program for stable PAH patients is receiving recognition and support. The effects of monitored exercise training were investigated in a randomized study of 30 patients stable on PAH pharmacotherapy.[4] Patients who received exercise training demonstrated improvements in 6-minute walk distance (6MWD), quality of life (QOL), functional class (FC), and peak oxygen consumption. Low-intensity level graded aerobic exercise, such as walking as tolerated, has been recommended for all stable patients on PAH-directed therapy. Conversely, heavy physical exertion or isometric activity, which involves straining against a fixed resistance, should be avoided, as such activity may result in exertional syncope.[5] Strict adherence to monitored sodium diet, at a minimum of less than 2400 mg per day (or less depending on the severity of PAH and right ventricular dysfunction), is important in managing volume status. Compliance with immunizations, such as those against influenza and pneumococcal pneumonia, are strongly recommended.[5] Current guidelines state that pregnancy be avoided, and if an unplanned pregnancy occurs early termination is advised, given a maternal mortality rate of 30% to 40%.[6] Although experts have differing opinions regarding the best mode of contraception, educating women with childbearing potential regarding the serious hazards of pregnancy and the importance of using dual methods of contraception (such as hormonal plus barrier methods) is critically important.[7]

Diuretics

The physiologic hallmarks of PAH are an increase in right ventricular (RV) afterload and an elevated pulmonary vascular resistance. For those patients with compensated PAH with low filling pressures and absent RV failure, diuretics are typically not required for symptom control. Over time, because of its propensity to progress, PAH often leads to RV failure and systemic venous congestion. In patients exhibiting signs and symptoms of right heart failure, loop diuretics are typically used as first-line therapies. Essential in diuretic therapy is adequate dosing, and routine monitoring of renal function and electrolytes. Diuretic resistance, leading to escalating dose requirements and use of synergistic diuretic combinations with metolazone, usually constitutes a sign of worsening right-sided heart failure and should prompt reassessment of disease status. In patients hospitalized with right-sided heart failure, bowel edema may limit oral absorption, and intravenous administration is often necessary. Spironolactone, an oral potassium-sparing aldosterone antagonist, may be considered for patients with problematic hypokalemia or prominent symptoms of ascites.[8]

Oxygen

Hypoxia leads to regional vasoconstriction within the pulmonary circulation, and may result in elevations in pulmonary vascular resistance and subsequent increased afterload on the right ventricle. There are multiple mechanisms of hypoxemia in PAH, including ventilation/perfusion mismatch, right-to-left shunting, hypoventilation, and reductions in diffusion capacity. Oxygen is frequently used to treat hypoxia in group III PH, and the benefits are believed to apply to those with PAH, although robust data supporting this hypothesis are lacking. It is generally advisable to maintain oxygen saturation at greater than 90% at rest and with ambulation.[5,9] Profound hypoxia is distinctly uncommon in PAH, and its presence should prompt a search for intracardiac or intrapulmonary shunting, pulmonary embolism, or parenchymal lung disease.

Anticoagulation

The rationale for anticoagulant therapy in patients with PAH stems from pathologic data demonstrating pulmonary arteriopathy with thrombotic lesions.[10] In addition, abnormalities of coagulation and fibrinolysis have been reported in PAH.[11,12] Anticoagulation with warfarin has been examined in 3 noncontrolled observational studies and has been found to be associated with improved survival in mostly idiopathic PAH (IPAH) patients.[3,10,13] These studies were performed before approval of PAH-specific treatments, and whether anticoagulation further improves survival in those patients on disease-specific therapy is unknown. For patients with APAH, a careful assessment of potential bleeding risk must be weighed against the benefits before therapy initiation. It is recommended that anticoagulation be instituted in those patients with advanced disease, such as those requiring intravenous treatments, in the absence of contraindications.[5] In suitable candidates, warfarin therapy with an international normalized ratio target range of 1.5 to 2.5 is advisable.[5] There are no data investigating the new oral anticoagulants, such as factor Xa inhibitors and the direct thrombin inhibitors, in pulmonary vascular disease.

Digoxin

Digoxin is not routinely used for the management of PAH. For patients with problematic supraventricular arrhythmias and concomitant RV failure, there may be a therapeutic role. The published literature studying digoxin in RV failure is limited to one study of intravenous digoxin that demonstrated improved cardiac output.[14] However, the potential to breach the narrow therapeutic safety window must be carefully assessed before initiation, particularly in women and in those patients with concomitant kidney disease and electrolyte abnormalities.

Calcium-Channel Blockers

Calcium-channel blockers (CCBs) were the first widely accepted therapy for PAH. Initial experience demonstrated a remarkable 95% intermediate-term survival in IPAH patients with a positive vasodilator response.[3] The techniques and definitions used to perform and define vasoreactive PAH are described elsewhere in this issue. A larger, more recent retrospective study by Sitbon and colleagues[15] identified the prevalence of a positive vasodilator response as 13% in IPAH, and of this group approximately half the patients were found to maintain functional improvement at 1 year. Based on this analysis, the current definition of a response is a decrease in mean pulmonary artery pressure (mPAP) of greater than or equal to 10 mm Hg down to an mPAP less than or equal to 40 mm Hg, with an unchanged or increased cardiac output.[5,15] Patients who meet these criteria and are considered for treatment with CCBs must be monitored closely for both safety and efficacy of CCBs, because recurrence of disease can occur with resultant deterioration after initial response. Long-acting nifedipine, diltiazem, or amlodipine are typically recommended, and use of verapamil is discouraged because of its potential negative inotropic effects. If a patient fails to improve to FC I or II on CCBs, the patient cannot be considered a chronic responder, and PAH-specific treatment should be implemented.

PAH-SPECIFIC THERAPY: AN OVERVIEW OF COMMERCIALLY AVAILABLE THERAPIES

Although the pathobiology of PAH remains incompletely understood, irrespective of the etiology several common abnormal pathways and molecular imbalances are present. Specifically, deficiencies of the endogenous vasodilators prostacyclin and nitric oxide (NO) and overabundance of the vasoconstrictive peptide endothelin have been identified as key mechanisms. Currently available pharmacotherapy targets these pathways, and is directed at restoring the balance between these factors.[16] **Table 1** summarizes these approved therapies and their side effects, and **Table 2** reviews the pivotal studies that led to drug approval.

Prostacyclin Therapies

Prostacyclin analogues induce vasodilatation, inhibit platelet activation, and demonstrate antiproliferative effects. Currently available therapies all target the prostaglandin I receptor located on endothelial cells within the pulmonary vasculature, and exhibit their effects via a second-messenger system, leading to increased intracellular cyclic adenosine monophosphate.[17] Irrespective of the mode of delivery, these modalities all exert their beneficial effects via this mechanism. A side-effect profile including headaches, flushing, jaw pain, calf pain, and diarrhea is common to all prostacyclins.

Epoprostenol

Intravenous epoprostenol (Flolan) was the first PAH-specific therapy approved by the Food and Drug Administration (FDA), in 1996. The landmark clinical trial randomized 81 patients with FC III or IV advanced IPAH to intravenous epoprostenol plus conventional therapy, versus conventional therapy alone. Despite a relatively short study duration of 12 weeks, the treatment group demonstrated improvement in 6MWD, hemodynamics, and QOL, as well as survival benefit.[18] Eight patients died during the study, all of whom were receiving conventional therapy (P = .003). Additional studies have expanded the benefit of intravenous epoprostenol to patients with systemic sclerosis, and have confirmed symptomatic and hemodynamic benefits.[19] Epoprostenol has also been studied in PAH associated with HIV, congenital heart disease, and portopulmonary hypertension.[20–22] The long-term treatment benefits among IPAH patients were reported from 2 large centers, showing improvements in FC, 6MWD, hemodynamics, and survival (compared with historical or calculated survival data).[23,24]

Intravenous epoprostenol is very effective, and remains the best studied agent in patients with class IV symptoms, but successful implementation requires a highly motivated patient and an experienced medical team. The short half-life (<6 minutes) requires continuous intravenous infusion via a tunneled catheter, and interruptions in therapy, due to pump or catheter malfunctions, can lead to potentially life-threatening hemodynamic compromise. The greatest risk involves catheter-related infections and malfunction, which can cause significant morbidity (0.1–0.6 cases per patient-year).[24] The molecule remains unstable at room temperature, and requires an ice pack. Epoprostenol that is stable at room temperature (Veletri) has been developed and is approved by the FDA. A multicenter registry collecting data regarding its use is being collected, and initial experiences suggest comparable dosing and efficacy to epoprostenol; published data are pending. The drug needs to be started in a closely monitored inpatient setting at 1 to 2 ng/kg/min and is titrated following efficacy and side effects commonly seen with all prostanoids, including headache, flushing, diarrhea, and nausea. Dosing needs to be highly individualized but most experts agree that for most patients, the optimal dose for chronic therapy is between 25 and 40 ng/kg/min. Chronic overdose can lead to high output failure, and it is recommended that patients undergo periodic RHC to ensure optimal dosing.[25]

Treprostinil

Treprostinil (Remodulin) is a prostacyclin analogue with half-life of 4 to 5 hours. Treprostinil can be delivered subcutaneously or intravenously, or be directly inhaled via a specialized hand-held device. Subcutaneous treprostinil was the first modality to receive FDA approval after demonstrating a modest increase in 6MWD during a 12-week, placebo-controlled randomized trial.[26] The major impediment using the subcutaneous delivery mode comes from the pain and erythema at the site of subcutaneous infusion, which was reported in 85% of the patients in the pivotal clinical trial. The site pain deterred proper dose escalation because it was initially believed to be dose related. Long-term experience has demonstrated that site pain is not related to dose and that most patients are able to manage the site discomfort after proper dose titration to alleviate the PAH symptoms. Management by an experienced PH multidisciplinary program, which includes patient support and education on catheter care, are vital to ensure patient compliance. Long-term results have been reported, demonstrating improvements in exercise capacity with survival benefits.[27,28]

To circumvent the limitations posed by subcutaneous mode, treprostinil was studied using an intravenous delivery system in a small study, which demonstrated safety and efficacy.[29] Pharmacokinetic studies confirm equivalent bioavailability of intravenous and subcutaneous delivery.[30] Intravenous treprostinil demonstrated marked functional improvement and a trend toward increased survival benefit in a recently published, randomized, placebo-controlled clinical trial.[31] This study is the

Table 1
Approved PAH treatments and their common side effects

Drug Class	Name, Year Approved	Route/Dose	Side Effects	Comments
Prostanoids	Epoprostenol (Flolan), 1995	Continuous IV Initiate 1–2 ng/kg/min and titrate to efficacy and side effects	Hickman catheter infection and malfunction Side effects related to prostacyclin[a]	Therapy complicated; it is recommended patients be referred to PAH treating centers for initiation and management Effective in patients with severe PAH and RHF Agent most frequently used as rescue therapy Long-term survival data available
	Epoprostenol (Generic), 2008	Reported to be same as Flolan	Reported to be same as Flolan	
	Epoprostenol (Veletri), 2010	Reported to be same as Flolan	Reported to be same as Flolan	
	Treprostinil (Remodulin SC), 2002	Continuous SC Initiate 1.25–2.5 ng/kg/min SC	Injection site pain Side effects related to prostacyclin	Effective for PAH but site pain affects most patients Experienced centers have reported successful outcome in managing patients with site pain issues Long-term survival data available
	Treprostinil (Remodulin IV), 2004	Continuous IV Initiate 1–2 ng/kg/min IV	Hickman catheter infection and malfunction Side effects related to prostacyclin[a] Leg pain	Therapy less complicated to manage than Flolan Need higher dose than Flolan for transitioning patients to achieve similar efficacy Long-term data not yet available
	Iloprost (Ventavis), 2004	Inhaled 6–9 inhalations per day while awake 2.5 and 5.0 µg	Cough, some jaw pain and headache	Selective delivery of prostacyclin to lungs Compliance can be an issue with need for frequent treatments Used as combination treatment with oral therapies

(continued on next page)

Table 1
(*continued*)

Drug Class	Name, Year Approved	Route/Dose	Side Effects	Comments
	Treprostinil (Tyvaso), 2009	Inhaled 4 treatments per day while awake; titrate to 12 puffs per treatment	Cough, jaw pain, headache	Selective delivery of prostacyclin to lungs Used as combination treatment with oral therapies
PDE-5 inhibitors	Sildenafil (Revatio), 2005	Oral 20 mg TID	Epistaxis, headache, flushing, diarrhea	Contraindicated with nitrates Some patients may need up titration of dose
	Tadalafil (Adcirca), 2009	Oral 40 mg daily	Headache, nasal congestion, flushing	Contraindicated with nitrates
ERA	Bosentan (Tracleer), 2001	Oral 62.5 and 125 mg BID	Headache, dizziness, edema	Need LFTs checked monthly Most effective in non–FC-IV patients Contraindicated with cyclosporine and glyburide Decreases effectiveness of oral hormonal contraceptives Long-term observed survival data available
	Ambrisentan (Letairis), 2007	Oral 5 and 10 mg QD	Peripheral edema, nasal congestion, sinusitis	More reported incidence of edema compared with other ERAs Decreases effectiveness of oral hormonal contraceptives

Abbreviations: BID, twice per day; ERA, endothelin receptor antagonists; FC-IV, functional class IV; IV, intravenous; LFTs, liver function tests; PDE-5, phosphodiesterase-5; RHF, right-side heart failure; QD, every day; SC, subcutaneous; TID, three times per day.

[a] Side effects related to prostacyclin: jaw pain, diarrhea, flushing, headache, nausea.

only placebo-controlled one involving intravenous PAH therapy, which raised some ethical concerns regarding placebo-controlled trials in PAH and the designs of future clinical studies.[32] Initial reports involving higher incidence of gram-negative infections in patients receiving intravenous treprostinil resulted in revision in recommendations regarding tunneled catheter care and using epoprostenol diluents.[33,34] Transition from intravenous epoprostenol to intravenous treprostonil have been shown overall to be safe and well tolerated, although the dose of treprostinil is typically higher, ranging from 1.5 to 2 times the original epoprostenol dose.[35] Similar to epoprostenol, maximal doses of intravenous or subcutaneous treprostinil have not been established and are patient dependent; intermittent increases in dose are required to maintain stable functional status. Side effects overall are similar to epoprostenol.

Inhaled treprostinil (Tyvaso) has demonstrated symptomatic and hemodynamic benefit in patients on oral background PAH therapy.[36] The pivotal TRIUMPH study randomized 235 patients on stable oral background therapy with either sildenafil or bosentan. The study demonstrated an increase in 6MWD at 12 weeks of 20 m, but no improvements in secondary end points, including time to clinical worsening, Borg dyspnea score, New York Heart Association FC. This drug is dosed 4 times daily via a special inhalation device. Two-year outcomes from an open-label extension of the TRIUMPH study have been published, demonstrating maintenance of 6MWD improvement and clinical stability, with two-thirds of patients not experiencing any clinical worsening.[37]

Iloprost

Iloprost is a prostacyclin analogue that is available as an inhaled therapy in the United States. A randomized controlled study of iloprost versus placebo in 207 patients with FC III and IV symptoms from PAH and CTEPH were enrolled in a 12-week study, demonstrating improvements in 6MWD, FC, and hemodynamics.[38] The study used a novel composite primary end point of absence of deterioration, improvement in FC, and greater than 10% improvement in 6MWT, which was met by 16% of the active treatment group and 4.9% of the placebo group (P = .007). Although generally well tolerated, a frequent dosing schedule (recommended 6–9 treatments while awake) coupled with a specialized delivery device requiring meticulous care affect patient compliance and feasibility. The REVEAL registry data demonstrate that inhaled iloprost is almost always used in combination with oral PAH treatments, with dosing frequency ranging from 4 to 6 times a day.[39] The availability of the 20-µg disk has significantly shortened treatment times (approximately 5 minutes per session). Longer-term outcome reports with iloprost monotherapy have been conflicting.[40,41] The iloprost inhalation device uses a novel technology that allows electronic transmission of daily dosing and treatment times, providing the physician with additional tools to identify and correct barriers to drug compliance. Common side effects include cough, headache, flushing, and jaw pain.

Phosphodiesterase Inhibitors

NO is released by the vascular endothelium, and results in pulmonary arterial vasodilatation mediated by increased production of cyclic guanosine monophosphate (cGMP). NO production is reduced in PAH owing to decreased expression of the enzyme NO synthase.[42] Phosphodiesterase type 5 (PDE-5) is abundant in the pulmonary vasculature, and its inhibitors prevent degradation of cGMP, thereby enhancing the downstream effects of NO. Side effects of PDE-5 inhibitors include headaches, flushing, and epistaxis, and concomitant nitrate therapy is absolutely contraindicated.

Sildenafil

Sildenafil (Revatio) was studied among 278 patients with IPAH or APAH in a 12-week prospective, placebo-controlled, randomized clinical trial (SUPER-1).[43] Treatment resulted in similar improvements in 6MWD among the 3 doses studied (45, 46, and 50 m for 20, 40, and 80 mg, respectively). Sildenafil is approved by the FDA to improve exercise ability at a dose of 20 mg 3 times daily. All treatment doses improved hemodynamics and FC. Of note, sildenafil treatment did not affect clinical worsening. Cessation of therapy in previously stable patients may lead to functional deteration.[44]

Patients completing the SUPER-1 study were eligible to enroll in an open-label long-term extension study investigating the 80-mg thrice-daily dose.[45] Results of this study were recently published and demonstrated that at 3 years, the majority of patients maintained functional status and approximately half of the patients improved or maintained their 6MWD. Some of the reported side effects include headache and epistaxis, although the drug was well tolerated overall. Reports regarding visual disturbances have raised some concerns, especially among diabetics and patients with cardiovascular risk factors. Sildenafil use is absolutely contraindicated with concomitant nitrate administration because of the risk of precipitating hypotension.

Tadalafil

Tadalafil (Adcirca) was studied in a 16-week placebo-controlled trial among 392 PAH patients (PHIRST).[46] The treated groups received doses of 2.5, 10, 20, and 40 mg. Tadalafil increased 6MWD in a dose-dependent manner, and treatment with 40 mg resulted in a statistically significant increase in 6MWD. Furthermore, the 40-mg dose group demonstrated improvement in the time to clinical worsening. Approximately half of the patients enrolled were on background therapy with bosentan, and this group of patients had a lower (23 m vs 44 m), but statistically significant, improvement in placebo-subtracted 6MWD. Tadalafil is approved by the FDA to improve exercise capacity at a dose of 40 mg once daily. Frequently encountered side effects included headache, myalgias, and flushing.

Endothelin Receptor Antagonists

Endothelin (ET-1) is overexpressed in various forms of pulmonary vascular disease. In PAH the plasma level of ET-1 is increased, and its level has been shown to be inversely proportional to the magnitude of the pulmonary blood flow and cardiac output.[42,47,48] The biological effects of endothelin are mediated by 2 receptors, ET_A (located on smooth muscle cells) and ET_B is located on

Table 2
Summary of pivotal clinical trials in pulmonary arterial hypertension

Drug Studied	Year Published	No. of Patients	Duration of Study (wk)	FC of Patients	Group of PAH Patients	Background Therapy	Primary End Point 6MWD Improvement	Comments
Epoprostenol[48]	1996	81	12	III/IV	IPAH	No	47 m (placebo corrected)	Only PAH trial demonstrating survival benefit
Epoprostenol[49]	2000	111	12	III/IV	PAH associated with scleroderma	No	108 m (placebo corrected)	Resulted in expansion of approved indication for epoprostenol to include CTD patients
Treprostinil SC[55]	2002	470	12	II/III/IV	IPAH, CTD, CHD	No	16 m (median; all in treatment group; unchanged in placebo)	Increase in 6MWD correlated with dose; patients underdosed due to site pain development
Bosentan[64] (BREATHE-1)	2002	213	16	III/IV	IPAH, CTD	No	44 m (placebo corrected)	Fist study to assess composite end point of time to clinical worsening
Iloprost[62] (AIR Study)	2002	203	12	III/IV	IPAH, CTD, appetite suppressants, CTEPH	No	36 m (placebo corrected)	Novel composite end point used as primary end point

Sildenafil (SUPER-1)	2005	278	12	II/III	IPAH, CTD, CHD	No	45 m (placebo corrected)	Did not meet delay in time to clinical worsening
Ambrisentan (ARIES 1 and 2)	2008	202 192	12	II/III	IPAH, CTD, appetite suppressants, HIV	No	31 m (5 mg) and 51 m (10 mg) for ARIES-1 32 m (2.5 mg) and 59 m (5 mg) for ARIES-2	Delayed time to clinical worsening for both ARIES trials
Tadalafil (PHIRST)	2009	405	16	II/III	IPAH, CTD, CHD, appetite suppressants	~50% on bosentan	33 m (placebo corrected)	40-mg group met the prespecified level of statistical significance
Treprostinil inhaled[61] (Triumph-1)	2010	235	12	III/IV	IPAH and all APAH	Yes	19 m (median)	Studied only as add-on combination therapy; improves QOL, but no impact on clinical worsening or functional class

Abbreviations: 6MWD, 6-minute walking distance; APAH, associated pulmonary arterial hypertension; CTD, connective tissue disease; CHD, congenital heart disease; CTEPH, chronic thromboembolic pulmonary hypertension; HIV, human immunodeficiency virus; IPAH, idiopathic pulmonary arterial hypertension; QOL, quality of life.

endothelial cells.[49] Activation of the ET_A and ET_B receptors on smooth muscle cells induces vasoconstriction, cellular proliferation, and hypertrophy. By contrast, stimulation of ET_B receptors on endothelial cells results in production of vasodilators and is involved in the clearance of ET-1 from the circulatory system.[49] The clinical significance of endothelin specificity in PAH is unclear. Murine data have suggested a theoretical benefit to selective ET_A blockade, but this has not translated clinically.[50,51]

Bosentan

Bosentan (Tracleer), a dual ET_A and ET_B receptor blocker, was the first oral PAH-specific therapy to be approved for PAH. The pivotal, randomized, placebo-controlled BREATHE-1 study conducted in 213 patients with FC-III to FC-IV PAH demonstrated improvements in exercise capacity and FC associated with bosentan therapy.[52] The BREATHE study was the first to report the time to clinical worsening as a secondary end point, a combined morbidity and mortality end point defined as time to death, lung transplantation, hospitalization for PH, lack of clinical improvement or worsening leading to discontinuation, need for epoprostenol therapy, or atrial septostomy. The time to clinical worsening was delayed by bosentan in comparison with placebo ($P = .0015$). In addition to IPAH, bosentan has been studied in APAH, specifically Eisenmenger syndrome and HIV, with functional improvements noted in these populations.[53,54] A randomized study that focused solely on FC II patients showed that 6 months of bosentan therapy was associated with hemodynamic improvements and a significant reduction in clinical worsening, which expanded the indications for this therapy.[55] Long-term observational findings of patients treated with bosentan as first-line therapy have shown improved survival compared with historical controls.[56]

The primary safety issue in using bosentan involves its effect on the hepatic function, because it is primarily metabolized through the P450 enzyme systems. Bosentan therapy requires monthly monitoring of liver function tests, as transaminase elevation, which is dose dependent and reversible, occurs in up to 10% to 12% of patients.[52] Hemoglobin should be checked every 3 months because bosentan therapy has been associated with anemia. The other side effect is edema, which can be transient to requiring diuretic treatments in some patients. Other side effects include headaches, flushing, and dizziness. Bosentan is teratogenic and may decrease the efficacy of hormonal contraception, so women of child-bearing age must be counseled to use dual contraception methods for birth control. Hormonal birth control may be less effective, and barrier contraception is advised. Glyburide and cyclosporine A are contraindicated with bosentan because of significant interaction and the potential for significant liver damage. There is no significant interaction between warfarin and bosentan.

Ambrisentan

Ambrisentan (Letaris) is a selective ET_A antagonist, approved by the FDA in 2007 for the treatment of mild to moderately symptomatic PAH.[57] The pivotal clinical trials, ARIES-1 and ARIES-2 conducted in the United States and Europe/South America, respectively, enrolled approximately 400 patients in a placebo-controlled 12-week study, which demonstrated that ambrisentan significantly improved 6MWD and delayed clinical worsening and improvement in FC. Two-year open-label extension results from the ARIES clinical studies were recently published, showing that improvements in exercise capacity and FC were sustained, with a low risk of clinical worsening.[58] Ambrisentan is approved to improve exercise capacity and delay clinical worsening at a dose of 5 or 10 mg daily.

Ambrisentan has fewer drug interactions than bosentan. When approved, the FDA required monthly liver function test monitoring; however, given reported safety with postmarketing experience, this monitoring requirement has now been removed although most centers perform scheduled intermittent laboratory monitoring. Ambrisentan is teratogenic; monthly pregnancy monitoring is required, and women of child-bearing potential must use adequate contraception. Similar recommendations regarding monitoring of hemoglobin is recommended, because its use is also associated with a decrease in hemoglobin. Edema is common, particularly in the elderly, and may require diuretic dosing adjustments. Nasopharyngitis is often encountered with this therapy.

GOALS OF TREATMENT

Although the primary end point of the pivotal clinical trials focused on improvement in 6MWD as the primary end point, successful therapy requires much more than symptomatic improvement. Therapeutic goals deserving consideration include increasing functional capacity, mitigating disease progression, reducing hospitalizations, and improving QOL and survival (**Table 3**).

Are these goals being achieved? Although the outcome for PAH patients has unequivocally improved with current therapies, the majority of patients enrolled in clinical trials failed to improve their FC by one grade, and approximately one-third to one-half failed to achieve a 6MWD greater

Table 3	
Treatment goals in PAH	
Objective Assessments	**Goals of Therapy**
WHO functional class	I or II
6MWD	>380 m; stable to increasing
Hemodynamics	RAP <10 mm Hg and CI >2.5 L/min/m^2
BNP	Normal to near normal; decreasing

Abbreviations: BNP, brain natriuretic peptide; CI, cardiac index; 6MWD, 6-minute walk distance; RAP, right atrial pressure; WHO, World Health Organization.

than 380 m, a distance that has been shown to correlate with improved outcome. Although disagreements may exist regarding optimal goals of therapy, it is clear that multiple parameters must be monitored for each patient and be incorporated into a global risk assessment, and focusing solely on FC or hemodynamic parameters is most likely inadequate.

CHOOSING THE INITIAL THERAPY

The authors support the American College of Cardiology/American Heart Association consensus treatment recommendations (**Fig. 2**). Patients with IPAH and select patients with APAH without clinical evidence of RV failure should undergo acute vasoreactivity testing at the time of RHC. Responders should be treated with a CCB and be carefully monitored for clinical deterioration. For most patients who are nonresponders, a careful categorization of patient FC and thorough risk assessment is required, comprising integration of hemodynamic, biomarker, imaging, and patient clinical data (**Table 4**). For those patients who do not respond to vasodilator testing, or those who progress in FC despite CCB therapy and are categorized as FC II to FC III, initiation with an oral therapy, either a PDE-5 inhibitor or an endothelin receptor antagonist (ERA), is recommended.[5]

It is important to recognize that no head-to-head studies have been performed comparing either classes of oral drugs or specific drugs within each class. In addition, none of the pivotal trials for these agents have looked at end points of morbidity or mortality, and no oral drugs have

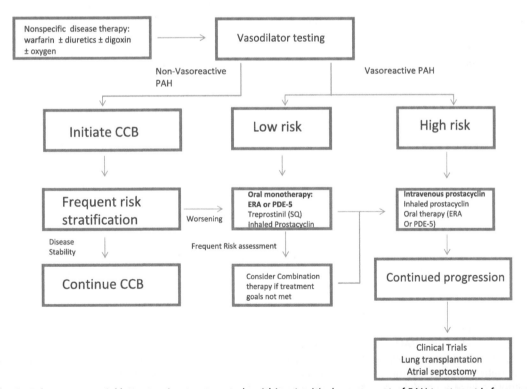

Fig. 2. Pulmonary arterial hypertension treatment algorithim. A critical component of PAH treatment is frequent re-assessment for clinical worsening, which may prompt therapeutic modifications. (*From* McLaughlin VV, Archer SL, Badesch DB, et al. ACCF/AHA expert consensus document on pulmonary hypertension. J Am Coll Cardiol 2009;53:1573–619; with permission.)

Table 4
Clinical features used for risk assessment in PAH

Clinical Feature	Low Risk	High Risk
Disease Progression	Slow	Rapid
WHO functional class	I, II, III	IV
6MWD	>380 m	<330 m
BNP	Near normal, Decreasing	Persistently elevated/increasing
Hemodynamics	Low RA pressure, normal cardiac index	Elevated RA pressure, low cardiac index
Imaging	Near normal RV size/function	Abnormal RV size/function, pericardial effusion

Abbreviations: RA, right atrium; RV, right ventricle.
Data from McLaughlin VV, McGoon MD. Pulmonary arterial hypertension. Circulation 2006;114:1417–31.

been prospectively studied to improve survival. Consequently, the decision to choose a specific ERA or specific PDE-5 inhibitor should be focused on patient side-effect profile, perceived compliance with therapy, and provider experience. For example, those patients with preexisting lower extremity edema or higher filling pressures at the time of RHC may have worsening symptoms with an ERA, or may have a higher likelihood of maintaining therapy with a PDE-5 inhibitor. Alternatively, in those patients with compensated PAH or those with headaches and comorbid conditions requiring intermittent nitrate use, an ERA should be considered.

Patients with FC-IV symptoms are best treated with intravenous prostacyclin therapy, and for patients who progress to worsening RV failure, escalation of therapy to prostacyclin deserves consideration.

COMMON DILEMMAS IN THE TREATMENT OF PAH

Should Patients with FC-I Symptoms Receive PAH Pharmacotherapy?

Initial studies of PAH patients included only those with FC-III to FC-IV symptoms. Later studies expanded enrollment to those with FC-II symptoms, and found significant improvement in exercise capacity and reductions in clinical worsenimg.[43,55,57] At present, no studies have enrolled significant numbers patients with FC-I symptoms. However, PAH is a progressive, incurable, chronic disease. Despite the lack of clinical trial data, even in asymptomatic patients, the authors advise a careful risk assessment, and in patients who manifest some markers of increased risk, even in the absence of subjective symptoms, initiation of oral therapy is advocated. If a more conservative watch-and-wait approach is chosen, careful follow-up is mandatory. Regardless of the chosen strategy, the patient must be carefully counseled regarding risks and benefits of either approach.

For Patients Who Progress on Oral Monotherapy, Should Add-On Continuous-Infusion Prostacyclin Therapy be Prescribed, or Combination Oral/Inhaled Therapy?

As in many chronic conditions such as systemic hypertension and diabetes, monotherapy is often inadequate in achieving desired end points, and a combination of drugs exerting desirable benefits targeting different pathways is used. Studies of combination therapy are limited to variable end points, entry criteria, and randomization (**Table 5**). In addition, suitable end points for "successful" PAH therapy, such as for other chronic diseases such as hyperlipidemia, diabetes, or systemic hypertension, have yet to be defined. Clearly the ideal patient would be one who maintains a 6MWD greater than 400 m, exhibits normalization of brain natriuretic peptide levels, and good hemodynamics; such a patient would be considered "at goal," and would not require escalation of therapy. Patients who have 1 or 2 of these features, but not all of them, may be considered at increased risk and require additional therapy, or a change in therapy to continuous-infusion prostacyclins.

The largest study of combination therapy assessed high-dose sildenafil therapy (80 mg 3 times daily) added to background epoprostenol therapy, and showed a significant increase in 6MWD and hemodynamic improvement.[59] Smaller studies, such as the STEP study, suggested safety and hemodynamic improvement with addition of inhaled iloprost to bosentan treatment, with a trend

Table 5
Combination therapy studies in pulmonary arterial hypertension

	Baseline Therapy	Add-On Therapy	No. of Patients	Study Duration	End Point	Completed?	Results
AMBITION	Ambrisentan vs tadalafil vs combination	Other therapy	300	Event driven	Morbidity/mortality	No	
COMPASS 2	Sildenafil	Bosentan	250	Eventdriven	Morbidity/mortality	No	
COMPASS 1[65]	Bosentan	Sildenafil	45	Single dose	PVR	Yes	Significant reduction in PVR
ATHENA	Sildenafil or tadalafil	Ambrisentan	40	24 wk	PVR	Yes	Improved hemodynamics; publication pending
PACES[59]	Epoprostenol	Sildenafil	267	16 wk	6MWD	Yes	28 m improvement in 6MWD
STEP[60]	Bosentan	Iloprost	67	12 wk	Safety; 6MWD	Yes	Improved FC; trend toward improved 6MWD
BREATHE-2[63]	Intravenous epoprostenol	Bosentan	33	16 wk	6MWD	Yes	No improvement with simultaneous bosentan initiation

Abbreviations: FC, functional class; PVR, pulmonary vascular resistance.

Table 6
Newer therapy studies in pulmonary arterial hypertension

	Baseline Therapy	Add-On Therapy	No. of Patients	Study Duration	End Point	Completed?	Results
IMPRES	≥2 current therapies	Imatinib	200	24 wk	6MWD	Yes	Improved 6MWD; publication pending
GRIPHON	ERA, PDE-5, or both	Selexipag	670	Event driven	Morbidity/mortality	No	
SERAPHIN	Naïve/PDE-5 or prostacyclin	Macitentan	742	Event driven	Morbidity/mortality	No	Enrollment complete, results pending
FREEDOM-C	Bosentan and/or sildenafil	Oral treprostinil	300	16 wk	6MWD	Yes	Not significant; publication pending
PATENT	Naïve/ERA/PDE-5	Riociguat	462	16 wk	6MWD	No	

toward improvement in 6MWD.[60] Many studies are of small nature, but limited data have suggested symptomatic and hemodynamic benefit with the addition of sildenafil to background iloprost, with a mean 6MWD improvement of 93 m.[61] Several smaller studies have demonstrated safety and clinical benefits with the addition of sildenafil to bosentan monotherapy.[62] Multiple combination therapy studies are nearing completion or have recently been completed, and it is hoped that additional data will become available to answer these questions (see **Table 5**). The ongoing COMPASS-2 (Effect of combination of bosentan and sildenafil vs sildenafil monotherapy on morbidity and mortality in symptomatic patients with PAH-2) is randomizing symptomatic PAH patients on background sildenafil to bosentan or placebo, and assessing the time to the first morbidity/mortality event. This study will provide critical information in understanding the progression of disease on oral monotherapy versus combination therapy.

For patients who do not achieve the desired treatment goals but have not yet developed overt RV failure, the authors favor combination oral therapy or combination oral/inhaled therapy. However, for higher-risk patients continuous-infusion prostacyclin therapy is advised. For those patients who continue to deteriorate on therapy, lung transplantation or atrial septostomy should be considered. Multiple studies of combination pharmacotherapy are currently under way that will hopefully provide answers to these questions.

Should Upfront Combination Therapy be Considered in Higher-Risk Patients?

Despite tremendous progress over the past decade, a large number of patients still progress on monotherapy or fail to respond altogether. For patients with marked abnormalities in functional status, it could be predicted up front that monotherapy may not be sufficient in achieving desired 6MWD and other treatment goals. Given the progressive nature of the disease, it could be hypothesized that in the 12 to 16 weeks that a patient is on monotherapy there may be subtle, but irreversible, clinical worsening. Only the BREATHE-2 study investigated upfront addition of bosentan or placebo to patients started on epoprostenol, and no significant differences were seen in 6MWD, although a trend to reduction in pulmonary vascular resistance was seen in the combination-therapy group.[63] The current AMBITION study, conducting upfront therapy with PDE-5 versus ERA versus the combination of both drugs, should shed light on this question. Given the costs and uncertainties with this approach, the authors cannot at this time recommend upfront combination therapy.

FUTURE THERAPIES FOR PAH

Between 2001 and 2009 a therapeutic explosion occurred in the treatment of PAH, as 8 therapies were approved for PAH therapy. Unfortunately, no new drugs have gained approval over the past 3 years. Several factors may account for this current drought in drug development. It is evident from combination-therapy studies that although a benefit exists in combination PAH therapy, the symptomatic benefit of 2 drugs, as measured by 6MWD, is less than the sum of the individual benefit of each drug. Because placebo-controlled studies are no longer ethical in PAH, and an increasing number of studies permit 1 or 2 drugs at baseline, it is more difficult to show a benefit with therapy. In addition, similar to experience with chronic heart failure, a ceiling effect may exist to therapies targeting current pathways.

Current research focuses on drugs targeting conventional pathways as well as novel pathways (**Table 6**). Four therapies focusing on current pathways are under investigation. Macitentan is a tissue specific, dual endothelin receptor antagonist; selexipag is an oral prostacyclin receptor agonist; riociguat is a soluble guanylate cyclase stimulator (NO pathway); and treprostinil is an oral prostacyclin analogue. Therapies targeting alternative pathways include the tyrosine kinase inhibitor imatinib, which has shown promise in highly symptomatic and advanced PAH.

SUMMARY

A recent meta-analysis of 21 randomized controlled trials involving 3140 PAH patients between 1990 and 2008 found a 43% reduction in mortality and 61% reduction in hospitalizations following therapy with PAH-specific agents in comparison with placebo.[64] Contemporary PAH pharmacotherapy has clearly altered the trajectory of this rapidly progressive disease. Despite this tremendous progress, morbidity and mortality remain unacceptably high, and all current therapies suffer from inherent limitations. Additional studies are required to define optimal end points for study treatment, to guide combination-therapy decisions, and to identify alternative treatment pathways.

REFERENCES

1. Dresdale DT, Schultz M, Michtom RJ. Primary pulmonary hypertension: a clinical and hemodynamic study. Am J Med 1951;11:686–705.

2. D'Alonzon GG, Barst RJ, Ayres SM, et al. Survival in patients with primary pulmonary hypertension: results from a national prospective registry. Ann Intern Med 1991;115:343–9.

3. Rich S, Kaugmann E, Levy PS. The effect of high dose calcium-channel blockers on survival in primary pulmonary hypertension. N Engl J Med 1992;327:76–81.

4. Mereles D, Ehlken N, Kreuscher S, et al. Exercise and respiratory training improve exercise capacity and quality of life in patients with severe chronic pulmonary hypertension. Circulation 2006;114:1482–9.

5. McLaughlin VV, Archer SL, Badesch DB, et al. ACCF/AHA expert consensus document on pulmonary hypertension. J Am Coll Cardiol 2009;53: 1573–619.

6. Weiss BM, Zemp L, Seifert B, et al. Outcome of pulmonary vascular disease in pregnancy: a systematic overview from 1978 through 1996. J Am Coll Cardiol 1998;31:1650–7.

7. Badesch DB, Abman SH, Simmonneau G, et al. Medical therapy for pulmonary arterial hypertension: updated ACCP evidence-based clinical practice guidelines. Chest 2007;131:1917–28.

8. Fogel MR, Sawhney VK, Neal EA, et al. Diuresis in the ascitic patient: a randomized controlled trial of three regimens. J Clin Gastroenterol 1981;3(Suppl 1): 73–80.

9. Available at: http://www.amiservices.com/documents/ Oxygen.doc. Accessed February 21, 2011.

10. Fuster V, Steele PM, Edwards WD, et al. Primary pulmonary hypertension: natural history and the importance of thrombosis. Circulation 1984;70:580–7.

11. Bjornsson J, Edwards WD. Primary pulmonary hypertension: a histopathological study of 80 cases. Mayo Clin Proc 1985;60:16–25.

12. Huber K, Beckmann R, Frank H, et al. Fibrinogen, t-PA, and PAI-1 plasma levels in patients with pulmonary hypertension. Am J Respir Crit Care Med 1994; 150:929–33.

13. Frank H, Mlczoch J, Huber K, et al. The effect of anticoagulant therapy in primary and anorectic drug-induced pulmonary hypertension. Chest 1997;112: 714–21.

14. Rich S, Seidlitz M, Dodlin E, et al. The short term effects of digoxin in patients with right ventricular dysfunction from pulmonary hypertension. Chest 1998;114:787–92.

15. Sitbon O, Humbert M, Jais X, et al. Long-term response to calcium channel blockers in idiopathic pulmonary arterial hypertension. Circulation 2005; 111:3105–11.

16. Farber JW, Loscalzo J. Pulmonary arterial hypertension. N Engl J Med 2004;351:1655–65.

17. Gomberg-Maitland M, Olschewski H. Prostacyclin therapies for the treatment of pulmonary arterial hypertension. Eur Respir J 2008;31:891–901.

18. Barst RJ, Rubin LJ, Long WA, et al. A comparison of continuous intravenous epoprostenol with conventional therapy for primary pulmonary hypertension. The Primary Pulmonary Hypertension Study Group. N Engl J Med 1996;334:296–302.

19. Badesch DB, Tapson VF, McGoon MD, et al. Continuous intravenous epoprostenol for pulmonary hypertension due to the scleroderma spectrum of disease: a randomized, controlled trial. Ann Intern Med 2000;132:425–34.

20. Aguilar RV, Farber HW. Epoprostenol (prostacyclin) therapy in HIV-associated pulmonary hypertension. Am J Respir Crit Care Med 2000;162:1846–50.

21. Rosenzweig EB, Kerstein D, Barst RJ, et al. Long-term prostacyclin for pulmonary hypertension with associated congenital heart defects. Circulation 1999;99:1858–65.

22. Kuo PC, Johnson LB, Plotkin JS, et al. Continuous intravenous infusion of epoprostenol for the treatment of portopulmonary hypertension. Transplantation 1997;63:604–6.

23. Sitbon O, Humbert M, Nunes H, et al. Long-term intravenous epoprostenol infusion in primary pulmonary hypertension: prognostic factors and survival. J Am Coll Cardiol 2002;40:780–8.

24. McLaughlin VV, Shillington A, Rich S. Survival in primary pulmonary hypertension: the impact of epoprostenol therapy. Circulation 2002;106:1477–82.

25. Rich S, McLaughlin VV. Effects of chronic prostacyclin therapy on cardiac output and symptoms in primary pulmonary hypertension. J Am Coll Cardiol 1999;34:1184–7.

26. Simonneau G, Barst RJ, Galie N, et al. Continuous subcutaneous infusion of Treprostinil, a prostacyclin analogue, in patients with pulmonary arterial hypertension: a double-blind, randomized, placebo-controlled trial. Am J Respir Crit Care Med 2002; 165:800–4.

27. Lang I, Gomez-Sanchez M, Kneussl M, et al. Efficacy of long term subcutaneous treprostinil sodium therapy in pulmonary hypertension. Chest 2006; 129:1636–43.

28. Barst RJ, Galie N, Naeije R, et al. Long-term outcome in pulmonary arterial hypertension patients treated with subcutaneous treprostinil. Eur Respir J 2006;28:1195–203.

29. Tapson VF, Gombert-Maitland M, McLaughlin VV, et al. Safety and efficacy of IV Treprostinil for pulmonary arterial hypertension: a prospective, multicenter, open-labeled 12 week trial. Chest 2006; 129:683–8.

30. Laliberte K, Arneson C, Jeffs R, et al. Pharmacokinetics and steady-state bioequivalence of treprostinil sodium (Remodulin) administered by the intravenous and subcutaneous route to normal volunteers. J Cardiovasc Pharmacol 2004;44(2): 209–14.

31. Hiremath J, Thanikachalam S, Parikh K, et al. Exercise improvement and plasma biomarker changes with intravenous treprostinil therapy for pulmonary arterial hypertension: a placebo-controlled trial. J Heart Lung Transplant 2010;29:137–49.

32. Park MH, Rubin LJ. The globalization of clinical trials in pulmonary arterial hypertension. J Heart Lung Transplant 2010;29:157–8.

33. Centers for Disease Control and Prevention. Bloodstream infections among patients treated with intravenous epoprostenol or intravenous treprostinil for pulmonary arterial hypertension-seven sites, United States, 2003-2006. MMWR Morb Mortal Wkly Rep 2007;56:170–2.

34. Doran A, Ivy D, Barst RJ, et al. Guidelines for the prevention of central venous catheter-related bloodstream infections with prostanoid therapy for pulmonary arterial hypertension. Adv Pulm Hypertens 2008;7:245–8.

35. Gomberg-Maitland M, Tapson VF, Benza RL, et al. Transition from intravenous epoprostenol to intravenous Treprostinil in pulmonary hypertension. Am J Respir Crit Care Med 2005;172:1586–9.

36. Mclaughlin VV, Benza RL, Rubin LJ, et al. Addition of inhaled treprostinil to oral therapy for pulmonary arterial hypertension: a randomized controlled clinical trial. J Am Coll Cardiol 2010; 55:1915–22.

37. Benza RL, Weeger W, McLaughlin VV, et al. Long term effects of inhaled treprostinil in patients with pulmonary arterial hypertension. The TReprostinil sodium Inhalation Use in the Management of Pulmonary arterial Hypertension (TRIUMPH) study open-label extension. J Heart Lung Transplant 2011; 30(12):1327–33.

38. Olschewski H, Simonneau G, Galie N, et al. Inhaled iloprost for severe pulmonary hypertension. N Engl J Med 2002;347:322–9.

39. Badesch DB, Raskob GE, Elliot G, et al. Pulmonary arterial hypertension: Baseline characteristics from the REVEAL Registry. Chest 2010;137(2):376–87.

40. Hoeper MM, Shwartz M, Ehlerding S, et al. Long-term treatment of primary pulmonary hypertension with aerolized iloprost, a prostacyclin analogue. N Engl J Med 2000;342:1866–70.

41. Opitz CF, Wensel R, Winkler J, et al. Clinical efficacy and survival with first-line inhaled iloprost therapy in patients with idiopathic pulmonary arterial hypertension. Eur Heart J 2005;26:1895–902.

42. Gaid A, Saleh D. Reduced expression of endothelial nitric oxide synthase in the lungs of patients with pulmonary hypertension. N Engl J Med 1995;333: 214–21.

43. Galie N, Ghofrani HA, Torbicki A, et al. Sildenafil Use in Pulmonary arterial hypERtension (SUPER) Study Group. Sildenafil citrate therapy for pulmonary arterial hypertension. N Engl J Med 2005;353:2148–57.

44. Keogh AM, Jabbour A, Hayward CS, et al. Clinical deterioration after sildenafil cessation in patients with pulmonary hypertension. Vasc Health Risk Manag 2008;4:1111–3.

45. Rubin LJ, Badesch DB, Fleming TR, et al. Long term treatment with sildenafil citrate in pulmonary arterial hypertension. The SUPER-2 Study. Chest 2011; 140(5):1274–83.

46. Galie N, Brundage BH, Ghofrani HA, et al. Tadalafil therapy for pulmonary arterial hypertension. Circulation 2009;119:2894–903.

47. Giad A, Yanagisawa M, Langleben D, et al. Expression of endothelin-1 in the lungs of patients with pulmonary hypertension. N Engl J Med 1993;328: 1732–9.

48. Vincent JA, Ross RD, Kassab J, et al. Relation of elevated plasma endothelin in congenital heart disease to increased pulmonary blood flow. Am J Cardiol 1993;71:1204–7.

49. Ogawa Y, Nakao K, Arai H, et al. Molecular cloning of a non-isopeptide-selective human endothelin receptor. Biochem Biophys Res Commun 1991; 178:248–55.

50. Nishida M, Eshiro K, Oada Y, et al. Roles of endothelin ETA and ETB receptors in the pathogenesis of monocrotaline-induced pulmonary hypertension in rats. J Cardiovasc Pharmacol 2004;44:187–91.

51. Dupuis J, Hoeper MM. Endothelin receptor antagonists in pulmonary arterial hypertension. Eur Respir J 2008;31:407–15.

52. Rubin LJ, Badesch DB, Barst RJ, et al. Bosentan therapy for pulmonary arterial hypertension. N Engl J Med 2002;346:896–903.

53. Galie N, Beghetti M, Gatzoulis MA, et al. Bosentan therapy in patients with Eisenmenger syndrome. A multicenter, double-blind, randomized, placebo-controlled study. Circulation 2006;114:48–54.

54. Degano B, Yaici A, Le Pavec J, et al. Long-term effects of bosentan in patients with HIV associated pulmonary arterial hypertension. Eur Respir J 2009;33:92–8.

55. Galie N, Rubin LJ, Hoeper MM, et al. Treatment of patients with mildly symptomatic pulmonary arterial hypertension with bosentan (EARLY study): a double-blind, randomized controlled trial. Lancet 2008;317:2093–100.

56. Mclaughlin VV, Sitbon O, Badesch DB, et al. Survival with first-line bosentan in patients with primary pulmonary hypertension. Eur Respir J 2005;25:244–9.

57. Galie N, Olschewski H, Oudiz R, et al. Ambrisentan for the treatment of pulmonary arterial hypertension. Results of the ambrisentan in pulmonary arterial hypertension, randomized, double-blind, placebo-controlled multicenter efficacy (ARIES) study 1 and study 2. Circulation 2008;117:3010–9.

58. Oudiz R, Galie N, Olschewski H, et al. Long-term ambrisentan therapy for the treatment of pulmonary

arterial hypertension. J Am Coll Cardiol 2009;54(21): 1971–81.

59. Simonneau G, Rubin LJ, Galie N, et al. Addition of sildenafil to long term intravenous epoprostenol therapy in patients with pulmonary arterial hypertension. Ann Intern Med 2008;149:521–30.

60. McLaughlin VV, Oudiz RJ, Frost A, et al. Randomized study of adding inhaled iloprost to existing bosentan in pulmonary arterial hypertension. Am J Respir Crit Care Med 2006;174:1257–63.

61. Ghofrani HA, Rose F, Schermuly RT, et al. Oral sildenafil as long term adjunct therapy to inhaled iloprost in severe pulmonary arterial hypertension. J Am Coll Cardiol 2003;42:158–64.

62. Mathai SC, Girgis RE, Fisher MR, et al. Addition of sildenafil to bosentan monotherapy in pulmonary arterial hypertension. Eur Respir J 2007;29:469–75.

63. Humbert M, Barst RJ, Robbins IM, et al. Combination of bosentan with epoprostenol in pulmonary arterial hypertension. BREATHE-2. Eur Respir J 2004;24:353–9.

64. Galie N, Manes A, Negro L, et al. A meta-analysis of randomized controlled trials in pulmonary arterial hypertension. Eur Heart J 2009;30:394–403.

65. Gruenig E, Michelakis E, Vachiery Jean-Luc, et al. Acute hemodyamic effects of sildenafil when added to established bosentan therapy in patients with pulmonary arterial hypertension: results of the COMPASS-1 Study. J Clin Pharm 2009;49:1343–52.

Right Ventricular Remodeling in Pulmonary Hypertension

Veronica Franco, MD, MSPH

KEYWORDS

- Heart failure • Right ventricle • Pulmonary hypertension • Right-sided heart failure
- B-type natriuretic peptide • Echocardiography

KEY POINTS

- Right ventricular (RV) function determines the symptoms and survival of patients with pulmonary arterial hypertension (PAH).
- High pressure in the right atrium is a key marker of acute RV failure. It is one of the most important factors of poor long-term outcomes (and higher mortality) in patients with PAH and heart failure with depressed left ventricular (LV) ejection fraction.
- Cardiac magnetic resonance imaging has several advantages over echocardiography and is considered the gold standard for imaging the right side of the heart.
- The RV function is currently understudied. Clinical trials and guidelines in the management of this disease do not include RV function and pulmonary hemodynamics as end points or determinants of escalation of therapy.
- At present, lowering pulmonary pressure via vasodilation and antiproliferative properties is the therapy for pulmonary hypertension. Unlike LV dysfunction, there is no standard of care directly targeting the RV.

INTRODUCTION

The right ventricle (RV) is in charge of pumping blood to the lungs for oxygenation. Its role is restricted to a single organ and generally is not associated with systemic vascular diseases.[1] Historically the RV has been considered a mere bystander, a victim of processes affecting the cardiovascular system, and its function has been largely understudied. Consequently, in comparison with the left ventricle (LV), little attention has been devoted to how RV dysfunction may be best detected and measured, what specific molecular mechanisms maintain a failing RV, how RV dysfunction evolves, or what interventions might best preserve RV function. Nevertheless, recent studies have shown that RV function should be recognized as an important contributor and prognostic indicator of cardiopulmonary diseases,

such as pulmonary hypertension and advanced heart failure.[2,3] This chamber, at times termed the forgotten ventricle, is no longer considered an unnecessary part of the normal circulation or regarded as a passive conduit. High pressure in the right atrium (RA), a key marker of RV failure, is considered one of the most important factors of worse outcomes in pulmonary hypertension and after implantation of an LV assist device and cardiac transplantation.

THE NORMAL RV

The RV pumps the same stroke volume as the LV but with approximately 25% of the stroke work because of low resistance in the pulmonary vasculature.[1] Thus the right side of the heart is less muscular than the left side. The LV appears ellipsoidal, whereas the RV appears triangular when

Department of Cardiovascular Disease, Pulmonary Hypertension and Adult Congential Heart Disease Program, Advanced Heart Failure and Transplantation Program, The Ohio State University, 473 West 12th Avenue, Columbus, OH 43210, USA
E-mail address: veronica.franco@osumc.edu

Heart Failure Clin 8 (2012) 403–412
doi:10.1016/j.hfc.2012.04.005
1551-7136/12/$ – see front matter © 2012 Elsevier Inc. All rights reserved.

viewed from the side and crescent shaped when viewed in cross section. The complexity in the shape of the RV is ideally suited for pumping blood across a low-resistance system. The characteristics of RV contraction are largely dependent on its loading conditions. Longitudinal shortening is a greater contributor to RV stroke volume than short-axis (circumferential) shortening.[4] The RV is closely linked to the LV by the following: a shared wall (the septum), mutually encircling epicardial fibers, and sharing of the pericardial space.[1] The septum and free wall contribute equally to RV contraction. The blood supply to the RV free wall is predominantly from the right coronary artery, and it receives almost equal blood flow during both systole and diastole. The left anterior descending coronary artery supplies the anterior two-thirds of the septum, and the posterior descending artery supplies the inferoposterior one-third.

The concept of ventricular interdependence is also of importance, and although always present, it is most apparent with sudden volume changes.[5] A small change in intrapleural pressure leads to a significant increase venous return and RV preload. Consequently, the septum moves toward the LV in diastole. The LV end-diastolic volume either remains unaltered or decreases. This increase in filling pressure associated with a decrease in volume generates changes in LV distensibility. Thus diastolic interaction is always present, and the interactions are large enough to be of pathophysiologic importance.

THE RV IN PULMONARY HYPERTENSION

Pulmonary arterial hypertension (PAH) is characterized by high pulmonary vascular resistance (PVR) and vascular remodeling, which results in a striking increase in RV afterload and subsequent failure.[3] Contractile function is the inherent capacity of the myocardium to contract independently of changes in the preload and afterload,[6] and in the nonfailing heart the RV can overcome physiologic acute increases in PVR. An RV without preexisting hypertrophy could not generate a systolic pulmonary arterial pressure greater than 50 to 60 mm Hg or mean pressure greater than 40 mm Hg. Yet chronically, the RV must hypertrophy to overcome sustained PAH.[5,7] Hypertrophy is established when the thickness of the RV free wall is greater than 7 mm or the RV mass is greater than 56 g.[8]

An initial adaptive response to myocardial hypertrophy is followed by maladaptive retort and progressive contractile dysfunction.[1] Eventually, the RV pools more blood to allow for compensatory preload and maintain stroke volume despite reduced fractional shortening, resulting in chamber dilation. As contractile weakening progresses, decompensated RV failure is characterized by increase filling pressures, diastolic dysfunction, diminish cardiac output, and worsen tricuspid regurgitation due to annular dilatation and poor leaflet coaptation.[1,5] An increased PVR may cause progressive dilatation of pulmonary arteries, and a pulmonary trunk diameter greater than 29 mm is considered abnormal.[8] In contrast to the asymmetric growth noted in patients with chronic thromboemboli pulmonary hypertension, the enlargement of the pulmonary arteries in PAH is usually symmetric. A pulmonary artery diameter greater than 40 mm can cause compression of the left main coronary artery, leading to ischemia. Compression of the right coronary artery by hypertrophic myocardium is another cause of ischemia, which is directly related to RV mass.

Ventricular dyssynchrony is often observed in progressive stages of PAH-induced heart failure.[8,9] Mechanical interventricular dyssynchrony, which is easily recognized clinically by the paradoxic bulging of the septum into the LV, is associated with impaired RV systolic function. The dancing septum and severe leftward ventricular bowing (D-shaped LV) are considered an unfavorable prognosis in PAH (**Fig. 1**). The delayed onset of relaxation in the RV relative to the LV is responsible for such a shift. Furthermore, ventricular dyssynchrony is also thought to impair LV diastolic function through septum bulging.[1,10] Using cardiac magnetic resonance (CMR) images, it was demonstrated that the onset of shortenings occurs without delay for both PAH and normal control groups; however, there is a large delay in the time-to-peak shortening of the RV free wall relative to the LV free wall.[10] Therefore, the RV continues to contract for almost 100 milliseconds after the end of LV ejection into the early LV filling time. An inefficient late systole of the RV, struggling with its high load, further impairs LV filling by shifting the innocent, already relaxing, septum leftward. A sudden shift in LV volume by the leftward bowing septum jeopardizes LV filling by preventing the rapid inward mitral flow wave that is expected at that time, resulting in lower cardiac output.

Over the past 2 decades, there has been significant progress in the understanding of the pathology of pulmonary vascular diseases and an explosion of clinical therapeutic trials for PAH, yet the RV remains understudied. The specific mechanisms underlying the development of RV failure secondary to pulmonary hypertension remain unclear.[1] For example, it is uncertain whether some patients develop RV myocardial ischemia,

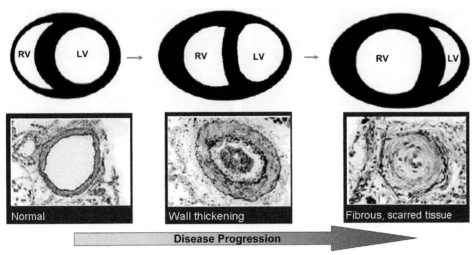

Fig. 1. RV is normally characterized by a crescent shape and is smaller in diameter than the LV. In pulmonary hypertension, there is increased end-diastolic volume and varying degrees of hypertrophy in the RV; subsequently, there is a change from the normal RV conformation to a spherical shape with a greater cross-sectional area than the LV. The more spherical RV results in abnormal septal function that also impairs the performance of the LV.

whether there is microvascular endothelial cell dysfunction, or whether myocytes undergo apoptosis. The mechanism by which a severely dilated end-stage RV repairs itself after lung transplantation is also uncertain.[11,12] Furthermore, it is becoming apparent that therapies improving or normalizing pulmonary pressure in patients with PAH do not necessarily lead to clinical improvement and prolonged survival unless accompanied by parallel improvement in RV hemodynamics and function. The degree of pulmonary hypertension does not strongly correlate with symptoms or survival because a hampered RV does not have the capacity to generate high pressures, but RV size and RA pressure foresee long-term outcomes.[3]

EVALUATION OF RV FUNCTION IN PAH
Laboratory Tests

B-type natriuretic peptide (BNP) is secreted by the ventricles in response to excessive stretching of the cardiomyocytes. BNP is cosecreted along with an N-terminal fragment (NT-proBNP), which is biologically inactive. The half-life of NT-proBNP is longer and the peptide has better stability than BNP, both in circulation and after sampling. Levels of BNP are a dynamic measurement of the degree of RV dysfunction in pulmonary hypertension. A study derived from REVEAL (Registry to Evaluate Early and Long-Term Pulmonary Arterial Hypertension Disease Management) showed a significant increase in the risk of death if patients had a BNP level greater than 180 pg/mL.[13] A BNP level of

less than 50 pg/mL was associated with increased 1-year survival. An NT-proBNP level of approximately 1400 pg/mL correlates with severe cardiac dysfunction.[3] These findings have been validated, and increases in natriuretic peptide levels during serial follow-up visits are associated with higher mortality in patients with idiopathic PAH and decreased functional capacity.[14–17] BNP and NT-proBNP have been proposed as vital end points for clinical trial designs in PAH[18,19] and as biomarkers to guide therapy.[3]

Echocardiography

Transthoracic echocardiography is a key tool in the evaluation of RV dysfunction. It is widely available and safe, and there are several echocardiographic indices and markers of poor long-term outcomes that guide patient therapeutic algorithms.[3,20–22] The major consequences of PAH are right-sided heart remodeling and impact on the left side of the heart. Patients with more severe PAH classically present with RA dilatation, hypertrophy and dilatation of the RV, evidence of RV remodeling (thickening of the moderator band), and systolic flattening of the interventricular septum, with a D-shaped deformity suggesting pressure overload (**Fig. 2**). There are 5 echocardiographic parameters that portray higher mortality in patients with PAH: presence of pericardial effusion,[3,13,23,24] RA area,[25,26] RV Tei index,[27,28] tricuspid annular plane systolic excursion (TAPSE),[29] and the eccentricity index.[24,30]

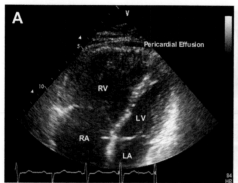 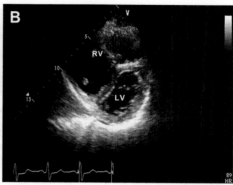

Fig. 2. (*A*) Typical echocardiographic features in a patient with severe PAH. Dilatation of the RV cavities, compression of the LV cavities, and presence of a pericardial effusion. (*B*) Evidence of LV compression and septal bowing due to end-stage right-sided heart failure as well as the presence of a prominent moderator band. LA, left atrium.

Dimensions of the RA

A simple echocardiographic parameter is the measurement of the dimensions of the RA, including the diameter of the RA and area measured on an apical 4-chamber view.[21] An RA area larger than 20 cm[2] is abnormal,[25] and an area larger than 27 cm[2] has been associated with worse prognosis.[26] RV measurements are challenging because of the frequent presence of large trabeculations, and the complex RV morphology is sometimes difficult to evaluate using echocardiography.[21,25] Measurement of the midcavity and basal RV diameters in the apical 4-chamber view at end-diastole is a simple method for quantification of RV size. The single-plane 2-dimensional (2D) approach to the calculation of RV volumes frequently results in volume underestimation. For this reason, there are no reference values for normal RV volume or areas measured by echocardiography. The ability of 3-dimensional (3D) echocardiographic imaging to directly measure RV volume has resulted in improved accuracy; however, RV volumes are still underestimated because of the effects of endocardial trabeculae in comparison with other techniques such as CMR imaging.[31] 3D echocardiography is not widely available and its use remains investigational. Besides, measurements of RV volume are not interchangeable between modalities and, therefore, serial evaluations should preferably be performed using the same imaging technique.[31]

Tei index

The precise estimation of the RV ejection fraction is subject to similar imaging limitations as mentioned earlier, and great attention has been paid to alternative techniques that measure RV function. The Tei index is derived solely by Doppler measurements and thus is not affected by RV geometry. The index assesses RV function quantitatively[27] and is

a predictor of mortality.[28] This global myocardial performance index requires the sum of RV isovolumetric contraction time and isovolumetric relaxation time, obtained by subtracting RV ejection time from the interval between cessation and onset of the tricuspid inflow velocities with pulsed-wave Doppler echocardiography. An index of combined RV systolic and diastolic functions was obtained by dividing the sum of both the isovolumetric intervals by ejection time (**Fig. 3**). The Tei index prolongs with more severe RV dysfunction. Results showed that the index was the single most powerful variable that differentiated patients with PAH from normal patients (0.93 ± 0.34 vs 0.28 ± 0.04; *P*<.001) and the strongest predictor of clinical status and survival. An increase of 0.1 in the index increased the risk of death by 1.3 times. The index has the advantage of being relatively independent of heart rate, RV pressure or dilatation, or tricuspid regurgitation.[27] The Tei index represents a global estimate of RV function independent of geometric assumptions but is limited by its mode of calculation being based on 2 different cardiac cycle measurements.[21]

More recent studies have shown that tissue Doppler imaging of the lateral tricuspid annulus allows simpler (and equally accurate) measurement of the RV Tei index.[32] This method eliminates the need for 2 separate Doppler interrogations and thereby reduces errors attributable to fluctuations in the heart rate. These parameters are not routinely calculated in clinical practice and entail postprocedure calculations. Furthermore, its precise measurement is infeasible in patients with atrial fibrillation, frequent premature ventricular contractions, disturbances of intraventricular or atrioventricular conduction, and a permanent pacemaker, or when Doppler images of sufficient quality cannot be acquired.[22] The calculation of this index based on short intervals

A

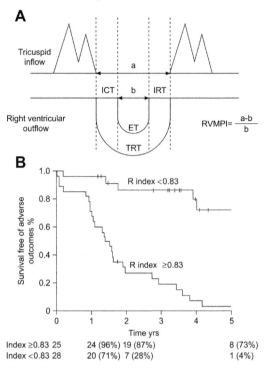

$$RVMPI = \frac{a-b}{b}$$

B

standard M-mode echocardiography of the RV annulus (**Fig. 4**). In comparison with a TAPSE value greater than 18 mm, a TAPSE value of 18 mm or less was associated with greater RV dysfunction (cardiac index [CI], 1.9 vs 2.7 L/min/m^2) and right-sided heart remodeling. Survival estimates at 1 and 2 years were 94% and 88%, respectively, in patients with PAH who had a TAPSE value greater than 18 mm, and 60% and 50%, respectively, in patients with a TAPSE value less than 18 mm. For every 1-mm decrease in the TAPSE value, the unadjusted risk of death increased by 17% (hazard ratio, 1.17; 95% confidence interval, 1.05–1.30; $P = .006$), which persisted even after adjusting other echocardiographic and hemodynamic variables and baseline treatment

| Index ≥0.83 25 | 24 (96%) 19 (87%) | 8 (73%) |
| Index <0.83 28 | 20 (71%) 7 (28%) | 1 (4%) |

Fig. 3. Assessment of the RV global performance by the Tei index. (*A*) Method of measurement of Tei index. RV myocardial performance index (RVMPI = [a − b]/b) is calculated by measuring 2 intervals: (1) *a* is the interval between cessation and onset of tricuspid inflow and (2) *b* is ejection time (ET) of RV outflow. ICT, isovolumetric contraction time; IRT, isovolumetric relaxation time; TRT, tricuspid regurgitation time. (*B*) Prognostic value of Tei index. (*Adapted from* Yeo TC, Dujardin KS, Tei C, et al. Value of a Doppler-derived index combining systolic and diastolic time intervals in predicting outcome in primary pulmonary hypertension. Am J Cardiol 1998;81:1157–61.)

requires very good–quality Doppler tracings, with special care for optimal visualization of isovolumic event timing. Shortcomings derive from its calculation based on different cardiac cycle measurements and being adversely affected by rhythm and conduction disturbances. In addition, when there is increased pressure in the RA, the Tei index may manifest a pseudonormalization effect resulting from a shortened isovolumic relaxation time.

TAPSE

The TAPSE measurement has become widely used as a marker of RV ejection fraction and is also an important prognostic marker in PAH.[29] The RV contraction is more related to longitudinal axis shortening (thus drawing the tricuspid annular plane toward the apex) than reduction in the cavity diameter, because the LV measurement is obtained by

A

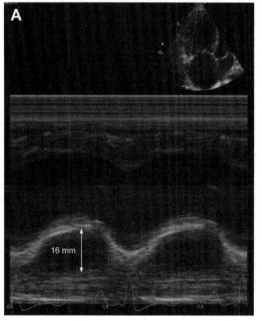

B

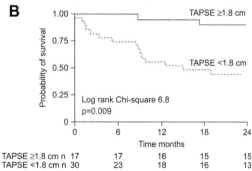

TAPSE ≥1.8 cm n 17	17	16	15	15
TAPSE <1.8 cm n 30	23	18	16	13

Fig. 4. Measurement of the TAPSE. (*A*) Method of measurement of TAPSE by M-mode echocardiography. (*B*) Prognostic value of TAPSE. (*Adapted from* Forfia PR, Fisher MR, Mathai SC, et al. Tricuspid annular displacement predicts survival in pulmonary hypertension. Am J Respir Crit Care Med 2006;174:1034–41.)

status. Nevertheless, TAPSE has several limitations[22] including angle and load dependency. TAPSE focuses only on a small part of the RV and may not be an appropriate surrogate for the entire RV. TAPSE ignores the outlet portion and septal contribution to RV ejection, which may be important to maintain overall RV function, especially when the longitudinal component decreases. Due to ventricular interdependence, the performances of both the RV and the LV may influence TAPSE values. In the recent PAH guidelines,[3] only pericardial effusion and a TAPSE value less than 15 mm were selected as major prognostic indications, on the basis that they were measured in most patients.

Compression of the LV

Compression of the LV is seen in patients with severe PAH and significant RV dilatation leading to abnormal LV filling, which is an additional factor that diminishes left cardiac output.[10] The compression carries prognostic value[24] and is estimated by the eccentricity index, which is a ratio of the long-axis to short-axis diameters of the LV, both in diastole and systole.[30] The eccentricity index is calculated on the 2D short-axis view of the LV and may discriminate between the RV volume and pressure overload states. Improvement in eccentricity index is seen with PAH-targeted treatment. However, there is the problem of different-level measurements affecting the results.[22] The other possible problem is identifying end diastole and end systole, which could also affect measurements.

Combination of parameters

At present, no echocardiographic parameter seems sufficient to give an adequate assessment of RV function; rather, a combination of the aforementioned parameters must be used to exclude heart failure. Among new echocardiographic techniques, strain imaging and 3D echocardiography have been shown to be potentially useful to assess RV function,[21] although these parameters warrant further validation in patients with PAH. There is substantial interest in exercise stress echocardiography, particularly in detecting early disease; however, this study is difficult to perform and interpret.

CMR Imaging

CMR imaging is renowned for its accuracy, lower operator dependency, interstudy variability,[33] and advantages over echocardiography, and is considered by some as the gold standard for imaging of the right side of the heart in patients with PAH.[18,19] CMR imaging yields high-quality images of the RV and is playing an emerging role in the evaluation of RV size, function, volume, mass, viability, interventricular septal configuration, and LV-RV relationships.[3,8,33–35] Furthermore, it allows for noninvasive assessment of blood flow, including stroke volume (measuring the volumetric flow in the main pulmonary artery), distensibility of pulmonary arteries, and all prognostic factors in patients with PAH-induced heart failure.

Increased RV end-diastolic volume may be the most appropriate marker for progressive RV failure.[3,33] A high RV end-diastolic volume index ($\geq$84 mL/m^2) and low LV end-diastolic volume index ($\leq$40 mL/m^2) are CMR imaging parameters independently associated with poor long-term outcome, treatment failure, and death in patients with PAH.[35] Lower LV volume might be due to a decrease in RV stroke volume or compression of the LV due to an increase in RV volume. Chronically high pulmonary pressures cause RV remodeling and hypertrophy. The degree of RV wall thickness is proportional to the level of PVR; however, it is not as significantly related to mortality as RV dilatation (**Fig. 5**).[35]

Contrast-enhancement techniques have revealed important cardiac structural abnormalities among patients with PAH.[34] Delayed contrast enhancement is believed to result from the delayed clearance of gadolinium from a relatively expanded extracellular volume within fibrotic, nonviable, or necrotic myocardial regions, and its presence is associated with worse prognosis.[8,36,37] Clearance is confined to the insertion points of the RV free wall in most patients with pulmonary hypertension. Some patients demonstrate extension of the process from the insertion points into the interventricular septum,[36] but none exhibit enhancement in the RV free wall.[8] The extent of delayed contrast enhancement is inversely related to the measure of RV systolic function ($r = -0.63$, $P = .001$) and RV stroke volume ($r = -0.67$, $P = .006$). The delayed enhancement mass correlates with increased RV remodeling indices, reduced eccentricity index, RV mass, and end-diastolic volume.[36,38] Furthermore, septal enhancement is associated with bowing of the RV to the left, and the extent of the process correlates with pulmonary hemodynamics (mean pulmonary arterial pressure and PVR).[37] Elevated mechanical wall stress (RV pressure) within these areas appears to be a precipitant of these focal myocardial abnormalities.

Tagged CMR imaging showed a significant interventricular asynchrony caused by a longer systolic contraction time in the RV than in the LV, presumably due to a decrease in electrical conductivity over the RV.[34] This ventricular asynchrony allows

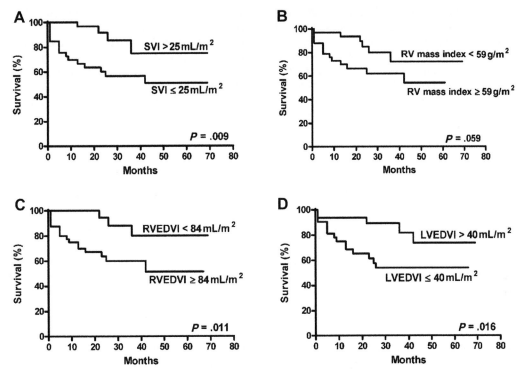

Fig. 5. Kaplan-Meier survival curves for baseline cardiac magnetic resonance imaging variables according to the median value in patients with pulmonary hypertension. (*A*) Stroke volume index (SVI) ≤25 mL/m², (*B*) RV mass index ≥59 g/m², (*C*) RV end-diastolic volume index (RVEDVI) ≥84 mL/m², and (*D*) LV end-diastolic volume index (LVEDVI) ≤40 mL/m² were predictors of mortality. (*From* von Wolferen SA, Marcus JT, Boonstra A, et al. Prognostic value of right ventricular mass, volume and function in idiopathic pulmonary arterial hypertension. Eur Heart J 2007;28:1255; with permission.)

for septal bowing, decreased RV function, and reduced left end-diastolic volume. Another application consists of CMR imaging analysis of main pulmonary artery distensibility, which was highly correlated with vasodilator response. Patients with PAH who have a positive hemodynamic response to vasodilators have significantly better long-term prognosis than nonresponders.[3] A cutoff value of 10% distensibility enables responders to be distinguished from nonresponders, with a sensitivity and specificity of 100% and 56%, respectively.[39]

The disadvantages of CMR imaging include long scan times, artifacts due to motion, inability to hold breath, and incompatibility with pacemakers, defibrillators, cochlear implants, and aneurysm clips.[34] Data acquisition and analysis tend to be more intensive, require more time, are not widely available, and are more expensive.[8]

Although CMR-based assessment is not yet ready to replace right-sided heart catheterization (RHC) with respect to confirmation of PAH diagnosis, it could be considered an alternative to RHC for follow-up purposes.[3,34] The high degree

of reproducibility of CMR imaging makes it an ideal tool to monitor changes in the RV and the impact of therapy. Progressive RV dilatation predicts RV failure at an early stage, which enables the prediction of treatment failure and thus offers an opportunity to change treatment or list for transplantation before fatal decompensation and death occur.[35] CMR imaging allows for the early identification of patients who are at a higher risk of clinical deterioration, allowing intensification and optimization of the therapy.[34] Although CMR imaging has been generally contested as a monitoring tool because of its complexity and cost, this may not hold true in patients with PAH.[33] The decision to continue or change the mode of therapy in a patient with PAH, sometimes evading the need to perform a RHC, usually has long-term consequences that markedly exceed the cost of CMR examination.

RHC

RHC is the gold standard for confirmation of PAH diagnosis. The importance of the progression of RV failure on the outcome of patients with PAH is confirmed by the prognostic impact of RA pressure and CI. Patients are considered stable and with better prognosis if their RA pressure is less than 8 mm Hg and their CI is less than 2.5 L/min/m^2.[3] Even with effective therapies, an RA pressure greater than 15 mm Hg and a CI less than or equal to 2.0 L/min/m^2 are harbingers of poor outcomes in patients with PAH.[3,13] A PVR greater than 32 Wood units foresees a 4-fold increase in the risk of death.[13] By contrast, the level of pulmonary arterial pressure only has modest prognostic significance, in part because pulmonary pressure levels drop as the RV approaches end stage.

Catheterization procedures, when performed in experienced centers, are associated with a low incidence of complications.[3] Nevertheless, the procedure is invasive and carries a small but real risk of morbidity and mortality, and serial hemodynamic assessments are not the norm. Furthermore, data are acquired in a supine resting position, and there are no standard guidelines for exercise hemodynamics despite dyspnea on exertion being the main complaint and symptom of patients with PAH. In addition, hemodynamic measurements could vary during consecutive measurements because of challenges in obtaining a precise wedge pressure, which is later used to calculate PVR.

Exercise Capacity

The peak oxygen consumption (pVo$_2$) is obtained during cardiopulmonary exercise testing and is a surrogate of cardiac output during maximal exercise. Its applications include estimating the risk and severity of disease, evaluating the effects of therapy, and estimating prognosis in patients with heart failure. The cardiac output response to exercise is a strong predictor of survival. Therefore, pVo$_2$ can be very useful when assessing the degree of cardiac dysfunction. Patients with PAH are considered stable and with better prognosis if their pVo$_2$ is greater than 15 mL/min/kg, and unstable and deteriorating if their pVo$_2$ is less than 12 mL/min/kg.[3]

In PAH, oxygen (O$_2$) uptake is reduced at the anaerobic threshold and during peak exercise in relation to disease severity, as are peak work rate, peak heart rate, O$_2$ pulse, and ventilatory efficiency. The walking distance and pVo$_2$ do correlate in PAH, but cardiopulmonary exercise testing failed to confirm improvements that were observed during 6-minute walk test (6MWT) in clinical trials.[3] Insufficient expertise in testing oxygen consumption was identified as the main reason for this discrepancy. At present, the 6MWT is the preferred and most widely used method to assess

functional capacity in patients with PAH.[3] Nevertheless, it is paramount to remember that treatment goals should be adjusted to the individual patient. For example, a 6-minute walking distance greater than 400 m is considered acceptable in patients with PAH. Younger patients are often capable of walking more than 500 m despite the presence of severe RV dysfunction. In these patients, guidelines recommend obtaining additional exercise testing and/or RHC for more reliable assessment of RV function.[3]

SUMMARY

Until the early 1990s, PAH was consistently fatal, with a median life expectancy of approximately 2.5 years. Over the past 2 decades, remarkable progress has been made in the treatment of PAH, and at present 4 different classes of medications (prostacyclins, endothelin receptor blockers, phosphodiesterase-5 inhibitors, and calcium antagonists) are available. However, PAH remains incurable and median survival is usually limited to 5 to 6 years.[3] PAH symptoms and prognosis are essentially determined by the state of the RV; yet clinical trials and current guidelines in the management of this disease do not include RV function and pulmonary hemodynamics as end points or determinants of escalation of therapy.

In patients with pulmonary hypertension, RHC and RV imaging studies, such as CMR imaging and echocardiography, should be seen as complementary procedures that determine outcomes and assist with monitoring the success of therapy. Furthermore, studies that understand the pathophysiology of RV dysfunction are pivotal. Current medications target the increased PVR in PAH, with subsequent reduction in RV load; however, determinants and management of right-sided heart failure remain poorly studied. There is still unexploited potential for therapies that directly target the RV, with the aim of supporting and protecting the right side of the heart, striving to prolong survival in patients with pulmonary hypertension.

REFERENCES

1. Voelkel NF, Quaife RA, Leinwand LA, et al. Right ventricular function and failure: report of a National Heart, Lung, and Blood Institute working group on cellular and molecular mechanisms of right heart failure. Circulation 2006;114:1883–91.
2. Costanzo MR, Dipchand A, Starling R, et al. The International Society of Heart and Lung Transplantation Guidelines for the care of heart transplant recipients. J Heart Lung Transplant 2010;29:914–56.

3. Galie N, Hoeper MM, Humbert M, et al. Guidelines for the diagnosis and treatment of pulmonary hypertension. The Task Force for the Diagnosis and Treatment of Pulmonary Hypertension of the European Society of Cardiology (ESC) and the European Respiratory Society (ERS), endorsed by the International Society of Heart and Lung Transplantation (ISHLT). Eur Heart J 2009;30:2493–537.

4. Kukulski T, Hubbert L, Arnold M, et al. Normal regional right ventricular function and its change with age: a Doppler myocardial imaging study. J Am Soc Echocardiogr 2000;13:194–204.

5. Brinker JA, Weiss JL, Lappe DL, et al. Leftward septal displacement during right ventricular loading in man. Circulation 1980;61:626–33.

6. Opie LH. Mechanisms of cardiac contraction and relaxation. In: Libby, Bonow, Mann, Zipes, editors. Braunwald's heart disease. Philadelphia (PA): Elsevier Saunders; 2008. p. 509–39.

7. Dias CA, Assad RS, Caneo LF, et al. Reversible pulmonary trunk banding. II. An experimental model for rapid pulmonary ventricular hypertrophy. J Thorac Cardiovasc Surg 2002;124:999–1006.

8. Marrone G, Mamone G, Luca A, et al. The role of 1.5T cardiac MRI in the diagnosis, prognosis and management of pulmonary arterial hypertension. Int J Cardiovasc Imaging 2010;26:665–81.

9. Roeleveld RJ, Marcus JT, Faes TJ, et al. Interventricular septal configuration at MR imaging and pulmonary arterial pressure in pulmonary hypertension. Radiology 2005;234:710–7.

10. Marcus JT, Gan CT, Zwanenburg JJ, et al. Interventricular mechanical asynchrony in pulmonary arterial hypertension: left-to-right delay in peak shortening is related to right ventricular overload and left ventricular underfilling. J Am Coll Cardiol 2008;51:750–7.

11. Ritchie M, Waggoner AD, Davila-Roman VG, et al. Echocardiographic characterization of the improvement in right ventricular function in patients with severe pulmonary hypertension after single-lung transplantation. J Am Coll Cardiol 1993;22:1170–4.

12. Schulman LL, Leibowitz DW, Anandarangam T, et al. Variability of right ventricular functional recovery after lung transplantation. Transplantation 1996;62:622–5.

13. Benza RL, Miller DP, Gomberg-Maitland M, et al. Predicting survival in pulmonary arterial hypertension: insights from the Registry to Evaluate Early and Long-Term Pulmonary Arterial Hypertension Disease Management (REVEAL). Circulation 2010;122:164–72.

14. Leuchte HH, Holzapfel M, Baumgartner RA, et al. Clinical significance of brain natriuretic peptide in primary pulmonary hypertension. J Am Coll Cardiol 2004;43:764–70.

15. Nagaya N, Nishikimi T, Uematsu M, et al. Plasma brain natriuretic peptide as a prognostic indicator in patients with primary pulmonary hypertension. Circulation 2000;102:865–70.

16. Park MH, Scott RL, Uber PA, et al. Usefulness of B-type natriuretic peptide as a predictor of treatment outcome in pulmonary arterial hypertension. Congest Heart Fail 2004;10:221–5.

17. Pruszczyk P. N-terminal pro-brain natriuretic peptide as an indicator of right ventricular dysfunction. J Card Fail 2005;11:S65–9.

18. McLaughlin VV, Badesch DB, Delcroix M, et al. End points and clinical trial design in pulmonary arterial hypertension. J Am Coll Cardiol 2009;54:S97–107.

19. Peacock AJ, Naeije R, Galie N, et al. End-points and clinical trial design in pulmonary arterial hypertension: have we made progress? Eur Respir J 2009;34:231–42.

20. Champion HC, Michelakis ED, Hassoun PM. Comprehensive invasive and noninvasive approach to the right ventricle-pulmonary circulation unit: state of the art and clinical and research implications. Circulation 2009;120:992–1007.

21. Habib G, Torbicki A. The role of echocardiography in the diagnosis and management of patients with pulmonary hypertension. Eur Respir Rev 2010;19(118):288–99.

22. Badano L, Ginghina C, Easaw J, et al. Right ventricle in pulmonary arterial hypertension: haemodynamics, structural changes, imaging, and proposal of a study protocol aimed to assess remodeling and treatment effects. Eur J Echocardiogr 2010;11:27–37.

23. Hinderliter AL, Willis PW IV, Barst RJ, et al. Effects of long-term infusion of prostacyclin (epoprostenol) on echocardiographic measures of right ventricular structure and function in primary pulmonary hypertension. Primary Pulmonary Hypertension Study Group. Circulation 1997;95:1479–86.

24. Raymond RJ, Hinderliter AL, Willis PW, et al. Echocardiographic predictors of adverse outcomes in primary pulmonary hypertension. J Am Coll Cardiol 2002;39:1214–9.

25. Lang RM, Bierig M, Devereux RB, et al. Recommendations for chamber quantification. Eur J Echocardiogr 2006;7:79–108.

26. Perrone S, De La Fuente RL, et al. Right atrial size and tricuspid regurgitation severity predict mortality or transplantation in primary pulmonary hypertension. J Am Soc Echocardiogr 2002;15:1160–4.

27. Tei C, Dujardin KS, Hodge DO, et al. Doppler echocardiographic index for assessment of global right ventricular function. J Am Soc Echocardiogr 1996;9:838–47.

28. Yeo TC, Dujardin KS, Tei C, et al. Value of a Doppler-derived index combining systolic and diastolic time intervals in predicting outcome in primary pulmonary hypertension. Am J Cardiol 1998;81:1157–61.

29. Forfia PR, Fisher MR, Mathai SC, et al. Tricuspid annular displacement predicts survival in pulmonary hypertension. Am J Respir Crit Care Med 2006;174:1034–41.

30. Ryan T, Petrovic O, Dillon JC, et al. An echocardio-graphic index for separation of right ventricular volume and pressure overload. J Am Coll Cardiol 1985;5:918–27.

31. Sugeng L, Mor-Avi V, Weinert L, et al. Multimodality comparison of quantitative volumetric analysis of the right ventricle. JACC Cardiovasc Imaging 2010;3:10–8.

32. Harada K, Tamura M, Toyono M, et al. Comparison of the right ventricular Tei index by tissue Doppler imaging to that obtained by pulsed Doppler in children without heart disease. Am J Cardiol 2002;90:566–9.

33. Torbicki A. Cardiac magnetic resonance in pulmo-nary arterial hypertension: a step in the right direc-tion. Eur Heart J 2007;28:1187–9.

34. Benza R, Biederman R, Murali S, et al. Role of cardiac magnetic resonance imaging in the management of patients with pulmonary arterial hypertension. J Am Coll Cardiol 2008;52:1683–92.

35. von Wolferen SA, Marcus JT, Boonstra A, et al. Prog-nostic value of right ventricular mass, volume and function in idiopathic pulmonary arterial hyperten-sion. Eur Heart J 2007;28:1250–7.

36. McCann GP, Gan CT, Beek AM, et al. Extent of MRI de-layed enhancement of myocardial mass is related to right ventricular dysfunction in pulmonary artery hyper-tension. AJR Am J Roentgenol 2007;188:349–55.

37. Blyth KG, Groenning BA, Martin TN, et al. Contrast enhancement-cardiovascular magnetic resonance imaging in patients with pulmonary hypertension. Eur Heart J 2005;26:1993–9.

38. Shehata ML, Lossnitzer D, Skrok J, et al. Myocardial delayed enhancement in pulmonary hypertension: pulmonary hemodynamics, right ventricular func-tion, and remodeling. AJR Am J Roentgenol 2011;196:87–94.

39. Jardim C, Rochitte CE, Humbert M, et al. Pulmonary artery distensibility in pulmonary arterial hyperten-sion: an MRI pilot study. Eur Respir J 2006;29:476–81.

Pulmonary Arterial Hypertension in Connective Tissue Diseases

Stephen C. Mathai, MD, MHS, Paul M. Hassoun, MD*

KEYWORDS

- Connective tissue disease • Pulmonary hypertension • Scleroderma
- Systemic lupus erythematosus • Mixed connective tissue disease • Therapy

KEY POINTS

- Pulmonary arterial hypertension (PAH) is a common complication of connective tissue diseases (CTDs), particularly scleroderma.
- When complicating CTD, PAH significantly worsens survival and is a leading cause of death in these patients.
- Scleroderma-associated PAH carries a significantly worse prognosis compared with other forms of PAH such as idiopathic PAH (IPAH).
- Standard PAH-specific therapy is not as effective in CTD-associated PAH in comparison with IPAH.
- There is a need for a better understanding of underlying mechanisms of CTD-associated PAH for the design of targeted therapy.

INTRODUCTION

Pulmonary arterial hypertension (PAH) is a progressive disease caused by a remodeling of precapillary arterioles that leads to a progressive increase in pulmonary vascular resistance and right ventricular failure. PAH is associated with significant morbidity and mortality, despite the advent of specific therapies that target pathobiologic pathways implicated in the disease process.[1–3] PAH can only be diagnosed by right heart catheterization (RHC), and is defined as a mean pulmonary artery pressure greater than 25 mm Hg in the absence of elevation of the pulmonary capillary wedge pressure. PAH includes a heterogeneous group of clinical entities sharing similar pathologic changes that have been subcategorized as idiopathic PAH (IPAH), familial PAH, and pulmonary hypertension associated with other diseases such as connective tissue diseases (CTDs), portopulmonary hypertension, and pulmonary hypertension related to human immunodeficiency virus infection, drugs, and toxins. An updated classification of all pulmonary hypertension syndromes has been recently published from the fourth World Symposium held at Dana Point, California, in 2008.[4]

The exact mechanisms involved in the pathogenesis of PAH remain vastly unknown but are likely to involve significant alterations in endothelial function,[5] an understanding of which has led over the past 2 decades to targeted therapy for this disease.[6] Several lines of evidence also support a role for autoimmunity in the development of the pulmonary vascular changes, including the presence of circulating autoantibodies,[7] proinflammatory cytokines (eg, interleukin [IL]-1 and IL-6),[8] and association of PAH with autoimmune diseases and CTDs such as systemic sclerosis (SSc), systemic lupus erythematosus (SLE), and mixed

Supported by: NHLBI K23 HL092287 (S.C.M.) and P50 HL084946 (P.M.H.).

The authors have nothing to disclose.

Pulmonary Hypertension Program, Division of Pulmonary and Critical Care Medicine, Department of Medicine, Johns Hopkins University, 1830 East Monument Street, Baltimore, MD 21205, USA

* Corresponding author.

E-mail address: phassoun@jhmi.edu

Heart Failure Clin 8 (2012) 413–425

doi:10.1016/j.hfc.2012.04.001

1551-7136/12/$ – see front matter © 2012 Elsevier Inc. All rights reserved.

connective tissue disease (MCTD). Despite the similarities in disease pathogenesis and hemodynamic perturbations, outcomes in patients with CTD-associated PAH differ significantly from other forms of PAH. In particular, patients with SSc-associated PAH (SSc-PAH) have a poorer response to therapy and significantly worse survival compared with IPAH patients.[9-11] There are serologic and pathologic features suggestive of inflammation in both IPAH and SSc-PAH, although inflammatory pathways and autoimmunity are likely more pronounced in SSc-PAH, perhaps explaining clinical discrepancies between the 2 syndromes.[9,10] Other CTDs such as SLE, MCTD, and to a lesser extent rheumatoid arthritis (RA), dermatomyositis, and Sjögren syndrome, can also be complicated by PAH and are discussed separately in this review.

SCLERODERMA

SSc is a heterogeneous disorder characterized by dysfunction of the endothelium, dysregulation of fibroblasts resulting in excessive production of collagen, and abnormalities of the immune system.[12] Progressive fibrosis of the skin and internal organs is a pathologic hallmark of the disease, resulting in major organ damage and failure and thus explaining the high morbidity and early death. Genetic and environmental factors are thought to contribute to host susceptibility[13] in the context of autoimmune dysregulation. Whether presenting in the limited or diffuse form, SSc is a systemic disease with the propensity to involve multiple organ systems such as the gastrointestinal tract, heart, kidneys, and lungs.[14] Pulmonary manifestations include PAH, interstitial fibrosis, and increased susceptibility to lung neoplasms.

The use of a standard classification system for SSc has allowed more accurate estimates of incidence and prevalence of SSc, which vary according to geographic location,[15] supporting a role for environmental factors in disease pathogenesis. Prevalence of SSc ranges from 30 to 70 cases per million in Europe and Japan[16-18] to approximately 240 cases per million in the United States.[15] Incidence varies similarly by geographic area, with the highest rates found in the United States (~19 persons per million per year).[19]

SCLERODERMA-ASSOCIATED PAH (SSc-PAH)

The prevalence of PAH in SSc patients, when the diagnosis is based on RHC for assessment of filling pressures, is about 8% to 14%.[20,21] Previous assessments based on echocardiographic measurements[22-25] have overestimated the true prevalence of SSc-PAH, and should not be relied on for establishing the diagnosis and initiating treatment. Echocardiography is limited in the diagnosis of PAH, because of the inaccuracy of the Doppler signal in assessing true right ventricular systolic pressure[26] and the frequent inability to obtain an adequate Doppler signal, particularly in patients with CTD. Furthermore, if estimated right ventricular pressure is indeed elevated, other diagnoses such as pulmonary venous hypertension cannot be excluded with certainty by echocardiography. However, while echocardiography overestimates the prevalence of PAH because of misclassification it is likely that SSc-PAH will remain underdiagnosed overall, as suggested by the lower than expected prevalence of the disease in the few registries available.[27-29]

Pathophysiology

There are early vascular changes in SSc,[30] which include gaps between endothelial cells,[31] cellular apoptosis,[32] endothelial activation with expression of cell adhesion molecules, inflammatory cell recruitment, a procoagulant state,[33] and remodeling of the small vessels with intimal proliferation and adventitial fibrosis leading to vessel obliteration. The extent of these vascular lesions in vital organs such as the lungs, kidneys, and heart defines the prognosis of patients with SSc.[34]

Specific endothelial injury is reflected by increased levels of soluble vascular cell adhesion molecule 1 (sVCAM-1),[35] disturbances in angiogenesis reflected by increased levels of circulating vascular endothelial growth factor (VEGF),[36,37] and the presence of angiostatic factors.[36,38] Increased VEGF may be a consequence of increased angiogenesis or profound disturbances in signaling in SSc. Dysregulated angiogenesis in SSc-PAH, exemplified by the upregulation of VEGF a glycoprotein with potent angiogenic and vascular permeability-enhancing properties, is a predominant pathologic feature of the disease and is a logical candidate for therapeutic targeting.

Autoantibodies

Several antibodies are frequently found in SSc-PAH, such as antifibrillarin antibodies (anti–U3-RNP)[39] and the poorly characterized antiendothelial antibodies (aECA), which correlate with digital infarcts.[40] Antibodies to fibrin-bound tissue plasminogen activator in patients with CREST syndrome (Calcinosis, Raynaud phenomenon, Esophageal dysmotility, Sclerodactyly, Telangiectasia)[41] and in IPAH patients with HLA-DQ7 antigen[42] and antitopoisomerase-IIα antibodies, particularly in association with HLA-B35 antigen,[43] have been reported in SSc-PAH. aECA antibodies, which can activate endothelial cells, induce the expression of adhesion molecules, and trigger apoptosis, are thought to play a role in the pathogenesis of PAH.[44]

Fibroblasts are essential components of the pulmonary vascular wall remodeling in PAH, and are found in the remodeled neointimal layer in both SSc-PAH and IPAH. In this regard, the detection of antifibroblast antibodies in the serum of SSc and IPAH patients[45,46] has significant pathogenic importance because these antibodies can activate fibroblasts and induce collagen synthesis, thus contributing potentially directly to the remodeling process. Antibodies from sera of patients with SSc induce a proadhesive and proinflammatory response in normal fibroblasts.[46] Antifibroblast antibodies from sera of IPAH and SSc-PAH patients have distinct reactivity profiles[47] and react with fibroblast proteins involved in the regulation of cytoskeletal function, cell contraction, cell and oxidative stress, cell energy metabolism, and different key cellular pathways.[48]

Taken together, particularly in light of the positive response to immunosuppressive therapy for some patients with PAH associated with SLE and MCTD,[49] these studies suggest that inflammation and autoimmunity play a major role in the pathogenesis of PAH, perhaps more specifically in CTD-associated PAH.

Genetic Factors

Polymorphisms involving the bone morphogenetic protein receptor-2 (*BMPRII*) are present in more than 80% of familial IPAH[50,51] and in up to 25% of sporadic[52,53] cases of IPAH. Additional candidate genes have been proposed to influence the pathogenesis of PAH.[54] Polymorphisms of the activin-receptor–like kinase 1 (*ALK1*) gene, another member of the transforming growth factor (TGF)-β receptor superfamily, have been reported in patients with hereditary hemorrhagic telangiectasia and PAH.[55] However, to date *BMPR2* mutations have not been identified in 2 small cohorts of SSc-PAH patients.[56,57]

Candidate genes associated with SSc have been reported in different populations, and include a variant in the promoter of monocyte chemotactic protein 1 (MCP-1)[58]; 2 variants in CD19 (−499G>T and a GT repeat polymorphism in the 3′-untranslated region)[59]; a promoter and coding polymorphism in TNFA (TNFA-238A>G, TNFA 489A>G)[60]; a variant in the promoter of the IL-1α gene (IL1A-889 T)[61,62]; and a haplotype with 3 single-nucleotide polymorphisms in IL-10.[63] A genome-wide association analysis

provided evidence for association to multiple loci in a Native American population.[64]

Recently, an association between an endoglin gene (*ENG*) polymorphism and SSc-related PAH was identified. Wipff and colleagues[65] demonstrated a significant lower frequency of the 6bINS allele in SSc-PAH patients compared with controls or patients with SSc but no PAH. Endoglin, a homodimeric membrane glycoprotein primarily present on human vascular endothelium, is part of the TGF-β receptor complex. The functional significance of the *ENG* polymorphism in SSc patients remains to be determined.

Thus, there are compelling data supporting a genetic basis for SSc. However, aside from the few examples cited here, the genes relevant to the pathogenesis and poor outcome associated with SSc-PAH have not been identified, and their definition will require robust, well-characterized, large patient populations to provide adequate power for analysis.

Clinical Features

Risk factors for the development of PAH in SSc patients include late-onset disease,[66] an isolated reduction in DL_{CO}, a percentage forced vital capacity/lung diffusing capacity for carbon monoxide ($FVC\%:DL_{CO}\%$) ratio greater than 1.6,[67,68] or a combined decreased DL_{CO}/alveolar volume with elevation of serum N-terminal pro–brain natriuretic peptide levels,[40,69,70] among others (**Box 1**). Typically patients with SSc-PAH are predominantly women, have limited sclerosis with predominantly anticentromere antibodies, are older, and have seemingly less severe hemodynamic impairment compared with IPAH patients.[10] Clinical symptoms are nonspecific, including dyspnea and functional limitation, which may be more severe than in IPAH owing to not only older age but also frequent involvement of the musculoskeletal system in these patients. SSc-PAH patients

---

Box 1
Clinical risk factors for the development of PAH in systemic sclerosis

Limited SSc

Late age of onset of SSc

Raynaud phenomenon

Number of telangiectasias

Decreased DL_{CO}

$FVC\%:DL_{CO}\% >1.6$

Increased N-terminal brain natriuretic peptide

Antibodies (eg, anti–U3-RNP)

also tend to have other organ involvement such as renal dysfunction and intrinsic heart disease. Indeed, patients with SSc (even in the absence of PAH) tend to have depressed right ventricular function[71,72] as well as left ventricular systolic and diastolic dysfunction.[73] Like IPAH patients, SSc-PAH patients already have severe right ventricular dysfunction at the time of presentation, but have more severely depressed right ventricular contractility compared with IPAH patients.[74] In addition, SSc-PAH patients are more likely to have left ventricular diastolic dysfunction and peri-cardial effusion (34% compared with 13% for IPAH).[10] In both groups, pericardial effusion portends a particularly poor prognosis.[10]

SSc-PAH patients also tend to have more severe hormonal and metabolic dysfunction such as high levels of N-terminal brain natriuretic peptide (N-TproBNP)[75] and hyponatremia.[76] Both N-TproBNP and hyponatremia have been shown, at baseline and with serial changes (for N-TproBNP[75]), to correlate with survival in PAH.[75,76]

Early Detection

Although IPAH is usually diagnosed late (patients presenting in World Health Organization functional status III and IV), a population at risk for PAH such as SSc theoretically allows establishing measures for early detection. An algorithm for early detection of PAH may be helpful if based on a combination of symptoms and screening echocardiography (**Fig. 1**), as exemplified by a recent large French registry, where patients with SSc with tricuspid regurgitation velocity (TRV) jet by transthoracic echocardiography greater than 3 m/s or between 2.5 and 3 m/s if accompanied by unexplained dyspnea, were systematically referred for RHC.[20] Investigators were able to detect incident cases of SSc-PAH with less severe disease (as judged on hemodynamic data) compared with patients with known disease. Therefore, unexplained dyspnea should prompt a search for PAH in these patients, in particular in the setting of a low single-breath DL_{CO} or declining DL_{CO} over time,[68] echo-cardiographic findings suggestive of the disease (elevated TRV jet or dilated right ventricle or right atrium), or elevated levels of N-TproBNP, which can reflect cardiac dysfunction and have been found to predict the presence of SSc-PAH.[75] Systematic screening should allow detection of early disease and prompt therapy, which may theoretically be beneficial from a prognostic standpoint.[77]

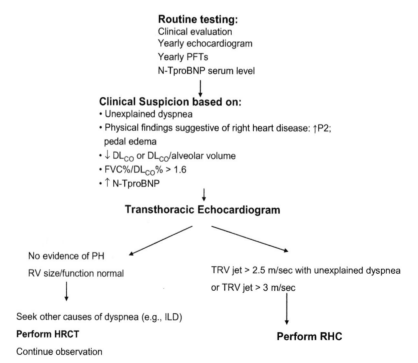

Routine testing:
Clinical evaluation
Yearly echocardiogram
Yearly PFTs
N-TproBNP serum level

Clinical Suspicion based on:
• Unexplained dyspnea
• Physical findings suggestive of right heart disease: ↑P2; pedal edema
• ↓ DL_{CO} or DL_{CO}/alveolar volume
• FVC%/DL_{CO}% > 1.6
• ↑ N-TproBNP

Transthoracic Echocardiogram

No evidence of PH
RV size/function normal

TRV jet > 2.5 m/sec with unexplained dyspnea
or TRV jet > 3 m/sec

Seek other causes of dyspnea (e.g., ILD)
Perform HRCT
Continue observation

Perform RHC

Fig. 1. Algorithm for detection of PAH in patients with systemic sclerosis, showing routine clinical tests in patients with systemic sclerosis aimed at early detection of pulmonary arterial hypertension or other causes of cardiac dysfunction (eg, left ventricular dysfunction). DL_{CO}, single-breath diffusing capacity to carbon monoxide; FVC, forced vital capacity; PFTs, pulmonary function tests; RHC, right heart catheterization; RV, right ventricle; TRV, tricuspid regurgitation jet.

Prognosis

Patients with SSc-PAH have a worse prognosis compared with patients with other forms of PAH such as IPAH. Indeed, 1-year survival rates for patients with SSc-PAH range from 50% to 81%,[9,11,21,25,78] considerably lower than the estimated 88% 1-year survival for IPAH.[79] Even when compared with patients with other forms of CTD-PAH, survival is markedly reduced in SSc-PAH (**Fig. 2**). In all patients with SSc, PAH significantly worsens survival and is one of the leading causes of mortality in these patients.[15,78,80]

PAH ASSOCIATED WITH OTHER CTDs

PAH can complicate any CTD, most frequently SSc as already discussed, but also SLE, MCTD, RA, or other diseases such as Sjögren syndrome and dermatomyositis.

Systemic Lupus Erythematosus

Pulmonary vascular involvement is common in SLE and, as in SSc, there is evidence of endothelial dysfunction with an imbalance between vasodilators and vasoconstrictors. Endothelin levels are high in patients with SLE, particularly in those patients with pulmonary hypertension. Other factors contributing to pulmonary vascular derangement in SLE include recurrent thromboembolic disease, particularly in patients with a hypercoagulable state from antiphospholipid antibodies that are present in up to 10% of patients with SLE,[81] pulmonary vasculitis, and parenchymal disease (eg, interstitial lung disease, and the shrinking lung syndrome from myositis of the diaphragm). Combined vasculitis and chronic hypoxia are frequent contributing offenders in these syndromes. Pulmonary venous hypertension may be a consequence of left ventricular dysfunction, myocarditis, or Libman-Sacks endocarditis.

The prevalence of PAH in SLE is unclear but is likely less than in SSc, affecting about 0.5% to 14% patients with SLE in a large review of the literature encompassing more than 100 patients.[82] The patients are predominantly female (90%), young (average age of 33 years at time of diagnosis), and often suffer from Raynaud phenomenon. The pathologic lesions are often indistinguishable from IPAH or SSc-PAH lesions, with intimal hyperplasia, smooth muscle cell hypertrophy, and medial thickening. Survival, which was quite poor (25%–50% at 2 years) even compared with SSc-PAH in studies antedating specific PAH therapy, is now improved and estimated at 75%.[11] It is also better than in SSc-PAH (see **Fig. 2**).

Mixed Connective Tissue Disease

Patients with MCTD have clinical features that overlap between those of SSc, SLE, RA, and polymyositis. The exact prevalence of PAH in MCTD is

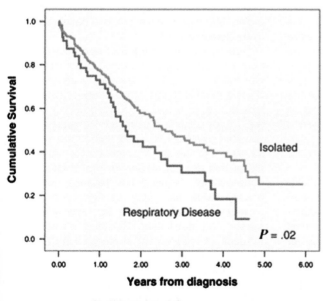

Fig. 2. Survival for patients diagnosed with PAH associated with SSc compared with patients diagnosed with PAH associated with SLE. (*From* Condliffe R, Kiely DG, Peacock AJ, et al. Connective tissue disease-associated pulmonary arterial hypertension in the modern treatment era. Am J Respir Crit Care Med 2009;179:151–7; with permission.)

Patients at risk

| 259 | 179 | 94 | 53 | 27 | 6 | Isolated |
| 56 | 38 | 18 | 10 | 3 | | Respiratory disease |

unknown but is thought to be as high as 50%.[83] PAH in these patients may occasionally respond to immunosuppressive drugs.[49]

Rheumatoid Arthritis

Both the prevalence and impact of PAH in patients with RA have not been well characterized, but are thought to be relatively low compared with other CTDs such as SSc, SLE, and MCTD.

Primary Sjögren Syndrome

Although primary Sjögren syndrome (pSS) is a relatively common autoimmune disease with glandular and extraglandular manifestations, it is very rarely complicated by PAH. In a recent review of patients with pSS and PAH by Launay and colleagues,[84] the mean age at diagnosis of PAH of these almost exclusively female patients was 50 years. Patients had severe functional class (FC III and FC IV), and hemodynamic impairment. Standard therapy (with endothelin receptor antagonists, phosphodiesterase inhibitors, or prostanoids) was typically ineffective despite an initial improvement. Some patients were reported to respond to immunosuppressive treatment. However, any conclusion regarding treatment is limited by the small size of this case report. Survival rate was low (66% at 3 years).

THERAPY FOR PAH RELATED TO CTD

Although randomized clinical trials of novel therapeutics for the treatment of PAH have included patients with PAH associated with CTD, the majority of the subjects included in trials were SSc-PAH. Given the differences in survival and potential differences in response to immunosuppressive therapy between the various forms of CTD-associated PAH, the generalizability of the results of the clinical trials may be limited to only SSc-PAH. However, the therapies discussed here are commonly used in all forms of CTD-associated PAH, although the evidence base for diseases other than SSc is lacking.

Evidence of chronically impaired endothelial function,[85–87] affecting vascular tone and remodeling, is the basis for current PAH therapy. Vasodilator therapy using high-dose calcium-channel blockers[88] is an effective long-term therapy for a minority of patients with IPAH who demonstrate acute and sustained vasodilation (eg, to nitric oxide or adenosine) during hemodynamic testing.[89] However, because most patients with CTD-associated PAH fail to demonstrate a vasodilator response to acute testing,[27] high-dose calcium-channel blocker therapy is usually not indicated

for these patients except at low dosage for Raynaud syndrome. Further, because the proportion of CTD patients who demonstrate a positive vasodilator response is so low, current guidelines recommend that vasodilator testing be performed on an individual basis in patients with CTD-associated PAH.[90]

Anti-Inflammatory Drugs

Inflammation may play a significant role in PAH associated with CTD. In this respect, it is interesting that occasional patients with severe PAH associated with some forms of CTD (such as SLE, pSS, and MCTD) have had dramatic improvement of their pulmonary vascular disease with corticosteroids and/or immunosuppressive therapy.[49] Unfortunately, this has not been the case for patients with SSc-PAH, whose PAH is usually notoriously refractory to immunosuppressive drugs.[49]

Prostaglandins

Prostacyclin (epoprostenol) has potent pulmonary vasodilatory, antiplatelet aggregating, and antiproliferative properties,[91] and has proved effective in improving exercise capacity, cardiopulmonary hemodynamics, New York Heart Association (NYHA) FC, symptoms, and survival in patients with PAH when given by continuous infusion.[92–94] In SSc-PAH, continuous intravenous epoprostenol improves exercise capacity and hemodynamics[95] compared with conventional therapy, and may have long-term beneficial effects,[96] although a clear effect on survival in these patients has yet to be demonstrated.

Treprostinil, an analogue of epoprostenol suitable for continuous subcutaneous administration, has modest effects on symptoms and hemodynamics in PAH.[97] In a small study of 16 patients (among whom 6 had CTD-related PAH), intravenous treprostinil improved the 6-minute walking distance (6MWD), FC, and hemodynamics after 12 weeks of therapy.[98] Although the safety profile of this drug is similar to that of intravenous epoprostenol, required maintenance doses are usually twice as much as for epoprostenol. However, for patients with SSc-PAH and often severe and debilitating Raynaud phenomenon, the lack of requirement of ice packing and less frequent mixing of the drug offer significant advantages.

Several reports of pulmonary edema in patients with SSc-PAH treated with prostaglandin derivatives, in both acute and chronic settings, have raised the suspicion of increased prevalence of veno-occlusive disease in these patients,[99,100] and concern about the usefulness of these drugs for this entity. Nevertheless, intravenous prostaglandin therapy remains an option for patients with CTD-PAH with NYHA class IV. Considering the frequent digital problems and disabilities that these patients often experience, this form of therapy can be quite challenging and may increase the already heavy burden of disease in these patients. In summary, both epoprostenol and treprostinil are approved by the Food and Drug Administration (FDA) for PAH, but are cumbersome therapies requiring continuous parenteral administration with the attendant numerous adverse effects (eg, infection and possibility of pump failure[101]), which make these drugs less than ideal.

Endothelin Receptor Antagonists

In randomized, placebo-controlled trials, bosentan therapy was shown to have a beneficial effect on FC, 6MWD, time to clinical worsening, and hemodynamics in PAH.[102,103] Roughly one-fifth of these patients consisted of SSc-PAH patients while a large majority had a diagnosis of IPAH. In a subgroup analysis, there was a nonsignificant trend toward a positive treatment effect on 6MWD among the SSc-PAH patients treated with bosentan compared with placebo.[103] At most, bosentan therapy prevented deterioration in these patients. Reasons for the less than optimal effect of therapy in patients with SSc-PAH are unknown, but may be related to the severity of PAH at time of presentation, as well as other factors such as potentially more severe right ventricular and pulmonary vascular dysfunction compared with patients with other forms of PAH (eg, IPAH).

In a recent analysis of patients with CTD-PAH (eg, patients with lupus, overlap syndrome, and other rheumatologic disorders) included in randomized clinical trials of bosentan, there was a trend toward improvement in 6MWD and improved survival compared with historical cohorts.[104] Single-center experience suggests that long-term outcome of first-line bosentan monotherapy is inferior in SSc-PAH compared with IPAH patients, with no change in FC and worse survival in the former group.[105] Because endothelin-1 seems to play an important pathogenic role in the development of SSc-PAH, contributing to vascular damage and fibrosis, inhibiting endothelin-1 remains a rational therapeutic strategy in these patients. As an example of the mechanistic effect, in a small study of 35 patients with SSc (10 of whom had SSc-PAH), bosentan treatment appeared to reduce endothelial cell (as determined by endothelial soluble

serum factors such as ICAM-1, VCAM-1, P-selectin, and PECAM-1) and T-cell subset (assessed by expression of lymphocyte function–associated antigen 1, very late antigen 4, and L-selectin on CD3 T cells) activation.[106] Aside from improving pulmonary hypertension, endothelin-1 receptor antagonists (specifically bosentan) cause significant reductions in the occurrence of new digital ulcerations; however, preexisting ulcers do not seem to improve with this therapy.[107]

In an effort to target the vasoconstrictive effects of endothelin while preserving its vasodilatory action, selective endothelin-A receptor antagonists have been developed. Sitaxsentan, which had been approved in Europe for the treatment of PAH, demonstrated exercise capacity, quality of life and hemodynamics in a post hoc analysis of a randomized controlled trial that included 42 patients with CTD-PAH.[108] However, recently this drug was removed from the market because of significant hepatotoxicity and death. A large placebo-controlled, randomized trial of ambrisentan, the only currently FDA-approved selective endothelin receptor antagonist, improved 6MWD in PAH patients at week 12 of treatment; however, the effect was larger in patients with IPAH than in patients with CTD-PAH (range of 50–60 m vs 15–23 m, respectively).[109] Ambrisentan is generally well tolerated, although peripheral edema (in up to 20% of patients[109]) and congestive heart failure have been reported.

Phosphodiesterase Inhibitors

Sildenafil, a phosphodiesterase type V inhibitor that reduces the catabolism of cyclic guanosine monophosphate, thereby enhancing the cellular effects mediated by nitric oxide, has become a widely used and highly efficacious therapy for PAH. The pivotal SUPER trial demonstrated that sildenafil therapy improved 6MWD in patients with IPAH, CTD-PAH, or PAH associated with repaired congenital heart disease (patients were predominantly FC II or III) at all 3 doses tested (20, 40, and 80 mg, given 3 times a day).[110] The current FDA recommended dose is 20 mg 3 times a day, because there were no significant differences in clinical effects and time to clinical worsening at week 12 between all doses tested. In a post hoc subgroup analysis of 84 patients with PAH related to CTD (45% of whom had SSc-PAH), data from the SUPER study suggest that sildenafil at a dose of 20 mg improved exercise capacity (6MWD), hemodynamic measures, and FC after 12 weeks of therapy.[111] However, there was no effect for the dose of 80 mg 3 times a day on hemodynamics in this subgroup of patients with CTD-related PAH.[111] For this reason and because of the potential for more side effects (such as bleeding from arteriovenous malformations) at high doses, a sildenafil dosage of 20 mg 3 times a day is recommended for patients with SSc-PAH (and patients with PAH associated with other forms of CTD) as standard therapy. Higher doses are occasionally attempted in cases of limited response. The impact of long-term sildenafil therapy on survival in these patients remains to be determined. Tadalafil, another phosphodiesterase inhibitor, has now been shown to be effective for PAH,[112] although subgroup analysis has not been performed as yet and thus its effects on CTD-PAH remain unclear. Tadalafil has the advantage over sildenafil of single daily dosage.

Combination Therapy

It is now common practice to add drugs when patients fail to improve on monotherapy. Adding inhaled iloprost to patients receiving bosentan has been shown to be beneficial in a small, randomized trial. Combining inhaled iloprost with sildenafil is mechanistically appealing and anecdotally efficacious,[113,114] as these drugs target separate, potentially synergistic pathways. Several multicenter trials are now exploring the efficacy of various combinations of 2 oral drugs or 1 oral and 1 inhaled drug. The recently published results of the PACES trial demonstrate that adding sildenafil (at a dose of 80 mg 3 times a day) to intravenous epoprostenol improves exercise capacity, hemodynamic measurements, time to clinical worsening, and quality of life.[115] About 21% of these patients had CTD, including 11% with SSc-PAH. Although no specific subgroup analysis is provided, improvement was apparently mainly in patients with IPAH. In a smaller single-center clinical trial, adding sildenafil to the regime of patients with IPAH or scleroderma-related PAH, after they failed initial monotherapy with bosentan, demonstrated that combination therapy improved the 6MWD and FC in IPAH patients. The outcome in patients with SSc-PAH was less favorable, although combination therapy may have halted clinical deterioration. In addition, there were more side effects reported in the SSc-PAH patients than in the IPAH patients, including hepatotoxicity that developed after addition of sildenafil to bosentan monotherapy.[116]

Anticoagulation

Based essentially on retrospective data showing a survival advantage,[87,117] anticoagulation is routinely recommended in the treatment of IPAH patients. However, the role of anticoagulation in other forms of PAH, in particular in CTD-PAH, is much less clear. Theoretically there is potential for increased bleeding in patients with CTD, particularly with SSc, in whom intestinal telangiectasias may be common. In the authors' experience, less than 50% of SSc-PAH patients started on anticoagulation remain on long-term therapy, because of bleeding complications (eg, often related to occult bleeding in the gastrointestinal tract) that are often difficult to diagnose.

Tyrosine Kinase Inhibitors

The finding that there is pathologically aberrant proliferation of endothelial and smooth muscle cells in PAH, as well increased expression of secreted growth factors such as VEGF and basic fibroblast growth factor, has caused a shift in paradigm in treatment strategies for this disease as some investigators have likened this condition to a neoplastic process reminiscent of advanced solid tumors.[118] As a result, antineoplastic drugs have been tested in experimental models.[119,120] The results of a phase II multicenter trial to evaluate the safety, tolerability, and efficacy of this drug in patients with PAH have recently published, and indicate that imatinib is well tolerated in PAH patients. Whereas there was no significant change in 6MWD (primary end point), there was a significant decrease in pulmonary vascular resistance and an increase in cardiac output in imatinib-treated patients compared with patients on placebo.[121] Whether these new antineoplastic drugs with antityrosine kinase activity will have a role in SSc (for which there is evidence for both dysregulated proliferation and increased expression of growth factors such as VEGF[122]) or in IPAH remains to be determined. A single case report suggests significant improvement of right ventricular function with imatinib treatment in a patient with SSc-PAH. Also of note is that imatinib is being investigated for SSc-related interstitial lung disease.[123]

Lung Transplantation

Lung transplantation (LT) is typically offered as a last resort to patients with PAH who fail medical therapy. CTD is not an absolute contraindication to LT; however, patients with CTD-PAH frequently suffer from associated morbidity and organ dysfunction other than the lung, which places them at a significantly increased risk for LT. Motility disorder of the esophagus and gastroesophageal reflux in patients with SSc significantly enhance the postoperative potential of aspiration and damage to the recipient lung. For these reasons, patients with SSc-PAH are often denied consideration for LT. However, if properly screened and approved for LT, patients with SSc experience similar rates of survival 2 years after the procedure in comparison with patients who receive LT for pulmonary fibrosis or IPAH.[124] In addition, a recent retrospective study suggests that the 1-year survival rate is similar for SSc patients (transplanted for respiratory failure related to PAH or interstitial lung disease) and patients with idiopathic pulmonary fibrosis, although acute rejection appears to be more common for the former group.[125]

SUMMARY

Pulmonary hypertension is a common complication of CTD, particularly SSc, for which it carries a very poor prognosis. Despite modern therapy for PAH, survival of patients with CTD-PAH remains unacceptably low. Possible reasons include an increased prevalence of pulmonary veno-occlusive lung disease in SSc-PAH patients,[126] or more severe vascular lesions affecting not only proximal and distal pulmonary vessels but also the heart (such as inflammatory myocarditis) in CTD. Thus, a better understanding of the underlying pathophysiology affecting the heart and pulmonary vessels in CTD is needed for better targeted therapy. Whether specific anti-inflammatory agents or drugs targeting tyrosine kinase activity will have any role in CTD-PAH is unclear at present, but needs to be explored.

REFERENCES

1. D'Alonzo GE, Barst RJ, Ayres SM, et al. Survival in patients with primary pulmonary hypertension. Results from a national prospective registry. Ann Intern Med 1991;115:343–9.
2. Gaine SP, Rubin LJ. Primary pulmonary hypertension. Lancet 1998;352:719–25.
3. Rich S, Dantzker DR, Ayres SM, et al. Primary pulmonary hypertension. A national prospective study. Ann Intern Med 1987;107:216–23.
4. Simonneau G, Robbins IM, Beghetti M, et al. Updated clinical classification of pulmonary hypertension. J Am Coll Cardiol 2009;54:S43–54.
5. Budhiraja R, Tuder RM, Hassoun PM. Endothelial dysfunction in pulmonary hypertension. Circulation 2004;109:159–65.
6. Humbert M, Sitbon O, Simonneau G. Treatment of pulmonary arterial hypertension. N Engl J Med 2004;351:1425–36.
7. Isern RA, Yaneva M, Weiner E, et al. Autoantibodies in patients with primary pulmonary hypertension: association with anti-Ku. Am J Med 1992;93:307–12.
8. Humbert M, Monti G, Brenot F, et al. Increased interleukin-1 and interleukin-6 serum concentrations in severe primary pulmonary hypertension. Am J Respir Crit Care Med 1995;151:1628–31.
9. Kawut SM, Taichman DB, Archer-Chicko CL, et al. Hemodynamics and survival in patients with pulmonary arterial hypertension related to systemic sclerosis. Chest 2003;123:344–50.
10. Fisher MR, Mathai SC, Champion HC, et al. Clinical differences between idiopathic and scleroderma-related pulmonary hypertension. Arthritis Rheum 2006;54:3043–50.
11. Condliffe R, Kiely DG, Peacock AJ, et al. Connective tissue disease-associated pulmonary arterial hypertension in the modern treatment era. Am J Respir Crit Care Med 2009;179:151–7.
12. Jimenez SA, Derk CT. Following the molecular pathways toward an understanding of the pathogenesis of systemic sclerosis. Ann Intern Med 2004;140:37–50.
13. Tan FK. Systemic sclerosis: the susceptible host (genetics and environment). Rheum Dis Clin North Am 2003;29:211–37.
14. LeRoy EC, Black C, Fleischmajer R, et al. Scleroderma (systemic sclerosis): classification, subsets and pathogenesis. J Rheumatol 1988;15:202–5.
15. Mayes MD. Scleroderma epidemiology. Rheum Dis Clin North Am 2003;29:239–54.
16. Silman A, Jannini S, Symmons D, et al. An epidemiological study of scleroderma in the West Midlands. Br J Rheumatol 1988;27:286–90.
17. Tamaki T, Mori S, Takehara K. Epidemiological study of patients with systemic sclerosis in Tokyo. Arch Dermatol Res 1991;283:366–71.
18. Allcock RJ, Forrest I, Corris PA, et al. A study of the prevalence of systemic sclerosis in northeast England. Rheumatology (Oxford) 2004;43: 596–602.
19. Mayes MD, Lacey JV Jr, Beebe-Dimmer J, et al. Prevalence, incidence, survival, and disease characteristics of systemic sclerosis in a large US population. Arthritis Rheum 2003;48:2246–55.
20. Hachulla E, Gressin V, Guillevin L, et al. Early detection of pulmonary arterial hypertension in systemic sclerosis: a French nationwide prospective multicenter study. Arthritis Rheum 2005;52: 3792–800.
21. Mukerjee D, St George D, Coleiro B, et al. Prevalence and outcome in systemic sclerosis associated pulmonary arterial hypertension: application of a registry approach. Ann Rheum Dis 2003;62: 1088–93.
22. Battle RW, Davitt MA, Cooper SM, et al. Prevalence of pulmonary hypertension in limited and diffuse scleroderma. Chest 1996;110:1515–9.

23. Stupi AM, Steen VD, Owens GR, et al. Pulmonary hypertension in the CREST syndrome variant of systemic sclerosis. Arthritis Rheum 1986;29: 515–24.

24. Sacks DG, Okano Y, Steen VD, et al. Isolated pulmonary hypertension in systemic sclerosis with diffuse cutaneous involvement: association with serum anti-U3RNP antibody. J Rheumatol 1996; 23:639–42.

25. MacGregor AJ, Canavan R, Knight C, et al. Pulmonary hypertension in systemic sclerosis: risk factors for progression and consequences for survival. Rheumatology (Oxford) 2001;40:453–9.

26. Fisher MR, Forfia PR, Chamera E, et al. Accuracy of Doppler echocardiography in the hemodynamic assessment of pulmonary hypertension. Am J Respir Crit Care Med 2009;179:615–21.

27. Humbert M, Sitbon O, Chaouat A, et al. Pulmonary arterial hypertension in France: results from a national registry. Am J Respir Crit Care Med 2006;173:1023–30.

28. Peacock AJ, Murphy NF, McMurray JJ, et al. An epidemiological study of pulmonary arterial hypertension. Eur Respir J 2007;30:104–9.

29. Badesch DB, Raskob GE, Elliott CG, et al. Pulmonary arterial hypertension: baseline characteristics from the REVEAL Registry. Chest 2010;137:376–87.

30. LeRoy EC. Systemic sclerosis. A vascular perspective. Rheum Dis Clin North Am 1996;22:675–94.

31. Fleischmajer R, Perlish JS. Capillary alterations in scleroderma. J Am Acad Dermatol 1980;2:161–70.

32. Sgonc R, Gruschwitz MS, Boeck G, et al. Endothelial cell apoptosis in systemic sclerosis is induced by antibody-dependent cell-mediated cytotoxicity via CD95. Arthritis Rheum 2000;43:2550–62.

33. Cerinic MM, Valentini G, Sorano GG, et al. Blood coagulation, fibrinolysis, and markers of endothelial dysfunction in systemic sclerosis. Semin Arthritis Rheum 2003;32:285–95.

34. Altman RD, Medsger TA Jr, Bloch DA, et al. Predictors of survival in systemic sclerosis (scleroderma). Arthritis Rheum 1991;34:403–13.

35. Denton CP, Bickerstaff MC, Shiwen X, et al. Serial circulating adhesion molecule levels reflect disease severity in systemic sclerosis. Br J Rheumatol 1995; 34:1048–54.

36. Distler O, Del Rosso A, Giacomelli R, et al. Angiogenic and angiostatic factors in systemic sclerosis: increased levels of vascular endothelial growth factor are a feature of the earliest disease stages and are associated with the absence of fingertip ulcers. Arthritis Res 2002;4:R11.

37. Choi JJ, Min DJ, Cho ML, et al. Elevated vascular endothelial growth factor in systemic sclerosis. J Rheumatol 2003;30:1529–33.

38. Hebbar M, Peyrat JP, Hornez L, et al. Increased concentrations of the circulating angiogenesis inhibitor endostatin in patients with systemic sclerosis. Arthritis Rheum 2000;43:889–93.

39. Okano Y, Steen VD, Medsger TA Jr. Autoantibody to U3 nucleolar ribonucleoprotein (fibrillarin) in patients with systemic sclerosis. Arthritis Rheum 1992;35:95–100.

40. Negi VS, Tripathy NK, Misra R, et al. Antiendothelial cell antibodies in scleroderma correlate with severe digital ischemia and pulmonary arterial hypertension. J Rheumatol 1998;25:462–6.

41. Fritzler MJ, Hart DA, Wilson D, et al. Antibodies to fibrin bound tissue type plasminogen activator in systemic sclerosis. J Rheumatol 1995;22:1688–93.

42. Morse JH, Barst RJ, Fotino M, et al. Primary pulmonary hypertension, tissue plasminogen activator antibodies, and HLA-DQ7. Am J Respir Crit Care Med 1997;155:274–8.

43. Grigolo B, Mazzetti I, Meliconi R, et al. Anti-topoisomerase II alpha autoantibodies in systemic sclerosis-association with pulmonary hypertension and HLA-B35. Clin Exp Immunol 2000;121:539–43.

44. Nicolls MR, Taraseviciene-Stewart L, Rai PR, et al. Autoimmunity and pulmonary hypertension: a perspective. Eur Respir J 2005;26:1110–8.

45. Tamby MC, Chanseaud Y, Humbert M, et al. Anti-endothelial cell antibodies in idiopathic and systemic sclerosis associated pulmonary arterial hypertension. Thorax 2005;60:765–72.

46. Chizzolini C, Raschi E, Rezzonico R, et al. Autoantibodies to fibroblasts induce a proadhesive and proinflammatory fibroblast phenotype in patients with systemic sclerosis. Arthritis Rheum 2002;46: 1602–13.

47. Tamby MC, Humbert M, Guilpain P, et al. Antibodies to fibroblasts in idiopathic and scleroderma-associated pulmonary hypertension. Eur Respir J 2006;28:799–807.

48. Terrier B, Tamby MC, Camoin L, et al. Identification of target antigens of antifibroblast antibodies in pulmonary arterial hypertension. Am J Respir Crit Care Med 2008;177:1128–34.

49. Sanchez O, Sitbon O, Jais X, et al. Immunosuppressive therapy in connective tissue diseases-associated pulmonary arterial hypertension. Chest 2006;130:182–9.

50. Deng Z, Morse JH, Slager SL, et al. Familial primary pulmonary hypertension (gene PPH1) is caused by mutations in the bone morphogenetic protein receptor-II gene. Am J Hum Genet 2000; 67:737–44.

51. Lane KB, Machado RD, Pauciulo MW, et al. Heterozygous germline mutations in BMPR2, encoding a TGF-beta receptor, cause familial primary pulmonary hypertension. The International PPH Consortium. Nat Genet 2000;26:81–4.

52. Newman JH, Trembath RC, Morse JA, et al. Genetic basis of pulmonary arterial hypertension:

current understanding and future directions. J Am Coll Cardiol 2004;43:33S–9S.

53. Koehler R, Grunig E, Pauciulo MW, et al. Low frequency of BMPR2 mutations in a German cohort of patients with sporadic idiopathic pulmonary arterial hypertension. J Med Genet 2004;41: e127.

54. Morse JH, Deng Z, Knowles JA. Genetic aspects of pulmonary arterial hypertension. Ann Med 2001; 33:596–603.

55. Trembath RC, Thomson JR, Machado RD, et al. Clinical and molecular genetic features of pulmonary hypertension in patients with hereditary hemorrhagic telangiectasia. N Engl J Med 2001; 345:325–34.

56. Morse J, Barst R, Horn E, et al. Pulmonary hypertension in scleroderma spectrum of disease: lack of bone morphogenetic protein receptor 2 mutations. J Rheumatol 2002;29:2379–81.

57. Tew MB, Arnett FC, Reveille JD, et al. Mutations of bone morphogenetic protein receptor type II are not found in patients with pulmonary hypertension and underlying connective tissue diseases. Arthritis Rheum 2002;46:2829–30.

58. Karrer S, Bosserhoff AK, Weiderer P, et al. The -2518 promoter polymorphism in the MCP-1 gene is associated with systemic sclerosis. J Invest Dermatol 2005;124(1):92–8.

59. Tsuchiya N, Kuroki K, Fujimoto M, et al. Association of a functional CD19 polymorphism with susceptibility to systemic sclerosis. Arthritis Rheum 2004; 50:4002–7.

60. Tolusso B, Fabris M, Caporali R, et al. -238 and +489 TNF-alpha along with TNF-RII gene polymorphisms associate with the diffuse phenotype in patients with systemic sclerosis. Immunol Lett 2005;96:103–8.

61. Kawaguchi Y, Tochimoto A, Ichikawa N, et al. Association of IL1A gene polymorphisms with susceptibility to and severity of systemic sclerosis in the Japanese population. Arthritis Rheum 2003;48: 186–92.

62. Hutyrova B, Lukac J, Bosak V, et al. Interleukin 1alpha single-nucleotide polymorphism associated with systemic sclerosis. J Rheumatol 2004;31: 81–4.

63. Crilly A, Hamilton J, Clark CJ, et al. Analysis of the 5' flanking region of the interleukin 10 gene in patients with systemic sclerosis. Rheumatology (Oxford) 2003;42:1295–8.

64. Zhou X, Tan FK, Wang N, et al. Genome-wide association study for regions of systemic sclerosis susceptibility in a Choctaw Indian population with high disease prevalence. Arthritis Rheum 2003; 48:2585–92.

65. Wipff J, Kahan A, Hachulla E, et al. Association between an endoglin gene polymorphism and systemic sclerosis-related pulmonary arterial hypertension. Rheumatology (Oxford) 2007;46: 622–5.

66. Schachna L, Wigley FM, Chang B, et al. Age and risk of pulmonary arterial hypertension in scleroderma. Chest 2003;124:2098–104.

67. Chang B, Schachna L, White B, et al. Natural history of mild-moderate pulmonary hypertension and the risk factors for severe pulmonary hypertension in scleroderma. J Rheumatol 2006;33:269–74.

68. Steen V, Medsger TA Jr. Predictors of isolated pulmonary hypertension in patients with systemic sclerosis and limited cutaneous involvement. Arthritis Rheum 2003;48:516–22.

69. Allanore Y, Borderie D, Avouac J, et al. High N-terminal pro-brain natriuretic peptide levels and low diffusing capacity for carbon monoxide as independent predictors of the occurrence of precapillary pulmonary arterial hypertension in patients with systemic sclerosis. Arthritis Rheum 2008;58:284–91.

70. Shah AA, Wigley FM, Hummers LK. Telangiectases in scleroderma: a potential clinical marker of pulmonary arterial hypertension. J Rheumatol 2010;37(1):98–104.

71. Hsiao SH, Lee CY, Chang SM, et al. Right heart function in scleroderma: insights from myocardial Doppler tissue imaging. J Am Soc Echocardiogr 2006;19:507–14.

72. Lee CY, Chang SM, Hsiao SH, et al. Right heart function and scleroderma: insights from tricuspid annular plane systolic excursion. Echocardiography 2007;24:118–25.

73. Meune C, Avouac J, Wahbi K, et al. Cardiac involvement in systemic sclerosis assessed by tissue-Doppler echocardiography during routine care: a controlled study of 100 consecutive patients. Arthritis Rheum 2008;58:1803–9.

74. Overbeek MJ, Lankhaar JW, Westerhof N, et al. Right ventricular contractility in systemic sclerosis-associated and idiopathic pulmonary arterial hypertension. Eur Respir J 2008;31:1160–6.

75. Williams MH, Handler CE, Akram R, et al. Role of N-terminal brain natriuretic peptide (N-TproBNP) in scleroderma-associated pulmonary arterial hypertension. Eur Heart J 2006;27:1485–94.

76. Forfia PR, Mathai SC, Fisher MR, et al. Hyponatremia predicts right heart failure and poor survival in pulmonary arterial hypertension. Am J Respir Crit Care Med 2008;177:1364–9.

77. Williams MH, Das C, Handler CE, et al. Systemic sclerosis associated pulmonary hypertension: improved survival in the current era. Heart 2006; 92:926–32.

78. Koh ET, Lee P, Gladman DD, et al. Pulmonary hypertension in systemic sclerosis: an analysis of 17 patients. Br J Rheumatol 1996;35:989–93.

79. McLaughlin VV, Shillington A, Rich S. Survival in primary pulmonary hypertension: the impact of epoprostenol therapy. Circulation 2002;106: 1477–82.

80. Steen VD, Medsger TA. Changes in causes of death in systemic sclerosis, 1972-2002. Ann Rheum Dis 2007;66:940–4.

81. Pope J. An update in pulmonary hypertension in systemic lupus erythematosus—do we need to know about it? Lupus 2008;17:274–7.

82. Haas C. Pulmonary hypertension associated with systemic lupus erythematosus. Bull Acad Natl Med 2004;188:985–97 [discussion: 997], [in French].

83. Sullivan WD, Hurst DJ, Harmon CE, et al. A prospective evaluation emphasizing pulmonary involvement in patients with mixed connective tissue disease. Medicine (Baltimore) 1984;63: 92–107.

84. Launay D, Hachulla E, Hatron PY, et al. Pulmonary arterial hypertension: a rare complication of primary Sjögren syndrome: report of 9 new cases and review of the literature. Medicine (Baltimore) 2007;86:299–315.

85. Giaid A, Saleh D. Reduced expression of endothelial nitric oxide synthase in the lungs of patients with pulmonary hypertension. N Engl J Med 1995; 333:214–21.

86. Tuder RM, Cool CD, Geraci MW, et al. Prostacyclin synthase expression is decreased in lungs from patients with severe pulmonary hypertension. Am J Respir Crit Care Med 1999;159:1925–32.

87. Giaid A, Yanagisawa M, Langleben D, et al. Expression of endothelin-1 in the lungs of patients with pulmonary hypertension. N Engl J Med 1993; 328:1732–9.

88. Rich S, Kaufmann E, Levy PS. The effect of high doses of calcium-channel blockers on survival in primary pulmonary hypertension. N Engl J Med 1992;327:76–81.

89. Sitbon O, Humbert M, Jais X, et al. Long-term response to calcium channel blockers in idiopathic pulmonary arterial hypertension. Circulation 2005; 111:3105–11.

90. McLaughlin VV, Archer SL, Badesch DB, et al. ACCF/AHA 2009 expert consensus document on pulmonary hypertension: a report of the American College of Cardiology Foundation Task Force on Expert Consensus Documents and the American Heart Association: developed in collaboration with the American College of Chest Physicians, American Thoracic Society, Inc, and the Pulmonary Hypertension Association. Circulation 2009; 119(16):2250–94.

91. Vane JR, Anggard EE, Botting RM. Regulatory functions of the vascular endothelium. N Engl J Med 1990;323:27–36.

92. Barst RJ, Rubin LJ, Long WA, et al. A comparison of continuous intravenous epoprostenol (prostacyclin) with conventional therapy for primary pulmonary hypertension. The Primary Pulmonary Hypertension Study Group. N Engl J Med 1996; 334:296–302.

93. McLaughlin VV, Genthner DE, Panella MM, et al. Reduction in pulmonary vascular resistance with long-term epoprostenol (prostacyclin) therapy in primary pulmonary hypertension. N Engl J Med 1998;338:273–7.

94. Rubin LJ, Mendoza J, Hood M, et al. Treatment of primary pulmonary hypertension with continuous intravenous prostacyclin (epoprostenol). Results of a randomized trial. Ann Intern Med 1990;112: 485–91.

95. Badesch DB, Tapson VF, McGoon MD, et al. Continuous intravenous epoprostenol for pulmonary hypertension due to the scleroderma spectrum of disease. A randomized, controlled trial. Ann Intern Med 2000;132:425–34.

96. Badesch DB, McGoon MD, Barst RJ, et al. Long-term survival among patients with scleroderma-associated pulmonary arterial hypertension treated with intravenous epoprostenol. J Rheumatol 2009; 36:2244–9.

97. Simonneau G, Barst RJ, Galie N, et al. Continuous subcutaneous infusion of treprostinil, a prostacyclin analogue, in patients with pulmonary arterial hypertension: a double-blind, randomized, placebo-controlled trial. Am J Respir Crit Care Med 2002; 165:800–4.

98. Tapson VF, Gomberg-Maitland M, McLaughlin VV, et al. Safety and efficacy of IV treprostinil for pulmonary arterial hypertension: a prospective, multicenter, open-label, 12-week trial. Chest 2006;129: 683–8.

99. Farber HW, Graven KK, Kokolski G, et al. Pulmonary edema during acute infusion of epoprostenol in a patient with pulmonary hypertension and limited scleroderma. J Rheumatol 1999;26:1195–6.

100. Palmer SM, Robinson LJ, Wang A, et al. Massive pulmonary edema and death after prostacyclin infusion in a patient with pulmonary veno-occlusive disease. Chest 1998;113:237–40.

101. Galie N, Manes A, Branzi A. Emerging medical therapies for pulmonary arterial hypertension. Prog Cardiovasc Dis 2002;45:213–24.

102. Channick RN, Simonneau G, Sitbon O, et al. Effects of the dual endothelin-receptor antagonist bosentan in patients with pulmonary hypertension: a randomised placebo-controlled study. Lancet 2001; 358:1119–23.

103. Rubin LJ, Badesch DB, Barst RJ, et al. Bosentan therapy for pulmonary arterial hypertension. N Engl J Med 2002;346:896–903.

104. Denton CP, Humbert M, Rubin L, et al. Bosentan treatment for pulmonary arterial hypertension related to connective tissue disease: a subgroup analysis of the pivotal clinical trials and their open-label extensions. Ann Rheum Dis 2006;65: 1336–40.

105. Girgis RE, Mathai SC, Krishnan JA, et al. Long-term outcome of bosentan treatment in idiopathic pulmonary arterial hypertension and pulmonary arterial hypertension associated with the scleroderma spectrum of diseases. J Heart Lung Transplant 2005;24:1626–31.

106. Iannone F, Riccardi MT, Guiducci S, et al. Bosentan regulates the expression of adhesion molecules on circulating T cells and serum soluble adhesion molecules in systemic sclerosis-associated pulmonary arterial hypertension. Ann Rheum Dis 2008; 67:1121–6.

107. Jain M, Varga J. Bosentan for the treatment of systemic sclerosis-associated pulmonary arterial hypertension, pulmonary fibrosis and digital ulcers. Expert Opin Pharmacother 2006;7: 1487–501.

108. Girgis RE, Frost AE, Hill NS, et al. Selective endothelin a receptor antagonism with sitaxsentan for pulmonary arterial hypertension associated with connective tissue disease. Ann. Rheum. Dis. 2007;66(11):1467–72.

109. Galie N, Olschewski H, Oudiz RJ, et al. Ambrisentan for the treatment of pulmonary arterial hypertension: results of the ambrisentan in pulmonary arterial hypertension, randomized, double-blind, placebo-controlled, multicenter, efficacy (ARIES) study 1 and 2. Circulation 2008;117:3010–9.

110. Galie N, Ghofrani HA, Torbicki A, et al. Sildenafil citrate therapy for pulmonary arterial hypertension. N Engl J Med 2005;353:2148–57.

111. Badesch DB, Hill NS, Burgess G, et al. Sildenafil for pulmonary arterial hypertension associated with connective tissue disease. J Rheumatol 2007;34: 2417–22.

112. Galie N, Brundage BH, Ghofrani HA, et al. Tadalafil therapy for pulmonary arterial hypertension. Circulation 2009;119:2894–903.

113. McLaughlin VV, Oudiz RJ, Frost A, et al. Randomized study of adding inhaled iloprost to existing bosentan in pulmonary arterial hypertension. Am J Respir Crit Care Med 2006;174:1257–63.

114. Hoeper MM, Faulenbach C, Golpon H, et al. Combination therapy with bosentan and sildenafil in idiopathic pulmonary arterial hypertension. Eur Respir J 2004;24:1007–10.

115. Simonneau G, Rubin LJ, Galie N, et al. Addition of sildenafil to long-term intravenous epoprostenol therapy in patients with pulmonary arterial hypertension: a randomized trial. Ann Intern Med 2008; 149:521–30.

116. Mathai SC, Girgis RE, Fisher MR, et al. Addition of sildenafil to bosentan monotherapy in pulmonary arterial hypertension. Eur Respir J 2007;29:469–75.

117. Fuster V, Steele PM, Edwards WD, et al. Primary pulmonary hypertension: natural history and the importance of thrombosis. Circulation 1984;70:580–7.

118. Adnot S. Lessons learned from cancer may help in the treatment of pulmonary hypertension. J Clin Invest 2005;115:1461–3.

119. Schermuly RT, Dony E, Ghofrani HA, et al. Reversal of experimental pulmonary hypertension by PDGF inhibition. J Clin Invest 2005;115:2811–21.

120. Moreno-Vinasco L, Gomberg-Maitland M, Maitland ML, et al. Genomic assessment of a multikinase inhibitor, sorafenib, in a rodent model of pulmonary hypertension. Physiol Genomics 2008; 33:278–91.

121. Ghofrani HA, Morrell NW, Hoeper MM, et al. Imatinib in pulmonary arterial hypertension patients with inadequate response to established therapy. Am J Respir Crit Care Med 2010;182(9):1171–7.

122. Grigoryev DN, Mathai SC, Fisher MR, et al. Identification of candidate genes in scleroderma-related pulmonary arterial hypertension. Transl Res 2008;151:197–207.

123. ten Freyhaus H, Dumitrescu D, Bovenschulte H, et al. Significant improvement of right ventricular function by imatinib mesylate in scleroderma-associated pulmonary arterial hypertension. Clin Res Cardiol 2009;98:265–7.

124. Schachna L, Medsger TA Jr, Dauber JH, et al. Lung transplantation in scleroderma compared with idiopathic pulmonary fibrosis and idiopathic pulmonary arterial hypertension. Arthritis Rheum 2006; 54:3954–61.

125. Saggar R, Khanna D, Furst DE, et al. Systemic sclerosis and bilateral lung transplantation: a single center experience. Eur Respir J 2010;36(4):893–900.

126. Dorfmuller P, Humbert M, Perros F, et al. Fibrous remodeling of the pulmonary venous system in pulmonary arterial hypertension associated with connective tissue diseases. Hum Pathol 2007;38: 893–902.

Congenital Heart Disease and Pulmonary Hypertension

Vedant Gupta, MD[a,b], Adriano R. Tonelli, MD[c],
Richard A. Krasuski, MD[d],*

KEYWORDS

- Congenital heart disease • Pulmonary hypertension • Eisenmenger syndrome • Management
- Treatment

KEY POINTS

- Pulmonary hypertension is common in patients with congenital heart disease, even in those patients with previously repaired lesions, and can lead to considerable symptoms, including exertional dyspnea.
- Pulmonary hypertension in these patients can be caused by pulmonary arterial or pulmonary venous causes and requires heart catheterization for accurate diagnosis.
- Some patients may be able to be treated with catheter-based or surgical interventions, particularly when the disease is reversible.
- Some patients with pulmonary arterial hypertension with unrepaired shunt lesions progress to Eisenmenger syndrome (pulmonary vascular disease with reversed [pulmonary-to-systemic] shunting). These patients have severe functional limitation and complications from systemic cyanosis.
- Successful treatment with each therapeutic class of selective pulmonary hypertension therapy (endothelin antagonists, phosphodiesterase-5 inhibitors and prostacyclin analogues) has been reported, although the BREATHE-5 (Bosentan Randomized Trial of Endothelin Antagonist Therapy-5) study, using bosentan, remains the only randomized trial of selective therapy in Eisenmenger syndrome.
- Prevention of pulmonary hypertension through early identification and repair of congenital heart defects is the ideal patient management.

INTRODUCTION

In 1897, Victor Eisenmenger described a patient with dyspnea since infancy who died of massive hemoptysis and was found on autopsy to have a large ventricular septal defect associated with abnormal pulmonary vasculature. This finding was not further characterized until nearly 60 years later. In the 1950s, more investigation gave further insight into the effect of congenital heart disease (CHD) on the pulmonary vasculature, and in 1958 Dr Paul Wood coined the term Eisenmenger syndrome to characterize patients with pulmonary hypertension (PH) caused by high pulmonary vascular resistance (PVR) associated with a large ventricular septal defect.[1] Multiple studies have

Disclosure: Dr Krasuski is on the speaker's bureau of Actelion Pharmaceuticals and Roche and has served as a consultant for Actelion Pharmaceuticals and Gilead. The other authors have no conflicts to disclose.
Funding support: None.
[a] Department of Internal Medicine, The Cleveland Clinic, 9500 Euclid Avenue, Cleveland, OH 44195, USA;
[b] Department of Medicine, The Cleveland Clinic, 9500 Euclid Avenue, Cleveland, OH 44195, USA; [c] Department of Pulmonary and Critical Care, Respiratory Institute, A90 Cleveland Clinic, 9500 Euclid Avenue, Cleveland, OH 44195, USA; [d] Department of Cardiovascular Medicine, Heart and Vascular Institute, The Cleveland Clinic, J2-4, 9500 Euclid Avenue, Cleveland, OH, USA
* Corresponding author.
E-mail address: krasusr@ccf.org

Heart Failure Clin 8 (2012) 427–445
doi:10.1016/j.hfc.2012.04.002
1551-7136/12/$ – see front matter © 2012 Elsevier Inc. All rights reserved.

since expanded our understanding of the syndrome to include other congenital heart defects.[2–19] CHD is one of the world's leading birth defects and pulmonary arterial hypertension (PAH) associated with CHD is one of the most common causes of morbidity and mortality in this group of patients.[20]

DEFINITION AND CLASSIFICATION

PH was most recently defined by the Fourth World Symposium on Pulmonary Hypertension as a mean pulmonary arterial pressure of 25 mm Hg or greater.[21] PAH is usually defined as the following: (1) mean pulmonary artery pressure of 25 mm Hg or greater and (2) either pulmonary capillary wedge pressure (PCWP) of 15 mm Hg or less or left ventricular end-diastolic pressure (LVEDP) of 15 mm Hg or less or measured left atrial pressure of less than 15 mm Hg and (3) PVR of 3 Wood units or greater.[22] It is inherent from these definitions that right heart catheterization is an essential test for the diagnosis of PAH.

The Fourth World Symposium on Pulmonary Hypertension in Dana Point, California, revised the classification of PH in 2008 (**Box 1**).[23] PH is classified into 5 different groups. The importance of the clinical system, as well as allowing a better understanding of pathophysiology, is to give a framework for understanding important branch points in the management and treatment of different conditions known to cause PH. Diseases that are predominantly associated with PAH are clustered in group 1, including idiopathic, heritable, drug-induced and toxin-induced and PAH associated with other conditions such as CHDs.[23] The reason for including CHDs in group 1 is because its histology and endothelial cell abnormalities are indistinguishable from other causes of PAH.[24]

Classically, all congenital conditions are grouped together when considered as a cause of PAH. However, it is important to identify the underlying congenital defect, because this has important prognostic implications. To help in this task, the Fourth World Symposium on Pulmonary Hypertension updated the anatomic and pathophysiologic classification of CHDs. This classification encompasses the type and dimension of the defect, direction of the shunt, associated cardiac and extracardiac abnormalities and repair status (**Box 2**).[23] Its use is helpful in providing a more detailed description for each particular condition.

PAH associated with CHD (PAH-CHD) is generally classified as PAH associated with small defects (ventricular or atrial septal defects less than 1 and 2 cm, respectively; presenting in similar fashion to idiopathic PAH), PAH associated with systemic-to-pulmonary shunts (moderate to large defects without cyanosis), Eisenmenger syndrome (large defects with severe increases in PVR and reversed or bidirectional shunting) and PAH after corrective surgery (PAH persists or recurs after surgery in the absence of postoperative residual lesions).[23]

Not all CHDs with systemic-to-pulmonary shunts lead to significant PH. Truncus arteriosus, ventricular septal defects, atrial septal defects, and patent ductus arteriosus are the mostly commonly identified lesions associated with severe PH and the development of Eisenmenger syndrome.

Eisenmenger syndrome is generally the result of systemic-to-pulmonary shunts caused by large congenital heart defects that with time lead to reversed (pulmonary-to-systemic) or bidirectional shunting accompanied by oxygen-unresponsive hypoxemia. It represents the most advanced form of PAH-CHD. This syndrome manifests as a disease process and not as an isolated condition. The clinical scenario includes reduced functional capacity, worsening hypoxia, cyanosis, erythrocytosis, and multiple organ system involvement.

UNIQUE CHARACTERISTICS COMPARED WITH OTHER CAUSES OF PAH

Although PAH-CHD is similar in many ways to other causes of PAH, there are some important differences. Unlike other causes of PAH, congenital left-to-right shunts lead to a more progressive increase of right ventricular pressures early in life, allowing the right ventricle to remodel and accommodate for the increased afterload. This chronic course allows patients to reset their normal level of activity, adjusting it to help compensate for the chronic hypoxia.[25–29] Therefore, they may not report the presence of significant symptoms with regular activity, underscoring the need for more objective assessment, as outlined later.

In addition, patients with PAH-CHD more commonly experience hemoptysis, cerebrovascular accidents, brain abscesses, erythrocytosis, coagulation abnormalities, and cardiac arrhythmias than other causes of PAH.[30] Adult patients with Eisenmenger syndrome have a more favorable hemodynamic profile and possibly a better prognosis than other groups of patients with PAH.[19]

EPIDEMIOLOGY

Congenital heart defects are usually reported in ~8 of 1000 live births.[31] Although the prevalence of CHD in the Western world has remained fairly constant, the number of adults with congenital heart lesions has gradually increased, as a result

Box 1
Updated clinical classification of PH (Dana Point, 2008)

1. PAH

    1.1. Idiopathic PAH

    1.2. Heritable

        1.2.1. BMPR2

        1.2.2. ALK1, endoglin (with or without hereditary hemorrhagic telangiectasia)

        1.2.3. Unknown

    1.3. Drug-induced and toxin-induced

    1.4. Associated with

        1.4.1. Connective tissue diseases

        1.4.2. Human immunodeficiency virus infection

        1.4.3. Portal hypertension

        1.4.4. CHDs

        1.4.5. Schistosomiasis

        1.4.6. Chronic hemolytic anemia

    1.5. Persistent PH of the newborn

    1.6. Pulmonary veno-occlusive disease or pulmonary capillary hemangiomatosis

2. PH caused by left heart disease

    2.1. Systolic dysfunction

    2.2. Diastolic dysfunction

    2.3. Valvular disease

3. PH caused by lung diseases or hypoxia

    3.1. Chronic obstructive pulmonary disease (COPD)

    3.2. Interstitial lung disease

    3.3. Other pulmonary diseases with mixed restrictive and obstructive pattern

    3.4. Sleep-disordered breathing

    3.5. Alveolar hypoventilation disorders

    3.6. Chronic exposure to high altitude

    3.7. Developmental abnormalities

4. Chronic thromboembolic PH

5. PH with unclear multifactorial mechanisms

    5.1. Hematologic disorders: myeloproliferative disorders, splenectomy

    5.2. Systemic disorders: sarcoidosis, pulmonary Langerhans cell histiocytosis: lymphangioleiomyomatosis, neurofibromatosis, vasculitis

    5.3. Metabolic disorders: glycogen storage disease, Gaucher disease, thyroid disorders

    5.4. Others: tumoral obstruction, fibrosing mediastinitis, chronic renal failure on dialysis

From Simonneau G, Robbins IM, Beghetti M, et al. Updated clinical classification of pulmonary hypertension. J Am Coll Cardiol 2009;54:S45; with permission.

of the development of successful operative repairs at an earlier age. There are now estimated to be nearly a million adults with CHD in North America, and, for the first time in medical history, more adults than children with congenital heart lesions.[32]

It is estimated that 5% to 10% of adults with CHD develop PAH.[22,33] Some studies estimate 4% to

Box 2
Anatomic-pathophysiologic classification of
congenital systemic-to-pulmonary shunts
associated with PAH

1. Type

  Simple pre-tricuspid shunts

    Atrial septal defect

      Ostium secundum

      Sinus venosus

      Ostium primum

    Total or partial unobstructed anomalous
    pulmonary venous return

  Simple post-tricuspid shunts

    Ventricular septal defect (VSD)

    Patent ductus arteriosus

  Combined shunts

  Complex congenital heart disease

    Complete atrioventricular septal defect

    Truncus arteriosus

    Single ventricle physiology with unob-
    structed pulmonary blood flow

    Transposition of the great arteries with
    VSD and/or patent ductus arteriosus

    Other

2. Dimension

  Hemodynamic

    Restrictive (pressure gradient across the
    defect)

    Nonrestrictive

  Anatomic

    Small to moderate (ASD $\leq$2 cm and VSD
    $\leq$1 cm)

    Large (ASD >2 cm and VSD >1 cm)

3. Direction of shunt

  Predominantly systemic-to-pulmonary

  Predominantly pulmonary-to-systemic

  Bidirectional

4. Associated cardiac and extracardiac abnor
   -malities

5. Repair status

  Unoperated

  Palliated

  Repaired

Adapted from Simonneau G, Robbins IM, Beghetti M,
et al. Updated clinical classification of pulmonary hypertension. J Am Coll Cardiol 2009;54:S47; with permission.

10% of all patients with CHD develop Eisenmenger syndrome; however, this increases to as high as 30% in patients with unrepaired congenital defects.[33–35] Worldwide, it is estimated that 3.2 million children are at risk for the development of PAH-CHD.[24] Most of them do not develop Eisenmenger syndrome, particularly if cardiac repair occurs within the first 2 years of life. Worldwide, because of inequality of access to medical care, only some patients (2%–15%) undergo reparative surgery.[24] A large outcome study in PAH-CHD showed a prevalence of PAH in CHD of 5.8% and its presence increased all-cause mortality and cardiac complications, including heart failure and arrhythmias, more than 2-fold and 3-fold, respectively.[36] In addition, the presence of PAH increased hospital days and intensive care unit days by more than 3-fold when compared with patients with CHD without PAH. Given the increased recognition of CHD in the pediatric population coupled with advances in surgical and medical management for congenital lesions, more patients with more complex congenital lesions are surviving to adulthood. These patients may present with various degrees of PAH in adulthood, underscoring the importance of adult cardiologists evolving their understanding of both CHD and PAH.

PATHOPHYSIOLOGY

Increased pulmonary blood flow from systemic-to-pulmonary shunts is responsible for initiating a series of events responsible for causing changes in the pulmonary vasculature that lead to pulmonary obstructive arteriopathy and to an increase in PVR and PAH.[10] Main risk factors for the development of PAH include the type and size of the underlying anatomic defect and magnitude of shunt. Initial dynamic PAH is reversible, if corrective surgery is performed before vascular changes become permanent. The potential for reversibility is difficult to assess, and there is a paucity of information in this regard.[2]

Most of the pathophysiologic processes in PAH-CHD seem similar to the pathogenesis implicated in the development of other forms of PAH. The pathogenesis of PAH is explained by a persistent high flow and pressure in the pulmonary vasculature that causes endothelial damage, leading to loss of endothelial barrier function and imbalance of vasoactive mediators that favor vasoconstriction, inflammation, thrombosis, cell proliferation, apoptosis, and fibrosis and result in pulmonary vascular remodeling and irreversible PAH.[37] A more detailed description of the mechanisms involved in the development of PAH helps to understand current and potential future therapeutic interventions.

The destruction of the vascular endothelial barrier causes degradation of the extracellular matrix as well as release of growth factors such as fibroblast growth factor, angiopoietin-1 and transforming growth factor β, which induces smooth muscle hypertrophy and proliferation.[38] In addition, endothelial dysfunction leads to activation of cytokines and localized inflammatory cascades.[39]

The pulmonary endothelium is responsible for the production of many vascular mediators. With endothelial cell dysfunction, there is a shift toward vasoconstriction, cellular proliferation, and apoptosis caused by increased production and decreased destruction of vasoconstrictors (ie, endothelin-1 and thromboxane A$_2$), as well as decreased production and increased destruction of vasodilators, such as nitric oxide (NO) and prostacyclin. Endothelin-1 is a potent vasoconstrictor that can cause smooth muscle proliferation as well, leading to vascular remodeling. Circulating endothelin levels have been found to correlate with disease severity and outcome in idiopathic PH,[40–42] although this mediator has been less extensively studied in Eisenmenger syndrome.[16,43–45]

The pulmonary endothelium is a major producer of NO. NO is endogenously synthesized by NO synthases and is a freely diffusible molecule that enters the pulmonary smooth muscle cells to produce guanosine 3′, 5′-cyclic monophosphate (cGMP), resulting in vasodilation, helping keep the pulmonary vascular circuit at low pressure.[46–48] Phosphodiesterases are responsible for breakdown of cGMP. With impaired production and normal degradation, cGMP levels decline, thereby decreasing cGMP-mediated vasodilation.[16,49,50] Endothelial damage also causes a decrease in prostacyclin production, a potent vasodilator that also inhibits platelet aggregation and smooth muscle cell proliferation by increasing cAMP levels.[8,16,21,51]

Recent research has revealed a genetic predisposition[52] (because not all patients with CHD develop PAH) and suggests the presence of other potential pathways involved in the pathogenesis of PAH-CHD, including downregulation of potassium channels,[53] increased matrix metalloproteinases,[54] decreased vasoactive intestinal peptide,[55] increased serotonin[56] and transforming growth factor β levels,[57] among others.[58] Potential new biomarkers and lines of therapies could result from these discoveries.[59]

CLINICAL PRESENTATION

The clinical presentation of PAH-CHD can be varied, and there is not a pathognomonic symptom pattern that can be easily identified. There are many different factors affecting the presenting symptoms: the underlying congenital defect, the repair status, and the degree of initial and residual shunting. Symptoms from PH itself are also nonspecific and include breathlessness, fatigue, chest pain, and syncope. Depending on the severity of PH, there may be cyanosis and clubbing. Most left-to-right congenital shunts do not initially have cyanosis, but its presence is often the harbinger of increasing pulmonary pressures and the development of Eisenmenger syndrome.[13,20,60] Complex congenital lesions may have some degree of chronic cyanosis, making the identification of worsening cyanosis difficult. In advanced stages, patients develop progressive right ventricular dysfunction, which may result in sudden death.

Exercise Intolerance

Dyspnea on exertion is the most common presenting symptom. Many patients with CHD have some degree of exercise intolerance, particularly those with PAH. Some estimates suggest that more than 90% of patients with PAH-CHD have New York Heart Association (NYHA) class II or worse symptoms. As mentioned earlier, these patients progressively restrict their regular activity, which complicates accurate estimation of their functional capacity.[61–64] Exercise intolerance is a nonspecific symptom, because it can represent PAH itself, hypoxemia, worsening heart failure, or deconditioning.

Hemoptysis

Hemoptysis is another common symptom in PAH-CHD, and is most often present in patients with Eisenmenger syndrome. Hemoptysis is caused by the development of bronchial collaterals in patients with long-standing cyanosis.[30] Case series and retrospective studies indicate that anywhere from 11% to 100% of patients present with hemoptysis.[1,25,65–67] Although unsettling for most patients, hemoptysis is generally not a cause of mortality for these patients.[25,65–67]

Pulmonary Embolism

Given the extensive strain on the pulmonary arterial system, as well as turbulent flow, there is a higher risk of pulmonary thromboembolism in patients with PAH-CHD. Some case series report that up to 30% of patients with Eisenmenger syndrome present with clinically detectable intrapulmonary thrombus, usually manifested by rapidly worsening dyspnea, hemoptysis, chest pain, and tachycardia.[68,69]

Hematologic Manifestations

There are a few major hematologic manifestations, including reactive or secondary erythrocytosis and chronic thrombocytopenia. Depending on the level of hypoxemia, patients with PAH-CHD develop compensatory erythrocytosis, which when severe can lead to hyperviscosity syndrome, the manifestations of which include headaches, blurry vision, dizziness, paresthesias, and myalgias.[70–74] Patients with Eisenmenger syndrome are generally iron deficient, and iron supplementation (oral or intravenous) is often necessary.

Because of the chronic hypoxemia, the presence of PAH and the use of epoprostenol, most patients with Eisenmenger syndrome have chronic thrombocytopenia, platelet dysfunction, and difficulties with clotting.[73–76] In addition, passive congestion of the liver because of worsening right heart failure can lead to deficiencies in clotting factor production. As a result, some patients may present with bleeding, although this is usually a late manifestation of the syndrome.

Infectious Considerations

Patients with congenital shunt lesions and coexistent cyanosis are at particularly high risk of bacterial endocarditis. Studies suggest that risk of development of endocarditis in unrepaired ventricular septal defects may be as high as 13% lifetime.[40] The risk in patients with Eisenmenger syndrome seems even more substantial (4% in 1 series over only 2 years of follow-up). Another infectious complication is cerebral abscess, presumably from septic emboli, with an incidence of more than 6% in patients with Eisenmenger syndrome followed for a 6-year period.[65]

Arrhythmias

Arrhythmias are often a late manifestation in patients with Eisenmenger syndrome and the most common cause of death. Patients with Eisenmenger syndrome are at significantly increased risk of sudden cardiac death,[66] with ventricular arrhythmias being the presumed cause. These arrhythmias result from a multitude of factors including structural heart lesions, electrolyte abnormalities, and worsening heart failure. Supraventricular arrhythmias are also common, with 1 study reporting supraventricular arrhythmias in 42% of patients on 24-hour Holter monitoring.

Other

Less frequently reported complications associated with PH in patients with CHD include bile stones, hyperuricemia and gout, acute renal injury associated with both hyperuricemia and glomerular injury, hepatic dysfunction, and cerebrovascular disease.[76–79]

DIAGNOSIS
History and Physical Examination

The history and physical examination are often insufficient to tease out PAH-CAD as the cause of PH. However, they are helpful in identifying when further investigation is necessary. It is important to inquire into the onset, severity, and progression of symptoms, because it may help to assess the severity of the condition.[20,60] In addition, associated symptoms may suggest a particular cause of PH.

Underlying conditions can give some insight into other causes of PH, such as a history of malignancy, which may be associated with chronic thromboembolic pulmonary disease, COPD, which can indicate PH associated with lung disease, and cardiovascular risk factors such as diabetes, which can point toward left heart failure. All of these conditions may also coexist with CHD.

Particular attention should be placed on determining the type of heart defect and the timing and nature of the corrective procedures, because these can alter the natural history of the disease. In general, patients with CHD have a more insidious course, thus a more insightful line of questioning may be necessary. For example, asking whether a patient is dyspneic may not be enough.[20,60] On the other hand, asking what activities the patient was able to do a few months ago but is not able to do now may provide more detailed information.

Physical examination in a patient with CHD may show cyanosis and clubbing of the fingernails and toenails. If the unrepaired defect is a patent ductus arteriosus, the feet may be cyanosed and clubbed, whereas the right and possibly also the left arm may be spared (pink and unclubbed), depending on the location of the duct. This finding is pathognomonic for an Eisenmenger ductus. There may be a prominent second pulmonic sound associated with increased pulmonary pressures, although this finding is often subtle. It is important to assess for S3 gallops, suggestive of heart failure and other valvular heart defects.[60] It is also important to perform a thorough cardiopulmonary examination, specifically looking for the typical findings found with atrial septal defects, ventricular septal defects, and patent ductus arteriosus, taking into account that as the PVR increases, the shunt decreases and most of the classic murmurs disappear.

Routine Laboratory Testing

Every patient with CHD should undergo routine laboratory evaluation, including complete blood counts, serum electrolytes, blood urea nitrogen, serum creatinine, and liver function tests. Specifically, it is important to assess for erythrocytosis, because a hematocrit level greater than 65% can be associated with hyperviscosity.[80] Given the propensity for arrhythmias, it is important to check for serum electrolytes, specifically potassium, magnesium, and calcium. Evaluation of the patient's renal function and liver function tests is also important for therapeutic monitoring.

Brain natriuretic peptide (BNP) and N-terminal pro-BNP have both been shown to be increased in pediatric and adult patients with CHD, both with and without PAH.[81,82] The lack of specificity makes these tests not particularly useful for the diagnosis of PAH. However; multiple studies have shown BNP to correlate with exercise capacity, response to therapy, and overall survival.[41,81]

Chest Radiography

The chest radiograph (CXR) is a sensitive, albeit nonspecific test. It is not particularly useful for diagnosis, prognosis, or treatment monitoring. Some studies have suggested that ~90% of patients with PAH have an abnormal CXR at the time of presentation, most often increased central pulmonary vascular congestion with loss of peripheral vessels.[83] On occasion, an abnormal CXR may reveal intrinsic lung disease that can motivate further evaluation.

Echocardiogram

Every patient with CHD should have at the least a transthoracic echocardiogram performed, ideally with a performing sonographer and an interpreting cardiologist with CHD experience. This test is important not only in the evaluation for congenital defects but also to estimate pulmonary pressure and assess for right ventricular strain. In addition, it assesses left ventricular function as a cause or contributor to PH and facilitates noninvasive monitoring after initiation of therapy or when symptoms progress.[22,84,85] Subcostal images from a transthoracic echocardiogram in **Fig. 1** show a large ventricular septal defect with evidence of bidirectional shunting, suggesting advanced PAH-CHD.

Cardiac Catheterization

Every patient with PH should be evaluated with a cardiac catheterization before initiation of PAH-specific therapy. The importance of this strategy is most evident in the CHD population, in whom pure PAH is often the exception rather than the rule. In the original Boston Adult Congenital Heart Cohort more than 80% of patients with CHD had coexistent triggers for increased pulmonary pressure outside PAH. These triggers included increased left-sided pressures, pulmonary artery or vein stenoses, and thromboembolic disease (Dr Michael J. Landzberg, personal communication, 2011). Similarly, in our cohort of patients with presumed PAH-CHD at the Cleveland Clinic, we have found other causes responsible for pulmonary pressure increase in more than one-third of patients. Empiric therapy with a selective pulmonary vasoactive therapy in lieu of catheterization in such patients may be detrimental. Certain patient populations such as those with repaired tetralogy of Fallot deserve closer attention when increased right-sided pressure is found on echocardiography. In such patients, a variety of other associated lesions can be responsible for increased right-sided pressures, including unexpected right ventricular outflow obstruction, peripheral pulmonic stenosis(es), and aortopulmonary collaterals.

The cardiac catheterization in the patient with PAH-CAD should include a full oximetry run to assess for the presence of shunting and to quantify the direction of this shunt. **Fig. 2** shows the stages of progression in a patient with a large ventricular septal defect, with notation made regarding the expected saturations in each heart chamber. Early in the disease process (see **Fig. 2**A) the shunt is left to right and large resulting in a significant step up in oxygenation at the level of the right ventricle. As the disease progresses (see **Fig. 2**B), the shunt progressively decreases as the PVR rises. Late in the disease process (see **Fig. 2**C), the PVR is large and the shunt reverses (becomes right to left). Also the cardiac output is reduced, as shown by the decreased saturation of the mixed venous (right atrial) blood.

Ideally, a vasodilator challenge should also be performed during catheterization, with careful attention to the impact on the amount and direction of the shunt. In some cases, balloon occlusion of the defect can be helpful to assess the impact on pulmonary pressures. In such cases, simultaneous measurement of pulmonary and systemic pressures during the occlusion is essential. We have found that a significant decrease in PVR identifies patients in whom repair is still feasible, whereas a decrease in systemic pressure during occlusion should be an ominous sign and absolute contraindication to defect repair.

The vasodilator challenge also seems to predict prognosis in patients with CHD. Inhaled NO

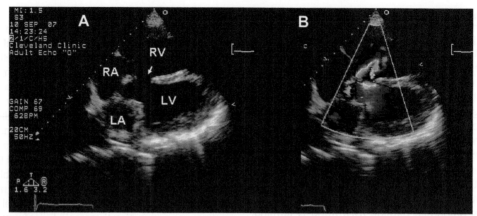

Fig. 1. Subcostal images from a transthoracic echocardiogram in a patient with a large ventricular septal defect (*arrow*) and PH. Images are without (*A*) and with (*B*) color Doppler applied. LA, left atrium; LV, left ventricle; RA, right atrium; RV, right ventricle.

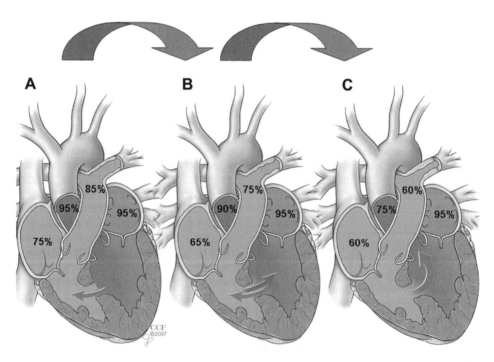

Fig. 2. The stages of progression of pulmonary vascular disease in a patient with a large ventricular septal defect (the arrows signify the flow of blood across the ventricular septal defect). The chambers are annotated with the oxygen saturations. Early in the disease process (*A*) the shunt is left to right and large. The right atrial saturation (equal to the mixed venous saturation) is 75% and increases to 85% beyond the right ventricle because of the shunt. The left atrial and aortic saturations are the same because no right to left shunt is present. As the disease progresses (*B*), the shunt is progressively reduced as the PVR rises. The cardiac output is starting to decrease as a result of the development of right ventricular dysfunction (decreased to 65%). There remains some left to right shunting (pulmonary artery saturation is 75%) but the aortic saturation (90%) is now lower than the left atrial saturation (95%) because some right to left shunting (bidirectional shunt) is present. Late in the disease process (*C*), the PVR is large and the shunt is fully reversed (right to left). The cardiac output is now even more reduced (right atrial saturation is 60%) and no step-up in saturation is now seen. A substantial decrease in aortic saturation (75%) is present as a result of the large right to left shunt. (*Courtesy of* Cleveland Clinic Foundation, Cleveland, OH; with permission.)

combined with oxygen can help identify candidates for corrective cardiac surgery and in addition identify patients with better long-term clinical outcome.[86–90]

Left heart catheterization may be necessary to confirm the LVEDP if the PCWP is difficult to obtain or interpret. Coronary angiography may also be needed to assess for atherosclerosis in older patients.

Current European and American College of Cardiology (ACC)/American Heart Association (AHA) guidelines strongly recommend a baseline right heart catheterization with a vasodilator challenge for both diagnostic purposes and before initiating therapy. In addition, monitoring for efficacy of PAH therapy invasively is suggested, although no time frame for repeating catheterization is provided.[22,84,85]

Exercise Testing

Formal exercise testing serves multiple purposes, which include assessing the severity of disease, determining prognosis, and evaluating the effectiveness of therapy. Two methods to assess exercise tolerance are the 6-minute walk test (6MWT) and cardiopulmonary exercise testing. Motivated by its simplicity, most studies in PH use the 6MWT to assess response to therapy.[62–64,91] Current guidelines recommend exercise testing before initiating therapy and at 3-month to 6-month intervals thereafter.[22,85]

Advanced Studies

More advanced studies such as transesophageal echocardiography, cardiac magnetic resonance imaging, V/Q scanning, and pulmonary function testing should be performed only if clinically indicated and if they are not part of the routine workup.[22,85]

TREATMENT
General Principles of Therapy

Patients with PAH-CHD should be monitored at regular intervals by experienced physicians to assess for changes in symptom profile, vital signs, complete blood counts, and electrolytes. The treatment strategy is for the most part based on clinical experience rather than being evidence-based.[30] Patients with Eisenmenger syndrome, in particular, should be managed in centers with experience in the treatment of this syndrome.[22]

A treatment approach for PAH-CHD similar to other causes of PAH has recently been proposed (**Fig. 3**).[92] Parts of this algorithm have been derived primarily from studies in idiopathic disease and

PAH associated with connective tissue disease, therefore care should be taken when extrapolating these data to PAH-CHD.[30]

Oxygen therapy
Most patients with CHD, depending on the degree of shunting, have a degree of chronic hypoxia. Oxygen therapy does not improve exercise tolerance or survival in these patients; however, some patients still receive oxygen to use with exertion or on a nocturnal basis, based on symptom relief.[93] Care should be exercised not to overoxygenate these patients, because this may depress their respiratory drive and lead to further hypoxia. Also because these patients are prone to bleeding, because of the hematologic issues mentioned earlier, high-flow nasal cannula oxygen can result in epistaxis, with all of its attendant problems.

Aerobic exercise
Aerobic exercise is often avoided by patients with CHD because of worsening dyspnea. However, it is important to encourage continued aerobic exercise to improve exercise tolerance. However, it is recommended to avoid strenuous exercise.[22]

Anticoagulation
There is a paucity of evidence regarding anticoagulation in patients with PAH-CHD. Therefore, current practice is varied and fragmented. Most centers anticoagulate these patients given their prothrombotic propensity.[25,68,69,73] However, because of the increased risk of hemorrhage and hemoptysis, anticoagulation should be carefully monitored.[22,25]

Antibiotic prophylaxis
Patients with CHD are at a markedly increased risk of infectious complications, specifically bacterial endocarditis.[40,66] Current ACC/AHA guidelines recommend antibiotic prophylaxis for invasive dental procedures (any procedure involving gum manipulation) in unrepaired patients with cyanotic CHD, patients with residual defects at the site or adjacent to the site of a prosthetic patch or prosthetic device that prevents endothelialization after repair, and for any patients within 6 months of surgical or percutaneous repairs using prosthetic materials or devices.[84,94,95] We further propose that any patient with CHD, repaired or unrepaired, who has associated PH should receive appropriate prophylactic antibiotics before dental procedures, given their complexity and poor clinical reserve.

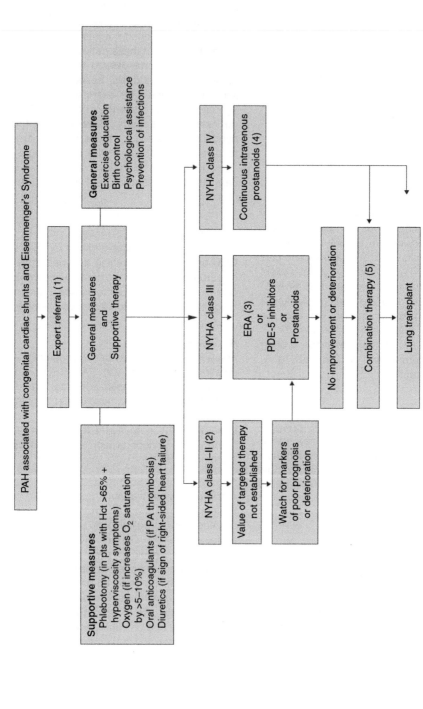

Fig. 3. Treatment algorithm for PAH-CHD. (1) Because of the complexity of the condition and the multiple treatment options available, expert referral is recommended. (2) Patients can remain clinically stable for prolonged periods and the efficacy/safety ratio of different therapies in these groups is not clear. (3) More evidence supports the use of bosentan. (4) Unstable patients should be treated with intravenous prostacyclin analogues, based on expert opinion. (5) In the absence of improvement or deterioration, combination therapy should be considered. (*Reproduced from* Galie N, Manes A, Palazzini M, et al. Management of pulmonary arterial hypertension associated with congenital systemic-to-pulmonary shunts and Eisenmenger's syndrome. Drugs 2008;68:1062; with permission.)

Diuretics, digitalis, antiarrhythmics, and calcium-channel blockers

Diuretics and digitalis are often used on an individual patient basis in Eisenmenger syndrome, with the precaution of avoiding dehydration, which can worsen hyperviscosity and produce hypotension.[29] Supraventricular and ventricular arrhythmias are common and may lead to hemodynamic decompensation and sudden death.[60] Amiodarone is often used, and the role of implantable defibrillators is unknown.[67] None of these approaches has significantly modified survival or risk of deterioration.[66] Calcium-channel blockers are generally contraindicated in patients with Eisenmenger syndrome because of their negative inotropic effects and systemic vasodilation (which increases right-to-left shunt and can worsen cyanosis).[22,92,96]

Treatment of hyperviscosity syndrome

Patients with hematocrit levels greater than 65% are at increased risk of hyperviscosity syndrome. When clinical judgment warrants phlebotomy for relief of symptoms of hyperviscosity, care needs to be taken to avoid air embolization and the risk of stroke.[70,73,77] Also, because these patients are sensitive to volume, adequate volume replacement is an important part of this therapy. Routine phlebotomy in cyanotic patients with CHD is associated with worsening exercise tolerance and increased risk of stroke, and therefore should be avoided.[70] In addition, monitoring for and treatment of iron deficiency is important, to ensure adequate hematopoiesis and erythrocytosis that is appropriate to the level of hypoxemia.[22,29]

Avoidance of pregnancy

CHD associated with PH is associated with a significantly increased risk of maternal and fetal morbidity and mortality. Some estimates suggest up to a 50% risk of maternal mortality and 40% risk of spontaneous abortion in patients with Eisenmenger syndrome.[97–99] These patients have an increased risk of cardiovascular events during birth, manifested as a higher incidence of arrhythmia, heart failure, and embolic events.[100] Therefore, pregnancy should be strongly discouraged in these patients. In individuals who become pregnant and do not wish to undergo elective abortion, careful monitoring and a multidisciplinary approach are essential.

For contraception, intrauterine devices impregnated with progesterone may be the best option, given theirs overall effectiveness and decreased risk of systemic thrombosis. Oral estrogen-based contraception is associated with an increased risk of thromboembolic events, and therefore is not ideal in these patients. Oral progesterone-based contraception has a high failure rate, and surgical options carry with them considerable perioperative risk.

Specific PH therapeutic options

Randomized controlled trials that have shown benefits of PH-specific therapies in patients with PAH have included a few individuals with Eisenmenger syndrome. This important limitation complicates the treatment strategy for these patients. PAH-specific therapies center around 3 major pathways: endothelin, NO, and prostacyclin.

Endothelin receptor antagonists Endothelin receptor antagonists (ERAs) are the most extensively studied class of medications for PAH-CHD. Three drugs in this class have been studied in patients with PAH: bosentan, ambrisentan, and sitaxsentan.[30] Bosentan (Tracleer) is a dual ERA that acts on both endothelin A and B receptors. Until recently, there had only been small-scale, open-label trials, which suggested efficacy of oral bosentan in patients with PAH-CHD.[87,101–108] The BREATHE-5 (Bosentan Randomized Trial of Endothelin Antagonist Therapy-5) trial was the first large (bosentan n = 37, placebo n = 17), randomized, double-blind, placebo-controlled trial looking at bosentan in World Health Organization (WHO) class III Eisenmenger syndrome. At 16 weeks, bosentan significantly improved exercise capacity (patients were able to walk 53.1 m more during 6MWT) and reduced PVR index (–472 dyn s/cm^5) and mean pulmonary artery pressure (–5.5 mm Hg) compared with placebo. In addition, bosentan did not worsen oxygen saturation.[109] A post hoc analysis showed no difference in efficacy within different types of congenital defects.[110] Long-term data have shown that the improvement on bosentan can be maintained without safety or tolerability issues.[111–116] A more recent randomized controlled trial of bosentan in patients with NYHA functional class II PAH included patients with PAH-CHD (n = 32 of 185 individuals). At 6 months, PVR significantly decreased from baseline but 6MWT distance change did not reach statistical significance (mean treatment effect 19.1 m, $P = .076$).[117] There appeared to be no difference in the short-term clinical response between adults and children with PAH associated with systemic-to-pulmonary shunts. Several studies have shown continued benefit in exercise tolerance (6MWT), NYHA functional class, and physical/mental health (Short Form-36 score), as far as 5 years from initiation of therapy. This benefit is more robust in patients with PAH-CHD without Down syndrome.[118–121] The predominant adverse reaction of bosentan is increased hepatic transaminases, which can be seen up to ~10% of patients.[105,116] However, the distinct benefit is that it is an oral agent and simple to administer. Dosage is generally initiated at 62.5 mg twice daily and uptitrated to 125 mg twice daily after 4 weeks.

Ambrisentan (Letaris) is a single ERA with preferential activity on the endothelin A receptor. It was studied in 2 large randomized, double-blind, placebo-controlled trials with improved exercise tolerance (6MWT), functional class (WHO), health survey score (Short Form-36 score), dyspnea score (Borg) and B-type natriuretic peptide in patients with PAH after 12 weeks of treatment.[122,123] Patients with PAH-CHD were excluded from this study; however, a recent single-center study involving 17 patients showed short-term (~6 months) improvement in exercise capacity (6MWT). This beneficial response diminished during long-term follow-up (~2.5 years).[124] Overall, there have been limited data with the use of this medication in PAH-CHD. Its benefits include better tolerance and less drug-to-drug interaction than other ERAs.[125]

Phosphodiesterase type-5 inhibitors Phosphodiesterase type-5 (PDE-5) inhibitors, such as sildenafil (Revatio) and tadalafil (Adcirca), inhibit the breakdown of cGMP in smooth muscle cells, leading to enhanced cGMP-mediated vasodilation. In a large randomized, placebo-controlled study, patients with PAH (including patients with PAH-CHD) reported improvements in exercise capacity, WHO function class, and hemodynamics after 12 weeks of treatment.[126] There have been limited data on PDE-5 inhibitors specifically in patients with Eisenmenger syndrome.[126–133] A recent large prospective, open-label trial of sildenafil in PAH showed significant improvements in functional class, oxygen saturations, and cardiopulmonary hemodynamics after 6 months of treatment.[127] Longer-term studies have suggested sustained benefits.

In a preliminary study, tadalafil showed efficacy and safety in a small group of symptomatic patients with Eisenmenger syndrome.[132] There have also been multiple small trials with sildenafil used in addition to prostanoids, with improved exercise capacity and hemodynamics shown as well.

Prostacyclin analogues Intravenous epoprostenol (Flolan) is the most extensively studied medication in patients with PAH-CHD, particularly in patients with Eisenmenger syndrome.[134,135] Several small studies have shown that continuous intravenous epoprostenol used in patients with Eisenmenger syndrome significantly improved function class, oxygen saturation, and exercise capacity and decreased PVR.[134–137] Treprostinil (Remodulin) is another effective therapy with an acceptable safety profile in patients with PAH. A randomized multicenter, double-blind study using treprostinil in PAH included 109 (of 469) patients with congenital systemic-to-pulmonary shunts. Improvement in exercise capacity was greater in sicker patients and was dose-related. Disease cause showed no significant interaction with the change in exercise capacity (+16 m on 6MWT).[138] Beraprost (an oral prostanoid that is not commercially available in the United States) showed no improvements in exercise capacity in PAH causes other than idiopathic PAH.[139]

Inhaled prostanoids are also available (iloprost [Ventavis] and treprostinil [Tyvaso]), which have improved safety profiles, but their efficacy in PAH-CAD has not been well established.[136,138–141] The use of subcutaneous or inhaled route of administration of prostanoids could prevent the risks associated with central lines in patients with Eisenmenger syndrome, including paradoxic embolism and sepsis, and deserves further study.[134,135]

Combination therapy A few studies have reported benefit to adding sildenafil to either bosentan[142] or prostacyclin analogues.[143–146] However, there has been no direct comparison among different classes of PH-specific therapies or between monotherapy or combined therapy in patients with Eisenmenger syndrome. Because of the limited data available, the use of combination therapy should be considered on a case-by-case basis.[92]

Transplantation

Transplant-free survival is difficult to predict in patients with Eisenmenger syndrome. Some patients have prolonged survival despite severe hypoxemia.[66] Before PAH-specific therapy became available, patients with Eisenmenger syndrome had improved survival compared with idiopathic PAH (3-year survival of 77% vs 35%).[27] This improved survival likely resulted from congenital adaptations of the right ventricle (the chamber remains hypertrophied after birth) and the presence of a shunt that prevented the development and limited the impact of suprasystemic pressures on the right ventricle.[26] Recent data from the US Registry to Evaluate Early and Long-Term PAH Disease Management (REVEAL) analyzed 1-year survival data from 2176 consecutive patients with PAH. Of patients with PAH, 11.8% had PAH-CHD. Overall 1-year survival was 91%, worse for patients with heritable, portopulmonary, and connective tissue disease-related PAH. CHD did not confer the expected survival advantage, regardless of the type of defect or the repair status.[147] This finding suggests that withholding PAH-specific therapy to patients with PAH-CHD because of presumed stability is a flawed strategy.

PAH-specific therapies seem to stabilize patients with PAH-CHD as assessed by 6MWT, mean pulmonary arterial pressure, and PVR.[148] Furthermore, 1 recent retrospective study has shown a substantial survival benefit (in both unadjusted and adjusted analyses) with PAH-specific therapies (73.5% of patients received bosentan, 25% sildenafil, and 1.5% epoprostenol) in patients with Eisenmenger syndrome followed in a large tertiary referral center. The overall 5-year mortality was 23.3%, and of the 52 patients who died, only 2 were on PAH-specific therapy.[149]

Perioperative mortality for transplantation is higher in CAD-PAH, but after this period some patients have an excellent response, with dramatic improvements in symptoms and quality of life.[42,150–152] Transplant options include heart-lung or lung transplantation, with concomitant heart defect repair. These options are reserved for special patients not responsive to medical treatment who have indicators of poor prognosis (syncope, refractory right heart failure, function class III/IV, or severe hypoxemia).[153] By the time patients with PAH-CHD are considered for transplantation, they are usually poor candidates because of multiple organ system failure.[29,154]

Shunt closure in patients with Eisenmenger syndrome

This is a controversial topic and there are only scatted case reports to assist in the decision of whether to close a hemodynamically significant shunt.[155] Potential candidates may be patients with right-to-left or neutral shunt that receive PAH-specific therapy and subsequently experience a reversal of shunt (becoming left-to-right) both at rest and during activities. This intervention (treat-and-repair) may improve oxygenation and pulmonary artery pressure at the expense of decreasing cardiac output. A careful selection of patients based on age, type of defect, resting, and exercise shunt hemodynamics is critical.[155,156] Some experts suggest a PVR less than 6 Wood units per m^2 and a PVR/systemic vascular resistance ratio of 0.3 or less, after initiation of PAH therapy, to consider shunt closure in previously inoperable CHD.[157] In our personal experience, we have yet to witness a patient with true Eisenmenger syndrome who improved with therapy to the point that their lesion could be successfully repaired.

Prevention

Access to medical therapy is the single most important factor to prevent the development of irreversible PH.[24] It is recommended that children with large left-to-right shunts or increased PVR undergo operative closure of the defect in the first 12 to 18 months of life to prevent development of Eisenmenger syndrome.[158] In children younger than 2 years, pulmonary vascular remodeling is usually reversible after the repair of the heart defect.[10] Some conditions such as truncus arteriosus or transposition of the great arteries with ventricular septal defect are repaired during the first months of life, because they have higher propensity to develop PAH.[24] The level of PVR that precludes the safe closure of a heart defect varies with the age of the patient, type of lesion, PVR, and the presence of vasoreactivity.[86,159–161] This topic remains a matter of significant controversy and outside the scope of this article.

SUMMARY

PAH-CHD is common among the different subtypes of PAH. Its severity depends on the type and size of the defect as well as the flow rate of the shunt. Cardiac catheterization is necessary for proper diagnosis and evaluation of severity. When reversibility is suspected, surgical or percutaneous correction is the treatment of choice. New PAH-specific therapies have proved beneficial, although further research is needed to determine optimal treatment of PAH-CHD. Lung or heart-lung transplantation remains an option for recalcitrant patients. More importantly, PAH may be preventable in many cases if the congenital heart defect(s) is identified and treated early.

REFERENCES

1. Wood P. The Eisenmenger syndrome or pulmonary hypertension with reversed central shunt. Br Med J 1958;2:755–62.
2. Steele PM, Fuster V, Cohen M, et al. Isolated atrial septal defect with pulmonary vascular obstructive disease–long-term follow-up and prediction of outcome after surgical correction. Circulation 1987;76:1037–42.
3. Evans W, Short DS. Pulmonary hypertension in congenital heart disease. Br Heart J 1958;20:529–51.
4. Cherian G, Uthaman CB, Durairaj M, et al. Pulmonary hypertension in isolated secundum atrial septal defect: high frequency in young patients. Am Heart J 1983;105:952–7.
5. Haworth SG. Pulmonary vascular bed in children with complete atrioventricular septal defect: relation between structural and hemodynamic abnormalities. Am J Cardiol 1986;57:833–9.

6. Newfeld EA, Sher M, Paul MH, et al. Pulmonary vascular disease in complete atrioventricular canal defect. Am J Cardiol 1977;39:721–6.

7. Campbell M. Natural history of ventricular septal defect. Br Heart J 1971;33:246–57.

8. Christman BW, McPherson CD, Newman JH, et al. An imbalance between the excretion of thromboxane and prostacyclin metabolites in pulmonary hypertension. N Engl J Med 1992;327:70–5.

9. Heath D, Edwards JE. The pathology of hypertensive pulmonary vascular disease; a description of six grades of structural changes in the pulmonary arteries with special reference to congenital cardiac septal defects. Circulation 1958;18:533–47.

10. Rabinovitch M, Haworth SG, Castaneda AR, et al. Lung biopsy in congenital heart disease: a morphometric approach to pulmonary vascular disease. Circulation 1978;58:1107–22.

11. Rabinovitch M, Keane JF, Norwood WI, et al. Vascular structure in lung tissue obtained at biopsy correlated with pulmonary hemodynamic findings after repair of congenital heart defects. Circulation 1984;69:655–67.

12. Besterman E. Atrial septal defect with pulmonary hypertension. Br Heart J 1961;23:587–98.

13. Diller GP, Gatzoulis MA. Pulmonary vascular disease in adults with congenital heart disease. Circulation 2007;115:1039–50.

14. Fasules JW, Tryka F, Chipman CW, et al. Pulmonary hypertension and arterial changes in calves with a systemic-to-left pulmonary artery connection. J Appl Physiol 1994;77:867–75.

15. Hoffman JI, Rudolph AM. The natural history of ventricular septal defects in infancy. Am J Cardiol 1965;16:634–53.

16. Humbert M, Morrell NW, Archer SL, et al. Cellular and molecular pathobiology of pulmonary arterial hypertension. J Am Coll Cardiol 2004;43: 13S–24S.

17. Kidd L, Driscoll DJ, Gersony WM, et al. Second natural history study of congenital heart defects. Results of treatment of patients with ventricular septal defects. Circulation 1993;87:I38–51.

18. Niwa K, Perloff JK, Kaplan S, et al. Eisenmenger syndrome in adults: ventricular septal defect, truncus arteriosus, univentricular heart. J Am Coll Cardiol 1999;34:223–32.

19. Vongpatanasin W, Brickner ME, Hillis LD, et al. The Eisenmenger syndrome in adults. Ann Intern Med 1998;128:745–55.

20. Diller GP, Dimopoulos K, Okonko D, et al. Exercise intolerance in adult congenital heart disease: comparative severity, correlates, and prognostic implication. Circulation 2005;112:828–35.

21. Badesch DB, Champion HC, Sanchez MA, et al. Diagnosis and assessment of pulmonary arterial hypertension. J Am Coll Cardiol 2009;54:S55–66.

22. Galie N, Hoeper MM, Humbert M, et al. Guidelines for the diagnosis and treatment of pulmonary hypertension: the Task Force for the Diagnosis and Treatment of Pulmonary Hypertension of the European Society of Cardiology (ESC) and the European Respiratory Society (ERS), endorsed by the International Society of Heart and Lung Transplantation (ISHLT). Eur Heart J 2009;30: 2493–537.

23. Simonneau G, Robbins IM, Beghetti M, et al. Updated clinical classification of pulmonary hypertension. J Am Coll Cardiol 2009;54:S43–54.

24. Adatia I, Kothari SS, Feinstein JA. Pulmonary hypertension associated with congenital heart disease: pulmonary vascular disease: the global perspective. Chest 2010;137:52S–61S.

25. Broberg C, Ujita M, Babu-Narayan S, et al. Massive pulmonary artery thrombosis with haemoptysis in adults with Eisenmenger's syndrome: a clinical dilemma. Heart 2004;90:e63.

26. Hopkins WE. The remarkable right ventricle of patients with Eisenmenger syndrome. Coron Artery Dis 2005;16:19–25.

27. Hopkins WE, Ochoa LL, Richardson GW, et al. Comparison of the hemodynamics and survival of adults with severe primary pulmonary hypertension or Eisenmenger syndrome. J Heart Lung Transplant 1996;15:100–5.

28. van Albada ME, Berger RM. Pulmonary arterial hypertension in congenital cardiac disease–the need for refinement of the Evian-Venice classification. Cardiol Young 2008;18:10–7.

29. Dimopoulos K, Giannakoulas G, Wort SJ, et al. Pulmonary arterial hypertension in adults with congenital heart disease: distinct differences from other causes of pulmonary arterial hypertension and management implications. Curr Opin Cardiol 2008;23:545–54.

30. Beghetti M, Galie N. Eisenmenger syndrome a clinical perspective in a new therapeutic era of pulmonary arterial hypertension. J Am Coll Cardiol 2009; 53:733–40.

31. Marelli AJ, Mackie AS, Ionescu-Ittu R, et al. Congenital heart disease in the general population: changing prevalence and age distribution. Circulation 2007;115:163–72.

32. Marelli AJ, Therrien J, Mackie AS, et al. Planning the specialized care of adult congenital heart disease patients: from numbers to guidelines; an epidemiologic approach. Am Heart J 2009;157:1–8.

33. Engelfriet PM, Duffels MG, Moller T, et al. Pulmonary arterial hypertension in adults born with a heart septal defect: the Euro Heart Survey on adult congenital heart disease. Heart 2007;93:682–7.

34. Friedman WF. Proceedings of National Heart, Lung, and Blood Institute pediatric cardiology

workshop: pulmonary hypertension. Pediatr Res 1986;20:811–24.

35. Duffels MG, Engelfriet PM, Berger RM, et al. Pulmonary arterial hypertension in congenital heart disease: an epidemiologic perspective from a Dutch registry. Int J Cardiol 2007;120:198–204.

36. Lowe BS, Therrien J, Ionescu-Ittu R, et al. Diagnosis of pulmonary hypertension in the congenital heart disease adult population impact on outcomes. J Am Coll Cardiol 2011;58:538–46.

37. Rabinovitch M. Pulmonary hypertension: pathophysiology as a basis for clinical decision making. J Heart Lung Transplant 1999;18:1041–53.

38. Du L, Sullivan CC, Chu D, et al. Signaling molecules in nonfamilial pulmonary hypertension. N Engl J Med 2003;348:500–9.

39. Diller GP, van Eijl S, Okonko DO, et al. Circulating endothelial progenitor cells in patients with Eisenmenger syndrome and idiopathic pulmonary arterial hypertension. Circulation 2008;117:3020–30.

40. Shah P, Singh WS, Rose V, et al. Incidence of bacterial endocarditis in ventricular septal defects. Circulation 1966;34:127–31.

41. Trojnarska O, Gwizdala A, Katarzynski S, et al. The BNP concentrations and exercise capacity assessment with cardiopulmonary stress test in cyanotic adult patients with congenital heart diseases. Int J Cardiol 2010;139:241–7.

42. Berman EB, Barst RJ. Eisenmenger's syndrome: current management. Prog Cardiovasc Dis 2002; 45:129–38.

43. Hassoun PM, Thappa V, Landman MJ, et al. Endothelin 1: mitogenic activity on pulmonary artery smooth muscle cells and release from hypoxic endothelial cells. Proc Soc Exp Biol Med 1992;199:165–70.

44. Zamora MR, Stelzner TJ, Webb S, et al. Overexpression of endothelin-1 and enhanced growth of pulmonary artery smooth muscle cells from fawn-hooded rats. Am J Physiol 1996;270:L101–9.

45. Cacoub P, Dorent R, Maistre G, et al. Endothelin-1 in primary pulmonary hypertension and the Eisenmenger syndrome. Am J Cardiol 1993;71:448–50.

46. Giaid A, Saleh D. Reduced expression of endothelial nitric oxide synthase in the lungs of patients with pulmonary hypertension. N Engl J Med 1995; 333:214–21.

47. Cooper CJ, Landzberg MJ, Anderson TJ, et al. Role of nitric oxide in the local regulation of pulmonary vascular resistance in humans. Circulation 1996;93:266–71.

48. Moncada S, Higgs A. The L-arginine-nitric oxide pathway. N Engl J Med 1993;329:2002–12.

49. Michelakis ED, Tymchak W, Noga M, et al. Long-term treatment with oral sildenafil is safe and improves functional capacity and hemodynamics in patients with pulmonary arterial hypertension. Circulation 2003;108:2066–9.

50. Rondelet B, Kerbaul F, Van Beneden R, et al. Signaling molecules in overcirculation-induced pulmonary hypertension in piglets: effects of sildenafil therapy. Circulation 2004;110:2220–5.

51. Tuder RM, Cool CD, Geraci MW, et al. Prostacyclin synthase expression is decreased in lungs from patients with severe pulmonary hypertension. Am J Respir Crit Care Med 1999;159:1925–32.

52. Roberts KE, McElroy JJ, Wong WP, et al. BMPR2 mutations in pulmonary arterial hypertension with congenital heart disease. Eur Respir J 2004;24: 371–4.

53. Newman JH, Fanburg BL, Archer SL, et al. Pulmonary arterial hypertension: future directions: report of a National Heart, Lung and Blood Institute/Office of Rare Diseases workshop. Circulation 2004;109: 2947–52.

54. Lepetit H, Eddahibi S, Fadel E, et al. Smooth muscle cell matrix metalloproteinases in idiopathic pulmonary arterial hypertension. Eur Respir J 2005; 25:834–42.

55. Petkov V, Mosgoeller W, Ziesche R, et al. Vasoactive intestinal peptide as a new drug for treatment of primary pulmonary hypertension. J Clin Invest 2003;111:1339–46.

56. Guignabert C, Izikki M, Tu LI, et al. Transgenic mice overexpressing the 5-hydroxytryptamine transporter gene in smooth muscle develop pulmonary hypertension. Circ Res 2006;98:1323–30.

57. Zaiman AL, Podowski M, Medicherla S, et al. Role of the TGF-beta/Alk5 signaling pathway in monocrotaline-induced pulmonary hypertension. Am J Respir Crit Care Med 2008;177:896–905.

58. Morrell NW, Adnot S, Archer SL, et al. Cellular and molecular basis of pulmonary arterial hypertension. J Am Coll Cardiol 2009;54:S20–31.

59. Erzurum S, Rounds SI, Stevens T, et al. Strategic plan for lung vascular research: an NHLBI-ORDR Workshop Report. Am J Respir Crit Care Med 2010;182:1554–62.

60. Diller GP, Dimopoulos K, Broberg CS, et al. Presentation, survival prospects, and predictors of death in Eisenmenger syndrome: a combined retrospective and case-control study. Eur Heart J 2006;27: 1737–42.

61. Dimopoulos K, Okonko DO, Diller GP, et al. Abnormal ventilatory response to exercise in adults with congenital heart disease relates to cyanosis and predicts survival. Circulation 2006;113:2796–802.

62. Paciocco G, Martinez FJ, Bossone E, et al. Oxygen desaturation on the six-minute walk test and mortality in untreated primary pulmonary hypertension. Eur Respir J 2001;17:647–52.

63. Miyamoto S, Nagaya N, Satoh T, et al. Clinical correlates and prognostic significance of six-minute walk test in patients with primary pulmonary hypertension. Comparison with cardiopulmonary

exercise testing. Am J Respir Crit Care Med 2000; 161:487–92.

64. Wensel R, Opitz CF, Anker SD, et al. Assessment of survival in patients with primary pulmonary hypertension: importance of cardiopulmonary exercise testing. Circulation 2002;106:319–24.

65. Cantor WJ, Harrison DA, Moussadji JS, et al. Determinants of survival and length of survival in adults with Eisenmenger syndrome. Am J Cardiol 1999; 84:677–81.

66. Daliento L, Somerville J, Presbitero P, et al. Eisenmenger syndrome. Factors relating to deterioration and death. Eur Heart J 1998;19:1845–55.

67. Sreeram N. Eisenmenger syndrome: towards identifying the risk factors for death. Eur Heart J 2006; 27:1644–5.

68. Broberg CS, Ujita M, Prasad S, et al. Pulmonary arterial thrombosis in eisenmenger syndrome is associated with biventricular dysfunction and decreased pulmonary flow velocity. J Am Coll Cardiol 2007;50:634–42.

69. Silversides CK, Granton JT, Konen E, et al. Pulmonary thrombosis in adults with Eisenmenger syndrome. J Am Coll Cardiol 2003;42: 1982–7.

70. Broberg CS, Bax BE, Okonko DO, et al. Blood viscosity and its relationship to iron deficiency, symptoms, and exercise capacity in adults with cyanotic congenital heart disease. J Am Coll Cardiol 2006;48:356–65.

71. Gidding SS, Stockman JA 3rd. Erythropoietin in cyanotic heart disease. Am Heart J 1988;116:128–32.

72. Kontras SB, Bodenbender JG, Craenen J, et al. Hyperviscosity in congenital heart disease. J Pediatr 1970;76:214–20.

73. Perloff JK, Rosove MH, Child JS, et al. Adults with cyanotic congenital heart disease: hematologic management. Ann Intern Med 1988;109: 406–13.

74. Rosove MH, Perloff JK, Hocking WG, et al. Chronic hypoxaemia and decompensated erythrocytosis in cyanotic congenital heart disease. Lancet 1986;2: 313–5.

75. Lill MC, Perloff JK, Child JS. Pathogenesis of thrombocytopenia in cyanotic congenital heart disease. Am J Cardiol 2006;98:254–8.

76. Perloff JK. Systemic complications of cyanosis in adults with congenital heart disease. Hematologic derangements, renal function, and urate metabolism. Cardiol Clin 1993;11:689–99.

77. Ammash N, Warnes CA. Cerebrovascular events in adult patients with cyanotic congenital heart disease. J Am Coll Cardiol 1996;28:768–72.

78. Perloff JK, Latta H, Barsotti P. Pathogenesis of the glomerular abnormality in cyanotic congenital heart disease. Am J Cardiol 2000; 86:1198–204.

79. Perloff JK, Marelli AJ, Miner PD. Risk of stroke in adults with cyanotic congenital heart disease. Circulation 1993;87:1954–9.

80. Kaemmerer H, Fratz S, Braun SL, et al. Erythrocyte indexes, iron metabolism, and hyperhomocysteinemia in adults with cyanotic congenital cardiac disease. Am J Cardiol 2004;94:825–8.

81. Diller GP, Alonso-Gonzalez R, Kempny A, et al. B type natriuretic peptide concentrations in contemporary Eisenmenger syndrome patients: predictive value and response to disease targeting therapy. Heart 2012;98(9):736–42.

82. Knirsch W, Hausermann E, Fasnacht M, et al. Plasma B-type natriuretic peptide levels in children with heart disease. Acta Paediatr 2011; 100:1213–6.

83. Sheehan R, Perloff JK, Fishbein MC, et al. Pulmonary neovascularity: a distinctive radiographic finding in Eisenmenger syndrome. Circulation 2005;112:2778–85.

84. Warnes CA, Williams RG, Bashore TM, et al. ACC/AHA 2008 Guidelines for the Management of Adults with Congenital Heart Disease: a report of the American College of Cardiology/American Heart Association Task Force on Practice Guidelines (writing committee to develop guidelines on the management of adults with congenital heart disease). Circulation 2008;118:e714–833.

85. McLaughlin VV, Archer SL, Badesch DB, et al. ACCF/AHA 2009 expert consensus document on pulmonary hypertension: a report of the American College of Cardiology Foundation Task Force on Expert Consensus Documents and the American Heart Association: developed in collaboration with the American College of Chest Physicians, American Thoracic Society, Inc., and the Pulmonary Hypertension Association. Circulation 2009;119: 2250–94.

86. Balzer DT, Kort HW, Day RW, et al. Inhaled nitric oxide as a preoperative test (INOP test I): the INOP Test Study Group. Circulation 2002;106:I76–81.

87. Post MC, Janssens S, Van de Werf F, et al. Responsiveness to inhaled nitric oxide is a predictor for mid-term survival in adult patients with congenital heart defects and pulmonary arterial hypertension. Eur Heart J 2004;25:1651–6.

88. D'Alto M, Romeo E, Argiento P, et al. Pulmonary vasoreactivity predicts long-term outcome in patients with Eisenmenger syndrome receiving bosentan therapy. Heart 2010;96:1475–9.

89. Budts W, Van Pelt N, Gillyns H, et al. Residual pulmonary vasoreactivity to inhaled nitric oxide in patients with severe obstructive pulmonary hypertension and Eisenmenger syndrome. Heart 2001; 86:553–8.

90. Goodwin TM, Gherman RB, Hameed A, et al. Favorable response of Eisenmenger syndrome to

inhaled nitric oxide during pregnancy. Am J Obstet Gynecol 1999;180:64–7.

91. ATS statement: guidelines for the six-minute walk test. Am J Respir Crit Care Med 2002;166:111–7.

92. Galie N, Manes A, Palazzini M, et al. Management of pulmonary arterial hypertension associated with congenital systemic-to-pulmonary shunts and Eisenmenger's syndrome. Drugs 2008;68:1049–66.

93. Deanfield J, Thaulow E, Warnes C, et al. Management of grown up congenital heart disease. Eur Heart J 2003;24:1035–84.

94. Antibiotic prophylaxis of infective endocarditis. Recommendations from the Endocarditis Working Party of the British Society for Antimicrobial Chemotherapy. Lancet 1990;335:88–9.

95. Wilson W, Taubert KA, Gewitz M, et al. Prevention of infective endocarditis: guidelines from the American Heart Association. Circulation 2007;116:1736–54.

96. Montani D, Savale L, Natali D, et al. Long-term response to calcium-channel blockers in non-idiopathic pulmonary arterial hypertension. Eur Heart J 2010;31:1898–907.

97. Avila WS, Grinberg M, Snitcowsky R, et al. Maternal and fetal outcome in pregnant women with Eisenmenger's syndrome. Eur Heart J 1995;16:460–4.

98. Uebing A, Steer PJ, Yentis SM, et al. Pregnancy and congenital heart disease. BMJ 2006;332:401–6.

99. Yentis SM, Steer PJ, Plaat F. Eisenmenger's syndrome in pregnancy: maternal and fetal mortality in the 1990s. Br J Obstet Gynaecol 1998;105:921–2.

100. Opotowsky AR, Siddiqi OK, D'Souza B, et al. Maternal cardiovascular events during childbirth among women with congenital heart disease. Heart 2012;98:145–51.

101. Apostolopoulou SC, Manginas A, Cokkinos DV, et al. Effect of the oral endothelin antagonist bosentan on the clinical, exercise, and haemodynamic status of patients with pulmonary arterial hypertension related to congenital heart disease. Heart 2005;91:1447–52.

102. Benza RL, Rayburn BK, Tallaj JA, et al. Efficacy of bosentan in a small cohort of adult patients with pulmonary arterial hypertension related to congenital heart disease. Chest 2006;129:1009–15.

103. Channick RN, Simonneau G, Sitbon O, et al. Effects of the dual endothelin-receptor antagonist bosentan in patients with pulmonary hypertension: a randomised placebo-controlled study. Lancet 2001;358:1119–23.

104. Christensen DD, McConnell ME, Book WM, et al. Initial experience with bosentan therapy in patients with the Eisenmenger syndrome. Am J Cardiol 2004;94:261–3.

105. Gatzoulis MA, Rogers P, Li W, et al. Safety and tolerability of bosentan in adults with Eisenmenger physiology. Int J Cardiol 2005;98:147–51.

106. Gilbert N, Luther YC, Miera O, et al. Initial experience with bosentan (Tracleer) as treatment for pulmonary arterial hypertension (PAH) due to congenital heart disease in infants and young children. Z Kardiol 2005;94:570–4.

107. Rubin LJ, Badesch DB, Barst RJ, et al. Bosentan therapy for pulmonary arterial hypertension. N Engl J Med 2002;346:896–903.

108. Schulze-Neick I, Gilbert N, Ewert R, et al. Adult patients with congenital heart disease and pulmonary arterial hypertension: first open prospective multicenter study of bosentan therapy. Am Heart J 2005;150:716.

109. Galie N, Beghetti M, Gatzoulis MA, et al. Bosentan therapy in patients with Eisenmenger syndrome: a multicenter, double-blind, randomized, placebo-controlled study. Circulation 2006;114:48–54.

110. Berger RM, Beghetti M, Galie N, et al. Atrial septal defects versus ventricular septal defects in BREATHE-5, a placebo-controlled study of pulmonary arterial hypertension related to Eisenmenger's syndrome: a subgroup analysis. Int J Cardiol 2010;144:373–8.

111. Gatzoulis MA, Beghetti M, Galie N, et al. Longer-term bosentan therapy improves functional capacity in Eisenmenger syndrome: results of the BREATHE-5 open-label extension study. Int J Cardiol 2008;127:27–32.

112. Apostolopoulou SC, Manginas A, Cokkinos DV, et al. Long-term oral bosentan treatment in patients with pulmonary arterial hypertension related to congenital heart disease: a 2-year study. Heart 2007;93:350–4.

113. D'Alto M, Vizza CD, Romeo E, et al. Long term effects of bosentan treatment in adult patients with pulmonary arterial hypertension related to congenital heart disease (Eisenmenger physiology): safety, tolerability, clinical, and haemodynamic effect. Heart 2007;93:621–5.

114. Diaz-Caraballo E, Gonzalez-Garcia AE, Renones M, et al. Long-term bosentan treatment of complex congenital heart disease and Eisenmenger's syndrome. Rev Esp Cardiol 2009;62:1046–9.

115. Diller GP, Dimopoulos K, Kaya MG, et al. Long-term safety, tolerability and efficacy of bosentan in adults with pulmonary arterial hypertension associated with congenital heart disease. Heart 2007;93:974–6.

116. Mehta PK, Simpson L, Lee EK, et al. Endothelin receptor antagonists improve exercise tolerance and oxygen saturations in patients with Eisenmenger syndrome and congenital heart defects. Tex Heart Inst J 2008;35:256–61.

117. Galie N, Rubin L, Hoeper M, et al. Treatment of patients with mildly symptomatic pulmonary arterial hypertension with bosentan (EARLY study): a double-blind, randomised controlled trial. Lancet 2008;371:2093–100.

118. Vis JC, Duffels MG, Mulder P, et al. Prolonged beneficial effect of bosentan treatment and 4-year survival rates in adult patients with pulmonary arterial hypertension associated with congenital heart disease. Int J Cardiol 2011. DOI:10.1016/j.ijcard.2011.06.064.

119. Avellana P, Segovia J, Sufrate E, et al. Long-term (5 years) effects of bosentan in patients with pulmonary arterial hypertension. Rev Esp Cardiol 2011; 64:667–73.

120. Monfredi O, Griffiths L, Clarke B, et al. Efficacy and safety of bosentan for pulmonary arterial hypertension in adults with congenital heart disease. Am J Cardiol 2011;108:1483–8.

121. van Loon RL, Hoendermis ES, Duffels MG, et al. Long-term effect of bosentan in adults versus children with pulmonary arterial hypertension associated with systemic-to-pulmonary shunt: does the beneficial effect persist? Am Heart J 2007;154:776–82.

122. Galie N, Olschewski H, Oudiz RJ, et al. Ambrisentan for the treatment of pulmonary arterial hypertension: results of the ambrisentan in pulmonary arterial hypertension, randomized, double-blind, placebo-controlled, multicenter, efficacy (ARIES) study 1 and 2. Circulation 2008;117:3010–9.

123. Oudiz RJ, Galie N, Olschewski H, et al. Long-term ambrisentan therapy for the treatment of pulmonary arterial hypertension. J Am Coll Cardiol 2009;54:1971–81.

124. Zuckerman WA, Leaderer D, Rowan CA, et al. Ambrisentan for pulmonary arterial hypertension due to congenital heart disease. Am J Cardiol 2011; 107:1381–5.

125. McGoon MD, Frost AE, Oudiz RJ, et al. Ambrisentan therapy in patients with pulmonary arterial hypertension who discontinued bosentan or sitaxsentan due to liver function test abnormalities. Chest 2009;135:122–9.

126. Galie N, Ghofrani HA, Torbicki A, et al. Sildenafil citrate therapy for pulmonary arterial hypertension. N Engl J Med 2005;353:2148–57.

127. Chau EM, Fan KY, Chow WH. Effects of chronic sildenafil in patients with Eisenmenger syndrome versus idiopathic pulmonary arterial hypertension. Int J Cardiol 2007;120:301–5.

128. Garg N, Sharma MK, Sinha N. Role of oral sildenafil in severe pulmonary arterial hypertension: clinical efficacy and dose response relationship. Int J Cardiol 2007;120:306–13.

129. Humpl T, Reyes JT, Holtby H, et al. Beneficial effect of oral sildenafil therapy on childhood pulmonary arterial hypertension: twelve-month clinical trial of a single-drug, open-label, pilot study. Circulation 2005;111:3274–80.

130. Lim ZS, Salmon AP, Vettukattil JJ, et al. Sildenafil therapy for pulmonary arterial hypertension associated with atrial septal defects. Int J Cardiol 2007; 118:178–82.

131. Mikhail GW, Prasad SK, Li W, et al. Clinical and haemodynamic effects of sildenafil in pulmonary hypertension: acute and mid-term effects. Eur Heart J 2004;25:431–6.

132. Mukhopadhyay S, Sharma M, Ramakrishnan S, et al. Phosphodiesterase-5 inhibitor in Eisenmenger syndrome: a preliminary observational study. Circulation 2006;114:1807–10.

133. Singh TP, Rohit M, Grover A, et al. A randomized, placebo-controlled, double-blind, crossover study to evaluate the efficacy of oral sildenafil therapy in severe pulmonary artery hypertension. Am Heart J 2006;151:851 e851–5.

134. Rosenzweig EB, Kerstein D, Barst RJ. Long-term prostacyclin for pulmonary hypertension with associated congenital heart defects. Circulation 1999; 99:1858–65.

135. Fernandes SM, Newburger JW, Lang P, et al. Usefulness of epoprostenol therapy in the severely ill adolescent/adult with Eisenmenger physiology. Am J Cardiol 2003;91:632–5.

136. Badesch DB, McLaughlin VV, Delcroix M, et al. Prostanoid therapy for pulmonary arterial hypertension. J Am Coll Cardiol 2004;43:56S–61S.

137. Frost AE, Quinones MA, Zoghbi WA, et al. Reversal of pulmonary hypertension and subsequent repair of atrial septal defect after treatment with continuous intravenous epoprostenol. J Heart Lung Transplant 2005;24:501–3.

138. Simonneau G, Barst RJ, Galie N, et al. Continuous subcutaneous infusion of treprostinil, a prostacyclin analogue, in patients with pulmonary arterial hypertension: a double-blind, randomized, placebo-controlled trial. Am J Respir Crit Care Med 2002;165:800–4.

139. Barst RJ, McGoon M, McLaughlin V, et al. Beraprost therapy for pulmonary arterial hypertension. J Am Coll Cardiol 2003;41:2119–25.

140. Galie N, Humbert M, Vachiery JL, et al. Effects of beraprost sodium, an oral prostacyclin analogue, in patients with pulmonary arterial hypertension: a randomized, double-blind, placebo-controlled trial. J Am Coll Cardiol 2002;39:1496–502.

141. Oudiz RJ, Schilz RJ, Barst RJ, et al. Treprostinil, a prostacyclin analogue, in pulmonary arterial hypertension associated with connective tissue disease. Chest 2004;126:420–7.

142. D'Alto M, Romeo E, Argiento P, et al. Bosentan-sildenafil association in patients with congenital heart disease-related pulmonary arterial hypertension and Eisenmenger physiology. Int J Cardiol 2012; 155(3):378–82.

143. Hoeper MM, Markevych I, Spiekerkoetter E, et al. Goal-oriented treatment and combination therapy for pulmonary arterial hypertension. Eur Respir J 2005;26:858–63.

144. Lunze K, Gilbert N, Mebus S, et al. First experience with an oral combination therapy using bosentan

and sildenafil for pulmonary arterial hypertension. Eur J Clin Invest 2006;36(Suppl 3):32–8.

145. McLaughlin VV, Oudiz RJ, Frost A, et al. Randomized study of adding inhaled iloprost to existing bosentan in pulmonary arterial hypertension. Am J Respir Crit Care Med 2006;174:1257–63.

146. Okyay K, Cemri M, Boyac B, et al. Use of long-term combined therapy with inhaled iloprost and oral sildenafil in an adult patient with eisenmenger syndrome. Cardiol Rev 2005;13:312–4.

147. Benza RL, Miller DP, Gomberg-Maitland M, et al. Predicting survival in pulmonary arterial hypertension: insights from the Registry to Evaluate Early and Long-Term Pulmonary Arterial Hypertension Disease Management (REVEAL). Circulation 2010;122:164–72.

148. Duffels M, van Loon L, Berger R, et al. Pulmonary arterial hypertension associated with a congenital heart defect: advanced medium-term medical treatment stabilizes clinical condition. Congenit Heart Dis 2007;2:242–9.

149. Dimopoulos K, Inuzuka R, Goletto S, et al. Improved survival among patients with Eisenmenger syndrome receiving advanced therapy for pulmonary arterial hypertension. Circulation 2010;121: 20–5.

150. Trulock EP. Lung transplantation for primary pulmonary hypertension. Clin Chest Med 2001;22:583–93.

151. Stoica SC, McNeil KD, Perreas K, et al. Heart-lung transplantation for Eisenmenger syndrome: early and long-term results. Ann Thorac Surg 2001;72: 1887–91.

152. Waddell TK, Bennett L, Kennedy R, et al. Heart-lung or lung transplantation for Eisenmenger syndrome. J Heart Lung Transplant 2002;21:731–7.

153. Klepetko W, Mayer E, Sandoval J, et al. Interventional and surgical modalities of treatment for pulmonary arterial hypertension. J Am Coll Cardiol 2004;43:73S–80S.

154. Dimopoulos K, Diller GP, Koltsida E, et al. Prevalence, predictors, and prognostic value of renal dysfunction in adults with congenital heart disease. Circulation 2008;117:2320–8.

155. Dimopoulos K, Peset A, Gatzoulis MA. Evaluating operability in adults with congenital heart disease and the role of pretreatment with targeted pulmonary arterial hypertension therapy. Int J Cardiol 2008;129:163–71.

156. Rame JE. Pulmonary hypertension complicating congenital heart disease. Curr Cardiol Rep 2009; 11:314–20.

157. Beghetti M, Galie N, Bonnet D. Can "inoperable" congenital heart defects become operable in patients with pulmonary arterial hypertension? Dream or reality? Congenit Heart Dis 2012;7:3–11.

158. Kidd L, Rose V, Collins G, et al. The hemodynamics in ventricular septal defect in childhood. Am Heart J 1965;70:732–8.

159. Yeager SB, Freed MD, Keane JF, et al. Primary surgical closure of ventricular septal defect in the first year of life: results in 128 infants. J Am Coll Cardiol 1984;3:1269–76.

160. Moller JH, Patton C, Varco RL, et al. Late results (30 to 35 years) after operative closure of isolated ventricular septal defect from 1954 to 1960. Am J Cardiol 1991;68:1491–7.

161. Neutze JM, Ishikawa T, Clarkson PM, et al. Assessment and follow-up of patients with ventricular septal defect and elevated pulmonary vascular resistance. Am J Cardiol 1989;63:327–31.

Pulmonary Hypertension Associated with Left-Sided Heart Disease

Christopher F. Barnett, MD, MPH[a], Teresa De Marco, MD[b],*

KEYWORDS

- Pulmonary hypertension • Heart failure • Heart transplant

KEY POINTS

- Pulmonary hypertension occurs commonly in patients with left-sided heart failure and is associated with higher morbidity and mortality.
- The diagnostic approach to patients undergoing evaluation for pulmonary hypertension should include a careful assessment to exclude the presence of unrecognized left-sided heart failure.
- The Approach to the treatment of pulmonary hypertension resulting from left-sided heart failure is optimal management of left-sided heart failure. For heart failure with reduced ejection fraction, evidence-based therapies including diuretics, β-blockers, angiotensin-converting enzyme inhibitors, aldosterone antagonists, and devices should be optimized.
- Results of ongoing well-designed larger prospective trials of phosphodiesterase inhibitors are needed before routine use of these agents in the treatment of pulmonary hypertension from left-sided heart failure.

INTRODUCTION

Pulmonary hypertension (PH) is characterized hemodynamically by significantly elevated pulmonary arterial pressure, which, if sustained, can result in clinical deterioration due to progressive right-sided heart failure and death. Elevated pulmonary arterial pressure that results from abnormalities localized to the precapillary pulmonary arterioles is referred to as pulmonary arterial hypertension (PAH). Abnormalities of the left side of the heart that raise left-sided filling pressure may cause pulmonary venous hypertension (PVH) resulting from passive congestion that resolves when pulmonary venous pressure is normalized. Long-standing PVH may induce abnormalities in pulmonary artery endothelial function and upregulation of neurohormones, cytokines, and other mediators leading to reactive vasoconstriction and, in certain instances, significant vascular remodeling such that pulmonary arterial pressure fails to decrease when pulmonary venous pressure is normalized. The classification scheme for PH was recently revised and provides a useful framework to identify the underlying disease process.[1] In some cases, such as in sickle cell disease, PH may result from simultaneous primary abnormalities of both the pulmonary arteries and the left-sided heart disease.[2]

Disclosures: Research grants: Novartis; Speaker's Bureau: Actelion, United Therapeutics; Consultant: Actelion, Gilead, United Therapeutics.
[a] Division of Cardiology, University of California, San Francisco, San Francisco General Hospital, 1001 Potrero Avenue, San Francisco, CA 94110, USA; [b] Heart Failure and Pulmonary Hypertension Program, Heart Transplantation, Division of Cardiology, University of California, San Francisco, Medical Center, 505 Parnassus Avenue, 1180-M, San Francisco, CA 94143-0124, USA
* Corresponding author.
E-mail address: demarco@medicine.ucsf.edu

Heart Failure Clin 8 (2012) 447–459
doi:10.1016/j.hfc.2012.04.009
1551-7136/12/$ – see front matter © 2012 Published by Elsevier Inc.

LEFT-SIDED HEART FAILURE AS A CAUSE OF PH

PH may complicate heart failure from left ventricular systolic dysfunction (heart failure with reduced ejection fraction [HFrEF]), diastolic dysfunction (heart failure with preserved ejection fraction [HFpEF]), and valvular heart disease (World Health Organization [WHO] Group II). Recent estimates report a high prevalence of left-sided heart failure (LHF) in 1% to 2% of the population, most commonly occurring in patients older than 65 years.[3] PH may occur in up to 60% of patients with severe systolic dysfunction. In a recent report, mixed PH (elevated pulmonary vascular resistance [PVR]>3 Wood units) occurred in 47% of hospitalized patients with decompensated heart failure enrolled in the invasive monitoring arm of the Evaluation Study of Congestive Heart Failure and Pulmonary Artery Catheterization Effectiveness (ESCAPE) trial.[4] PH has also been noted in 80% of patients with diastolic dysfunction[5] and in up to 50% of patients undergoing heart transplant evaluation,[6] making left-sided heart failure one of the most common causes of PH in developed countries. Valvular heart disease, especially mitral valve disease, is also an important cause of PH, and the presence of PH is an important factor in determining the timing of surgical repair of the mitral valve.[7,8]

HFpEF represents a particularly underrecognized cause of PH secondary to left-sided heart disease. HFpEF may be more common than generally appreciated, with diastolic dysfunction found in up to 25% of otherwise healthy European subjects.[9] Criteria for the diagnosis of HFpEF are not well established, and the evaluation of diastolic function is difficult, even during invasive hemodynamic monitoring.[10] In fact in a community-based study of 244 patients clinically diagnosed with HFpEF compared with 719 patients with systemic hypertension only, the presence of elevated pulmonary arterial pressures on echocardiography was found to be both sensitive and specific for the diagnosis of HFpEF.[5] The REVEAL (Registry to Evaluate Early and Long-term Pulmonary Arterial Hypertension Disease Management) probably also included a significant number of patients with left-sided heart disease because patients diagnosed with PAH in the setting of elevated pulmonary artery wedge pressure (PAWP) (16–18 mm Hg) were included in the registry. Of 2967 adult patients enrolled, 239 had an elevated PAWP. Not surprisingly, these patients were significantly older, more likely of the female gender, obese, diabetic, and hypertensive and had renal impairment and sleep apnea, characteristics that are also associated with a diagnosis of HFpEF. These data suggest either that a significant number of patients diagnosed as having PAH may in fact have PVH from HFpEF or that coexistent left-sided heart disease is common among patients referred for management of PAH.

SIGNIFICANCE OF PH IN LEFT-SIDED HEART FAILURE

It is now well established that PH in patients with LHF is associated with increased mortality and morbidity, worse exercise tolerance, and adverse outcomes after heart transplantation. In an early study of 28 patients with ischemic or idiopathic dilated cardiomyopathy and an ejection fraction (EF) less than 20%, those with a tricuspid regurgitant jet velocity (TRV) greater than 2.5 m/s after 28 months of follow-up had a mortality rate of 57%, 40% higher than patients with a TRV of 2.5 m/s or less. Eighty-nine percent of the patients died or were hospitalized in comparison with 32% of patients with a low TRV.[11] In a logistic regression model, a TRV greater than 2.5 m/s was the best predictor of mortality. Recently, an analysis of patients with decompensated heart failure monitored with a pulmonary artery catheter and treated for 48 hours with nesiritide, nitroglycerin, or placebo showed that mean pulmonary artery pressure (MPAP) less than 25 mm Hg, MPAP greater than 25 mm Hg/PAWP less than 15 mm Hg, and MPAP greater than 25 mm Hg/PAWP greater than 15 mm Hg were associated with a 6-month mortality of 8.6%, 21.8%, and 48.3% respectively.[12,13] Another study followed up 1134 patients with cardiomyopathy for an average of 4.4 years to determine the prognostic utility of the MPAP and examine the association between hemodynamics and outcome for various underlying causes of cardiomyopathy.[14] In multivariate Cox regression analysis, the mean arterial pressure (MAP) and the MPAP emerged as the only 2 significant predictors of mortality. For every 5 mm Hg increase in the MPAP, the hazard of death increased by 25%, and for every 5 mm Hg increase in the MAP, the hazard of death decreased by 11%. This relationship was most pronounced in patients with cardiomyopathy due to myocarditis, among whom an increase in MPAP of 23% was associated with an increase in the hazard of death of 85%. Although not significant in multivariate analysis, a nonlinear relationship between mortality and PVR was noted, with a doubling of the mortality rate in patients with a PVR more than 3 Wood units. A second large study evaluated the significance of an elevated echo-estimated pulmonary artery systolic pressure (PASP) in 1049 subjects with a diagnosis of heart failure. After controlling for age, sex, comorbidities, diastolic function, and EF, elevated PASP, depending on severity, was associated with a hazard ratio of death between 1.45 and 2.64. Addition of PASP to a prognostic model significantly improved the ability to predict 1-year all-cause and cardiovascular mortality.[15]

Exercise changes in MPAP may provide additional useful prognostic information beyond resting hemodynamics. In one recent report, invasive hemodynamic assessment was performed in 60 patients with HFrEF and 19 controls during graded exercise. Compared with controls, subjects with HFrEF had a greater increase in MPAP, transpulmonary gradient (TPG), and effective arterial elastance. In 65% of the subjects with HFrEF, a steady linear increase was seen in the MPAP with workload, whereas in 35%, the MPAP increased and then plateaued. Compared with the linear pattern, the plateau pattern was associated with reduced peak oxygen consumption, lower right ventricular stroke work index augmentation, and reduced survival. Resting hemodynamics was not predictive of the exercise hemodynamic pattern.[16]

In the setting of LHF from mitral regurgitation, the development of PH with a PASP greater than 50 mm Hg is a guideline-recommended criterion for mitral valve repair[7]; however, even lower levels of PH may be associated with a poor outcome. One registry study examined outcomes in 286 Korean patients with severe asymptomatic mitral regurgitation who did not meet American College of Cardiology/American Heart Association (ACC/AHA) criteria for surgery and were managed with watchful waiting versus early surgery. Early surgery was offered at the discretion of the treating physician for indications that could include mild to moderate PH. The 7-year cardiac mortality was 0% versus 5% in the early surgery group versus the watchful waiting group. Event-free survival (operative mortality, cardiac death, repeated mitral valve surgery, hospitalization for heart failure) was higher in patients undergoing early surgery (99% vs 85%, P = .001). Multivariate analysis of the watchful waiting group demonstrated that even mild PH at baseline independently predicted heart failure or the development of conventional surgical indications during follow-up.[17]

PH in the setting of heart transplantation is associated with a dramatic decrease in early and late posttransplant survival.[18] In one report, right ventricular failure was the source of 50% of all posttransplant complications and 20% of early posttransplant mortality.[19] A useful measure to characterize PH

due to LHF is the TPG, equal to the MPAP minus the PAWP. A TPG greater than or equal to 16 is thought to reflect reactive PH in excess of that produced by passive congestion and has been associated with increased right ventricular failure after heart transplant (**Box 1**).[20,21] Several studies have shown PH that is reversible with vasodilator challenge while maintaining systemic arterial pressure is associated with lower posttransplant mortality compared with irreversible or fixed PH.[6]

PATHOPHYSIOLOGY

Although the nomenclature, hemodynamic definitions, and criteria are quite variable in the literature, patients with PH and LHF have postcapillary PH with elevated left-sided filling pressures. However, this group presents with differing hemodynamic profiles. In many patients with PH and LHF, elevation in pulmonary artery pressure (PAP) results from elevated left-sided filling pressure that is passively transmitted retrograde to the pulmonary arterial tree. The TPG and the PVR are within normal to mildly elevated ranges. In the literature, this hemodynamic profile is referred to as passive PH or PVH. One study of 1000 patients undergoing evaluation for heart transplantation found that PASP was tightly correlated with PAWP ($r = 0.79$). A reduction in PASP was also correlated with a reduction in the PAWP

Box 1
Hemodynamic characteristics associated with a poor outcome after cardiac transplantation

1. PAH and elevated PVR should be considered as a relative contraindication to cardiac transplantation when the PVR is greater than 5 Woods units or the PVR index is greater than 6 or the TPG exceeds 16 to 20 mm Hg.

2. If the PASP exceeds 60 mm Hg in conjunction with any 1 of the preceding 3 variables, the risk of right-sided heart failure and early death is increased.

3. If the PVR can be reduced to less than 2.5 Woods units with a vasodilator but the systolic blood pressure decreases to less than 85 mm Hg, the patient remains at high risk of right-sided heart failure and mortality after cardiac transplantation.

Reproduced from Mandeep RM, Jon K, Randall S, et al. Listing criteria for heart transplantation: international society for heart and lung transplantation guidelines for the care of cardiac transplant candidates—2006. J Heart Lung Transplant 2006;25(9):1029; with permission.

(r = 0.67), suggesting that in this population of patients with advanced heart failure, elevations and changes in PAP were dependent largely on PAWP or left-sided heart filling pressures.[22]

In other patients with PH due to LHF, the hemodynamic profile is one of MPAP elevation out of proportion to the elevation in left-sided filling pressure, with significantly elevated TPG and PVR due to "reactive" vasoconstriction with or without vascular remodeling. This group has a mixed PH picture with hemodynamic features of both PAH and PVH. Response to preload reduction maneuvers, vasodilators, inodilators, and mechanical devices then defines reversible compared with irreversible/fixed PH due to LHF with variable hemodynamic response criteria defined in the literature (see **Box 1**). The pathophysiology of mixed PH in this setting is multifactorial and complex. Chronicity and severity of left-sided filling pressure elevation, mitral regurgitation, and extent of cardiac dysfunction with associated upregulation of neurohormones, cytokines, growth factors, and other mediators are likely to play a role. Central to the pathophysiology is pulmonary vascular endothelial dysfunction characterized by an imbalance of vasodilator-apoptotic (nitric oxide, prostacyclin) to vasoconstrictor-proliferative (endothelin) mediators leading to vasoconstriction and variable degrees of vascular remodeling.[23–25]

The contribution of neurohumoral activation mediated by the sympathetic nervous system and the renin-angiotensin-aldosterone system (RAAS) to the pathophysiologic changes in LHF is well established. RAAS activation may also play a causative role in the development of PH by mediating vasoconstriction and structural remodeling of the pulmonary vasculature. Evidence for this comes from a randomized blinded study in 10 healthy subjects treated with lisinopril or placebo before 30 minutes of hypoxemia with oxygen saturations of 75% to 80%. Subjects treated with lisinopril had a significantly lower MPAP during hypoxemia (13.4 vs 19.6 mm Hg) and total pulmonary resistance.[26] The beneficial effects of standard heart failure therapy in the treatment of PH associated with LHF have been demonstrated in studies showing a decrease in neurohumoral activation and reduced PVR after initiation of angiotensin-converting enzyme (ACE) inhibitors and β-blockers.[26–28] Recent data further implicate the RAAS system by demonstrating that activation of ACE-2 by a novel molecule reduced PAP and proinflammatory cytokine levels in a rat monocrotaline model of PH.[29]

Endothelin-1 (ET-1) is primarily produced by vascular endothelial and smooth muscle cells and likely represents a major mediator in the development of PH associated with LHF. Factors stimulating its production may include shear stress, pulsatile stress, angiotensin II, epinephrine, cortisol, thrombin, inflammatory cytokines, transforming growth factor β, and hypoxia. Smooth muscle cell ET_A and ET_B receptors mediate the vascular effects of ET-1. Although activation of ET_A receptors result primarily in vasoconstriction and cellular proliferation, ET_B receptors can mediate vasodilation (through nitric oxide and prostacyclin release) and clearance of endothelin, especially in the lung. Other than heart failure and PH, there is evidence for a major pathogenic role of ET-1 in systemic hypertension, atherosclerosis, myocardial infarction, and renal dysfunction (**Fig. 1**).

The importance of ET-1 in the development of WHO group I PAH is well established and supported by the well-described benefits from treatment with endothelial receptor antagonists (ERAs).[30] The known physiologic effects of ET-1 combined with evidence of increased ET activity and decreased clearance support a major role for ET in PH from LHF. The importance of ET in human heart failure was first suggested by a report that examined the relationship between plasma ET-1 levels and functional classification in 16 patients with idiopathic dilated cardiomyopathy.[31] ET-1 levels in patients were significantly higher than those in controls (7.1 pg/mL vs 1.6 pg/mL, $P<.001$), increased with worsening functional class, and were negatively correlated with echocardiographically determined left ventricular systolic function (r = −0.751, $P<.01$). A subsequent study sought a relationship between ET-1 levels and hemodynamics in cardiomyopathy. ET-1 levels were elevated in 20 patients with cardiomyopathy compared with that in controls (9.07 pg/mL vs 3.7 pg/mL, $P<.0001$) and was significantly correlated to the systolic pressure, diastolic pressure, and MPAP and the resistance ratio (PVR:systemic vascular resistance [SVR]). Based on the multiple regression analysis, the authors determined that 69% of the variance in the ET-1 level was related to the MPAP and the PAWP.[32]

Another study specifically evaluated the relationship between outcomes and levels of big ET-1 (the precursor of ET-1) in 113 patients with an EF less than 20%.[33] In a multivariate model, only functional classification and level of big ET-1 were predictive of mortality or transplant at 12 months of follow-up.

DIAGNOSTIC APPROACH

The prognosis and treatment of PH varies dramatically depending on the underlying etiology of the disease. Patients who have signs and symptoms

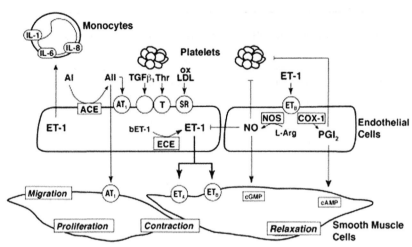

Fig. 1. The endothelin system in heart failure. ET-1 exerts vasoconstriction and proliferation via ET$_A$ receptors on smooth muscle cells. ET$_B$ receptors mediate vasodilation via release of nitric oxide (NO) and prostacyclin. ET$_B$ receptors in the lung clear ET-1 from plasma. AI/II, angiotensin I/II; AT, angiotensin receptor; cAMP, cyclic adenosine monophosphate; cGMP, cyclic guanosine monophosphate; COX, cyclooxygenase; ECE, endothelin-converting enzyme; IL, interleukin; L-Arg, L-arginine; NOS, nitric oxide synthase; oxLDL, oxidized low-density lipoprotein; PGI$_2$, prostacyclin; SR, scavenger receptor; T, thrombin receptor; TGF, transforming growth factor; Thr, thrombin. (*Reproduced from* Spieker LE, Noll G, Ruschitzka FT, et al. Endothelin receptor antagonists in congestive heart failure: a new therapeutic principle for the future? J Am Coll Cardiol 2001;37(6):1494; with permission.)

suggestive of PH should undergo a screening echocardiography. If consistent with a diagnosis of PH, a systematic, comprehensive, and exhaustive search for the underlying etiology of PH should be undertaken as recommended in the recently updated ACC/AHA guidelines.[1]

Patients may present with clinical features suggestive of LHF, including orthopnea, paroxysmal nocturnal dyspnea, murmurs consistent with valvular heart disease or gallop on auscultation, pulmonary edema or pleural effusion on chest radiography, or left atrial enlargement on electrocardiography (**Table 1**). The presence of systolic or diastolic dysfunction, significant valvular heart disease, left atrial myxoma with obstruction or cor triatriatum identified during echocardiography may point toward LHF as the etiology of PH and obviate further evaluation. Echocardiographic findings such as left atrial enlargement, abnormal mitral inflow, and left ventricular hypertrophy may suggest a diagnosis of HFpEF or other conditions such as constrictive pericarditis or restrictive/infiltrative cardiomyopathy that may present as PH.[34] Echocardiography, however, may not be adequately sensitive, and a high index of suspicion should be maintained in patients with clinical risk factors for HFpEF to avoid a misdiagnosis of PAH. Right heart catheterization is mandatory in all patients for whom a diagnosis of PAH is being considered regardless of the echocardiographic findings and to rule out the presence of occult left-sided heart disease.

Right-sided heart catheterization in patients with PH should be performed by a practitioner with an interest in PH and expertise in invasive hemodynamic assessment. When performed in a high-volume center, right-sided heart catheterization is safe, even in patients with severe PH.[35] There are currently no evidence-based guidelines or standards to guide practitioners during the performance of right-sided heart catheterization, and there is significant regional and institutional variation in the approach to data collection and interpretation. Training tools have been developed by professional societies that reflect expert opinion and are available online (Pulmonary Artery Catheter Education Project, www.pacep.org); however, evidence-based practice standards should be developed in the future.

Close attention should be paid to ensure proper leveling and zeroing of transducers during each study. An appropriate response on the monitor to vertical movement of the catheter is required before insertion into the patient, and a rapid flush test is performed after insertion. All waveforms are evaluated to ensure that they are of high quality, and all hemodynamic measurements are made at end expiration. Fick cardiac output (CO) and thermodilution CO are both performed and recorded. Obtaining a reliable PAWP may be particularly difficult in patients with PH. The PAWP waveform tracing must be carefully examined to ensure that reliable data are collected. If the validity of the PAWP is in question,

Table 1
Diagnostic evaluation in patients with PH suspected to be from left-sided heart disease

Evaluation	Findings
History taking and physical examination	History of hypertension, coronary artery disease, and risk factors; orthopnea; PND; pulmonary edema or effusions; cardiac enlargement; left-sided S3 or S4; murmurs of valvular disease
Laboratory testing	Testing to rule out anemia, renal or hepatic dysfunction, BNP
Echocardiography	Evaluation of left ventricular systolic and diastolic function and valvular function
Right- and left-sided heart catheterization	Measurement of pulmonary hemodynamics, evaluation for CAD and valvular disease, direct measurement of left-sided heart filling pressures, performance of provocative maneuvers (exercise or volume challenge) to elicit occult diastolic dysfunction
Vasoreactivity testing	Assessment of PH reversibility in cardiac transplant candidates

Abbreviations: BNP, B-type natriuretic peptide; CAD, coronary artery disease; PND, paroxysmal nocturnal dyspnea.

slow balloon inflation with manipulation of the catheter may be required. In addition, the catheter may be manipulated into another pulmonary artery segment or the oxygen saturation may be obtained of a blood sample withdrawn with the catheter in the wedge position while the balloon is inflated. In the absence of an intracardiac shunt, the oxygen saturation of blood withdrawn from the wedged catheter should be the same as the systemic arterial saturation. In our laboratory, we perform left-sided heart catheterization and measure left ventricular end-diastolic pressure (LVEDP) in any patient with an unreliable PAWP tracing, the wedged oxygen saturation not matching the systemic oxygen saturation, or a PAWP greater than 15 mm Hg.

In patients undergoing evaluation for heart transplant, acute vasodilator challenge is performed in those who have mixed PH to assess if PH is reversible and to identify patients at risk for posttransplant complications. The most commonly used measure of severity of PH in this population is the TPG. A variety of methods and agents are acceptable to perform vasodilator testing in candidates for transplantation.[20] More aggressive maneuvers may be instituted in patients who do not respond immediately to vasodilator challenge in the catheterization laboratory using various vasoactive and/or inodilator agents over a period of 72 hours or more chronically using IV inodilators, oral vasodilators, mechanical circulatory support devices, or a combination of these strategies (**Fig. 2**).

As previously discussed, patients with HFpEF may present with relatively normal hemodynamics during right-sided heart catheterization. This is especially true if they have been well diuresed, are undergoing catheterization after being made to fast overnight, and have received medications for moderate sedation. If clinical characteristics or echocardiographic findings suggest HFpEF, recent guidelines have recommended performing provocative maneuvers to elicit elevated left-sided filling pressures. Administration of a 250- to 500-mL bolus of normal saline or low workload upper extremity or supine bicycle exercise can be performed while monitoring for an increase in the PAWP or LVEDP that would be consistent with HFpEF.

TREATMENT

Although multiple agents for PAH are now available, none are currently approved by the Food and Drug Administration (FDA) for the treatment of PH resulting from LHF. In this setting, the initial approach in all patients should be optimal and aggressive management of the underlying heart disease (see **Fig. 2**) based on current published guidelines.[3] In many patients, PH is secondary to passive congestion, and correction of volume status, blood pressure, and valvular heart disease will lead to resolution or improvement of the PH. HFpEF may present a particularly difficult therapeutic challenge with little evidence base to guide treatment. HFpEF treatment of the underlying condition is recommended (ie, revascularization of coronary artery disease, surgery for valvular heart disease), and therapies targeted at

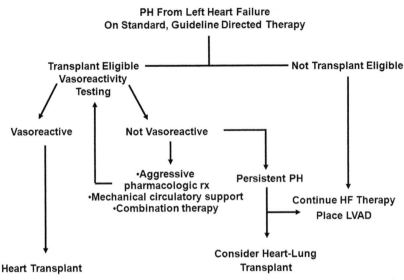

Fig. 2. Proposed strategy to manage PH in patients with LHF who are candidates for cardiac transplantation. HF, heart failure; LVAD, left ventricular assist device; rx, treatment.

comorbidities such as diabetes and hypertension should be maximized.[36]

Treatment with PAH-specific therapy in patients with mixed or out-of-proportion PH is conceptually appealing, and short-term studies have demonstrated favorable hemodynamic effects of PAH-specific agents (**Table 2**). No adequately powered, well-designed, prospective trial has yet demonstrated a benefit, and several trials have shown worsening morbidity or mortality in patients with systolic LHF.

Prostacyclin Analogues

Arterial vasodilation and a reduction in SVR by the prostacyclin analogue epoprostenol provided the rationale for clinical trials in systolic heart failure. The Flolan International Randomized Survival Trial (FIRST) included 471 patients with an EF less than 25% and with class III or IV heart failure maximized on ACE inhibitors, digoxin, and diuretics who were randomized to a continuous epoprostenol infusion

or standard care.[37] Short-term administration resulted in improvement in hemodynamics with a reduction in PVR and SVR, PAWP, and CO. After 36 weeks, however, there was no improvement in exercise tolerance in the epoprostenol group, and, subsequently, the trial was stopped early for a possible increase in mortality in the epoprostenol group.

Nesiritide

Nesiritide is a natriuretic peptide approved for the treatment of acute decompensated heart failure in 2004 after a large trial demonstrated an acute reduction in dyspnea and PAWP in patients treated with nesiritide compared with placebo. In this study, there was a significant reduction in PAWP, MPAP, systolic PAP and PVR.[38] A subsequent study of nesiritide in 10 patients with PAH and 10 patients with mixed PH due to LHF recapitulated the immediate hemodynamic benefits of nesiritide in patients with mixed PH but not in

Table 2
Effects of PAH-specific therapy in patients with PH from left heart disease

Agent	Acute Response	Long-Term Outcome
Prostacyclin[37]	↓PVR, ↓SVR, ↓PAWP, ↑CO	↑Mortality
Sildenafil[52,56–58,60–62]	↓PVR, ↓PAWP, ↓MPAP, ↑CO	Lower PAP, improved endothelial function and exercise tolerance
Bosentan[42–44]	↓PVR	↑Transaminases, ↑fluid retention,
Darusentan[48,49]	↓SVR	No benefit
Tezosentan[50]	↓PVR, ↓SVR, ↓PAWP, ↑CI	No benefit

Abbreviations: CI, cardiac index; SPAP, systolic PAP.

those with PAH.[39] Despite these promising results, a recently completed large randomized trial (ASCEND-HF [Acute Study of Clinical Effectiveness of Nesiritide in Decompensated Heart Failure] trial) has definitively shown that there is no long-term benefit of nesiritide for the treatment of decompensated LHF.[40] Future trials in PH secondary to LHF are unlikely.

Calcium Channel Blockers

In selected patients with PAH, improvement after treatment with calcium channel blockers portends an excellent outcome.[41] However, in patients with HFrEF, calcium channel blockers other than amlodipine worsen outcomes and should not be used.[3] In patients with HFpEF, depending on comorbid factors, calcium channel blockers may be a reasonable choice for the control of systemic hypertension or to slow heart rate in sinus tachycardia or atrial dysrhythmias.

Endothelin Receptor Antagonists

Identification of the vasoconstrictive and proliferative effects of ET and beneficial effects of ERAs on endothelial function, cardiac remodeling, and survival in animal models of heart failure[42] lead to human trials of ERAs with overall disappointing results.[43] None of these trials, however, has examined the effects of ERAs specifically in patients with PH associated with LHF.

Early acute hemodynamic trials of bosentan demonstrated favorable reductions in PVR prompting the performance of larger randomized trials.[44] The REACH-1 (Research on Endothelin Antagonism in Chronic Heart Failure) trial suggested a possible long-term benefit, although there was an early elevation in transaminase levels and worsening of heart failure.[42,45,46] The ENABLE-1 and ENABLE-2 (Endothelin Antagonist Bosentan for Lowering Cardiac Events) trials enrolled 1613 patients in the United States and Europe with New York Heart Association (NYHA) class IIIB or IV symptoms despite optimal medical therapy and randomized them to lower-dose bosentan at 125 mg daily or placebo. After a mean follow-up of 1.5 years, there was an increase in hospitalization for heart failure but no difference in mortality.[47] Liver function test abnormalities with elevations more than 3 times the normal level were more common with bosentan (2.7% with placebo, 9.5% with bosentan). Worsening lower extremity edema and fluid retention were noted in the treatment group despite increased diuretic usage.

The HEAT (Heart Failure ETA Receptor Blockade Trial) examined the hemodynamic and neurohumoral effects of 3 weeks of treatment with the selective ET_A receptor antagonist darusentan in patients with NYHA class III heart failure.[48] Short-term administration resulted in a nonsignificant increase in cardiac index (CI), which became significant after 3 weeks of therapy. SVR was significantly decreased, but PAP, PAWP, right atrial pressure, and PVR remained unchanged as did heart rate, systemic blood pressure, and plasma catecholamine levels. A nonsignificant trend toward harm was noted with higher dosages including increased heart failure exacerbations and death without further improvement in hemodynamic measures. The subsequent EARTH (Endothelin A Receptor Antagonist Trial in Heart Failure) study evaluated the effects of darusentan on cardiac remodeling and neurohumoral effects in 642 patients with moderate left ventricular systolic dysfunction and NYHA class II-IV symptoms on maximal standard heart failure treatment.[49] After 24 weeks of treatment with darusentan or placebo, there was no change in the primary end point of left ventricular end systolic volume. Also unchanged were secondary end points of serum concentration of norepinephrine, epinephrine, and aldosterone.

Results of the ENCOR (Enrasentan Cooperative Randomized Evaluation)[43] trial were presented in 2001 but have yet to be published. The study randomized 419 patients with stable NYHA class II or III LHF and an EF fraction less than 35% on standard therapies to 30, 60, or 90 mg of the dual-receptor ERA enrasentan. There was no benefit relative to placebo, and patients receiving active drug were more likely to be hospitalized. There was also a trend toward higher mortality and progressive left ventricular dysfunction with enrasentan.

The RITZ-5 (Randomized Intravenous Tezosentan) trial studied the effects of IV tezosentan[50] in 84 patients with severe acute pulmonary edema secondary to a heart failure exacerbation. In the treatment group, tezosentan was given as an IV bolus followed by a continuous drip. There was no difference between tezosentan and placebo in the primary end point of oxygen saturation after 60 minutes. In addition, hypotension was more common with tezosentan (38% vs 19% with placebo, $P = .05$) as was an increase in creatinine.

Phosphodiesterase Type 5 Inhibitors

Sildenafil is a phosphodiesterase type 5 (PDE5) inhibitor initially developed in 1986 for the treatment of hypertension and angina.[51] Nitric oxide induces the production of cyclic guanosine monophosphate (cGMP), which activates protein kinase G leading to vasodilation and inhibition of smooth muscle cell proliferation. Inhibition of PDE5 prevents degradation of cGMP in smooth muscle cells and prolongs the effects of nitric oxide. Recognition of the potential benefits in patients with PAH led to the SUPER-1[52] (Sildenafil Use in Pulmonary Arterial Hypertension) trial and FDA approval for improvement in exercise tolerance, followed more recently by approval of the longer-acting analogue tadalafil.[53] In addition to improvements in endothelial function and inhibition of remodeling, sildenafil may have additional benefits, and there has been much recent interest in sildenafil for the treatment of HFrEF and HFpEF.[54,55] Of note, these agents are contraindicated in patients who take nitrates for ischemic heart disease or LHF because the combination may precipitate severe hypotension.

Several studies demonstrating a favorable acute hemodynamic response to sildenafil have been published. In one trial 14 patients with advanced heart failure (average EF, 24%) undergoing right-sided heart catheterization for heart transplant evaluation received 25 or 50 mg of sildenafil every 8 hours for 3 or less doses. There was a significant reduction in MPAP (44 to 31 mm Hg), PAWP (25 to 18 mm Hg), and PVR (311 to 191 dyne·s/cm^5) and an increase in CI (2.4 to 2.8 L/min/m^2).[56] Another study examined the acute hemodynamic effects of sildenafil, nitric oxide, and both in 11 patients with idiopathic dilated cardiomyopathy and PH undergoing heart transplant evaluation.[57] Sildenafil alone decreased MPAP by 12%, PVR by 12%, SVR by 13%, and PAWP by 12% and increased CI by 14%. The combination of sildenafil and nitric oxide increased CI by 30% and decreased SVR by 24% and PVR by 50%, whereas the change in MPAP and LVEDP was similar to that resulting from sildenafil alone. The acute effects of sildenafil on exercise tolerance were studied in 13 patients with NYHA class III heart failure who underwent assessment of hemodynamics, gas exchange, and radionuclide ventriculography at rest and with cycle ergometry 60 minutes before and after administration of 50 mg of sildenafil.[58] Of the 13 patients, 7 had PH with a resting MPAP of 37 mm Hg. In these patients, sildenafil decreased the MPAP to 27 mm Hg without changing the PAWP or CO. Sildenafil reduced exercise MPAP by 15%, increased CI by 14%, and did not change the PAWP. It also improved right ventricular EF and ventilatory efficiency but only in patients with PH at baseline. There were not significant changes in exercise variables in patients without baseline PH.[58]

More recently, results of several trials examining the long-term effects of sildenafil in patients with LHF have been published. Forty-six male patients with LHF on a stable medical regimen were assigned to sildenafil, 50 mg 3 times daily, or placebo and followed up for 6 months.[59] Systolic PAP determined by echocardiography was significantly lower at 6 months in patients taking sildenafil versus placebo (23.9 vs 33.7 mm Hg). There were also significant improvements in measures of endothelial function and exercise tolerance, which, the authors hypothesize, were partly related to improved exercise hemodynamics. In a follow-up study, 45 patients with HFrEF were randomized to sildenafil, 50 mg 3 times daily, or placebo. At 1 year of follow-up, there was significant improvement in EF, diastolic function, left atrial size index, left ventricular mass index, peak exercise oxygen consumption, ventilation efficiency, and quality of life without significant adverse effects.[60] In another study the same authors tested the hypothesis that sildenafil would be beneficial in patients with heart failure with exercise oscillatory breathing (EOB), an abnormality thought secondary to pulmonary vasoconstriction. Thirty-two patients with EOB were randomized to sildenafil or placebo. After 1 year of follow-up, exercise breathing normalized in 15 patients in the sildenafil group in comparison with 2 in the placebo group. In addition, sildenafil significantly improved peak oxygen consumption and ventilation efficiency and decreased PCWP and MPAP in comparison with placebo.[61] Long-term improvement in MPAP, RV function, right atrial pressure, and left ventricular systolic and diastolic function was also seen at 1 year in a randomized trial of sildenafil versus placebo in patients with HFpEF.[62]

Biological plausibility, rapidly accumulating reports of hemodynamic and exercise benefits, and few adverse effects from PDE5 inhibitors suggest that they may represent a significant advance in the treatment of LHF. However, further, larger, well-designed prospective trials with appropriate outcome measures are required to evaluate the long-term effects of PDE5 inhibitors with respect to safety and efficacy in patients with LHF before they are routinely prescribed for this purpose. The RELAX (Phosphodiesterase-5 Inhibition to Improve Quality of Life And Exercise Capacity in Diastolic Heart Failure) trial in HFpEF and a proposed trial in HFrEF are likely to shed light on this issue.

Candidates for Cardiac Transplantation

PH in patients undergoing heart transplantation is associated with a poor outcome and is a contraindication to transplantation (see **Box 1**). Among transplant candidates with PH, a reduction in the MPAP and the TPG during the infusion of vasodilators identifies a subset of patients who may have mortality similar to those of patients without PH undergoing transplantation.[63,64] In patients with fixed PH, there are few data to guide management; however, some experts have advocated for aggressive, long-term hemodynamic support with inotropes/inodilators, which may restore vasoreactivity. There are also limited data that suggest treatment with sildenafil can restore vasoreactivity in heart transplant candidates (see **Fig. 2**).[65] Combined heart and lung transplantation is now infrequently performed but may provide an alternative for patients with fixed PH.[66,67] The procedure is most commonly reserved for patients with PAH or PH associated with congenital heart disease.

In some patients, therapy with a left ventricular assist device (LVAD) significantly improves pulmonary hemodynamics and permits transplantation.[64] In a recent study of 58 consecutive patients treated with LVAD support, pulmonary hemodynamics rapidly improved to a similar level in all patients after LVAD implantation regardless of severity of baseline abnormalities.[68] Several other studies have demonstrated dramatic improvements in pulmonary hemodynamics even in patients with fixed PH. One such study compared 26 patients with fixed PH treated with LVAD with 52 subjects without PH undergoing transplantation. All patients with PH underwent LVAD placement, with normalization of pulmonary hemodynamics by 6 weeks and successful heart transplantation. There was no difference in mortality between patients with and without PH before transplant.[69]

SUMMARY

PH associated with LHF is an increasingly recognized problem. It is clear that PH with LHF is associated with higher morbidity and mortality, worse exercise capacity, and adverse outcomes after heart transplantation. Hemodynamic derangements and activation of neurohormones, cytokines, and other mediators with endothelial dysfunction contribute to the development of mixed PH. In patients undergoing an evaluation for PH, a complete cardiac evaluation to exclude left-sided heart disease as a cause is mandatory. In patients with PH and LHF, appropriate maximal guideline-recommended medical and surgical management of the underlying heart disease is the mainstay of treatment. At present, none of the agents approved for the treatment of PAH have been shown to benefit patients with PH secondary to LHF and there is evidence that they may be harmful. Growing data suggest a possible benefit of the PDE5 inhibitor sildenafil in LHF, but appropriately designed larger-scale confirmatory trials have yet to be performed. Emerging data suggest a role for mechanical circulatory support alone or in combination with medical therapy. Heart-lung transplantation is an option for suitable candidates with persistent irreversible PH due to LHF. Future studies using standardized/consistent nomenclature, definitions, and hemodynamic criteria for PH due to LHF are warranted to better characterize the epidemiology, natural history, and response to therapy.

REFERENCES

1. Simonneau G, Robbins IM, Beghetti M, et al. Updated clinical classification of pulmonary hypertension. J Am Coll Cardiol 2009;54(Suppl 1):S43–54.
2. Gladwin MT, Sachdev V, Jison ML, et al. Pulmonary hypertension as a risk factor for death in patients with sickle cell disease. N Engl J Med 2004;350(9):886–95.
3. Hunt SA, Abraham WT, Chin MH, et al. 2009 focused update incorporated into the ACC/AHA 2005 Guidelines for the Diagnosis and Management of Heart Failure in Adults: a report of the American College of Cardiology Foundation/American Heart Association Task Force on Practice Guidelines: developed in collaboration with the International Society for Heart and Lung Transplantation. Circulation 2009;119(14):e391–479.
4. Khush KK, Tasissa G, Butler J, et al. Effect of pulmonary hypertension on clinical outcomes in advanced heart failure: analysis of the Evaluation Study of Congestive Heart Failure and Pulmonary Artery Catheterization Effectiveness (ESCAPE) database. Am Heart J 2009;157(6):1026–34.
5. Lam CS, Roger VL, Rodeheffer RJ, et al. Pulmonary hypertension in heart failure with preserved ejection fraction: a community-based study. J Am Coll Cardiol 2009;53(13):1119–26.
6. Costard-Jackle A, Fowler MB. Influence of preoperative pulmonary artery pressure on mortality after heart transplantation: testing of potential reversibility of pulmonary hypertension with nitroprusside is useful in defining a high risk group. J Am Coll Cardiol 1992;19(1):48–54.
7. Bonow RO, Carabello BA, Chatterjee K, et al. ACC/AHA 2006 guidelines for the management of patients with valvular heart disease: a report of the American College of Cardiology/American Heart Association Task Force on Practice Guidelines (writing committee to revise the 1998 Guidelines for the Management of Patients with Valvular Heart Disease) developed in collaboration with the Society of Cardiovascular Anesthesiologists endorsed by the Society for Cardiovascular Angiography and Interventions and the Society of Thoracic Surgeons. J Am Coll Cardiol 2006;48(3):e1–148.
8. Braunwald E, Braunwald NS, Ross J Jr, et al. Effects of mitral-valve replacement on the pulmonary

vascular dynamics of patients with pulmonary hypertension. N Engl J Med 1965;273:509–14.

9. Kuznetsova T, Herbots L, Lopez B, et al. Prevalence of left ventricular diastolic dysfunction in a general population. Circ Heart Fail 2009;2(2):105–12.

10. Pieske B. Heart failure with preserved ejection fraction—a growing epidemic or 'The Emperor's New Clothes?' Eur J Heart Fail 2011;13(1):11–3.

11. Abramson SV, Burke JF, Kelly JJ Jr, et al. Pulmonary hypertension predicts mortality and morbidity in patients with dilated cardiomyopathy. Ann Intern Med 1992;116(11):888–95.

12. Chatterjee NA, Lewis GD. What is the prognostic significance of pulmonary hypertension in heart failure? Circ Heart Fail 2011;4(5):541–5.

13. Aronson D, Eitan A, Dragu R, et al. The relationship between reactive pulmonary hypertension and mortality in patients with acute decompensated heart failure. Circ Heart Fail 2011;4(5):644–50.

14. Cappola TP, Felker GM, Kao WH, et al. Pulmonary hypertension and risk of death in cardiomyopathy: patients with myocarditis are at higher risk. Circulation 2002;105(14):1663–8.

15. Bursi F, McNallan SM, Redfield MM, et al. Pulmonary pressures and death in heart failure: a community study. J Am Coll Cardiol 2012;59(3):222–31.

16. Lewis GD, Murphy RM, Shah RV, et al. Pulmonary vascular response patterns during exercise in left ventricular systolic dysfunction predict exercise capacity and outcomes/clinical perspective. Circ Heart Fail 2011;4(3):276–85.

17. Kang DH, Kim JH, Rim JH, et al. Comparison of early surgery versus conventional treatment in asymptomatic severe mitral regurgitation. Circulation 2009; 119(6):797–804.

18. Chen JM, Levin HR, Michler RE, et al. Reevaluating the significance of pulmonary hypertension before cardiac transplantation: determination of optimal thresholds and quantification of the effect of reversibility on perioperative mortality. J Thorac Cardiovasc Surg 1997;114(4):627–34.

19. Erickson KW, Costanzo-Nordin MR, O'Sullivan EJ, et al. Influence of preoperative transpulmonary gradient on late mortality after orthotopic heart transplantation. J Heart Lung Transplant 1990;9(5): 526–37.

20. Mandeep RM, Jon K, Randall S, et al. Listing criteria for heart transplantation: international society for heart and lung transplantation guidelines for the care of cardiac transplant candidates—2006. J Heart Lung Transplant 2006;25(9):1024–42.

21. Butler J, Stankewicz MA, Wu J, et al. Pre-transplant reversible pulmonary hypertension predicts higher risk for mortality after cardiac transplantation. J Heart Lung Transplant 2005;24(2):170–7.

22. Drazner MH, Hamilton MA, Fonarow G, et al. Relationship between right and left-sided filling pressures in 1000 patients with advanced heart failure. J Heart Lung Transplant 1999;18(11):1126–32.

23. Delgado JF, Conde E, Sánchez V, et al. Pulmonary vascular remodeling in pulmonary hypertension due to chronic heart failure. Eur J Heart Fail 2005; 7(6):1011–6.

24. Moraes DL, Colucci WS, Givertz MM. Secondary pulmonary hypertension in chronic heart failure: the role of the endothelium in pathophysiology and management. Circulation 2000;102(14):1718–23.

25. Budhiraja R, Tuder RM, Hassoun PM. Endothelial dysfunction in pulmonary hypertension. Circulation 2004;109(2):159–65.

26. Cargill RI, Lipworth BJ. Lisinopril attenuates acute hypoxic pulmonary vasoconstriction in humans. Chest 1996;109(2):424–9.

27. Bristow MR. Beta-adrenergic receptor blockade in chronic heart failure. Circulation 2000;101(5):558–69.

28. A placebo-controlled trial of captopril in refractory chronic congestive heart failure. Captopril Multicenter Research Group. J Am Coll Cardiol 1983; 2(4):755–63.

29. Ferreira AJ, Shenoy V, Yamazato Y, et al. Evidence for angiotensin-converting enzyme 2 as a therapeutic target for the prevention of pulmonary hypertension. Am J Respir Crit Care Med 2009;179(11): 1048–54.

30. Rubin LJ, Badesch DB, Barst RJ, et al. Bosentan therapy for pulmonary arterial hypertension. N Engl J Med 2002;346(12):896–903.

31. Hiroe M, Hirata Y, Fujita N, et al. Plasma endothelin-1 levels in idiopathic dilated cardiomyopathy. Am J Cardiol 1991;68(10):1114–5.

32. Cody RJ, Haas GJ, Binkley PF, et al. Plasma endothelin correlates with the extent of pulmonary hypertension in patients with chronic congestive heart failure. Circulation 1992;85(2):504–9.

33. Pacher R, Stanek B, Hulsmann M, et al. Prognostic impact of big endothelin-1 plasma concentrations compared with invasive hemodynamic evaluation in severe heart failure. J Am Coll Cardiol 1996; 27(3):633–41.

34. Nagueh SF, Appleton CP, Gillebert TC, et al. Recommendations for the evaluation of left ventricular diastolic function by echocardiography. J Am Soc Echocardiogr 2009;22(2):107–33.

35. Hoeper MM, Lee SH, Voswinckel R, et al. Complications of right heart catheterization procedures in patients with pulmonary hypertension in experienced centers. J Am Coll Cardiol 2006;48(12): 2546–52.

36. Shah SJ, Gheorghiade M. Heart failure with preserved ejection fraction: treat now by treating comorbidities. JAMA 2008;300(4):431–3.

37. Califf RM, Adams KF, McKenna WJ, et al. A randomized controlled trial of epoprostenol therapy for severe congestive heart failure: the

Flolan International Randomized Survival Trial (FIRST). Am Heart J 1997;134(1):44–54.

38. Publication Committee for the VMAC Investigators (Vasodilatation in the Management of Acute CHF). Intravenous nesiritide vs nitroglycerin for treatment of decompensated congestive heart failure. JAMA 2002;287(12):1531–40.

39. Michaels AD, Chatterjee K, De Marco T. Effects of intravenous nesiritide on pulmonary vascular hemodynamics in pulmonary hypertension. J Card Fail 2005;11(6):425–31.

40. 2010 clinical trial/clinical science abstracts. Circulation 2010;122(21):2215–26.

41. Sitbon O, Humbert M, Jaïs X, et al. Long-term response to calcium channel blockers in idiopathic pulmonary arterial hypertension. Circulation 2005; 111(23):3105–11.

42. Cowburn PJ, Cleland JG. Endothelin antagonists for chronic heart failure: do they have a role? Eur Heart J 2001;22(19):1772–84.

43. Kelland NF, Webb DJ. Clinical trials of endothelin antagonists in heart failure: publication is good for the public health. Heart 2007;93(1):2–4.

44. Sutsch G, Kiowski W, Yan XW, et al. Short-term oral endothelin-receptor antagonist therapy in conventionally treated patients with symptomatic severe chronic heart failure. Circulation 1998;98(21):2262–8.

45. Packer M, McMurray J, Massie BM, et al. Clinical effects of endothelin receptor antagonism with bosentan in patients with severe chronic heart failure: results of a pilot study. J Card Fail 2005;11(1):12–20.

46. Teerlink JR. Recent heart failure trials of neurohormonal modulation (OVERTURE and ENABLE): approaching the asymptote of efficacy? J Card Fail 2002;8(3):124–7.

47. Kalra PR, Moon JC, Coats AJ. Do results of the ENABLE (Endothelin Antagonist Bosentan for Lowering Cardiac Events in Heart Failure) study spell the end for non-selective endothelin antagonism in heart failure? Int J Cardiol 2002;85(2–3):195–7.

48. Luscher TF, Enseleit F, Pacher R, et al. Hemodynamic and neurohumoral effects of selective endothelin A (ETA) receptor blockade in chronic heart failure: the heart failure ETA receptor blockade trial (HEAT). Circulation 2002;106(21):2666–72.

49. Anand PI, McMurray PJ, Cohn JN, et al. Long-term effects of darusentan on left-ventricular remodelling and clinical outcomes in the Endothelin A Receptor Antagonist Trial in Heart Failure (EARTH): randomised, double-blind, placebo-controlled trial. Lancet 2004;364(9431):347–54.

50. Kaluski E, Kobrin I, Zimlichman R, et al. RITZ-5: randomized intravenous TeZosentan (an endothelin-A/B antagonist) for the treatment of pulmonary edema: a prospective, multicenter, double-blind, placebo-controlled study. J Am Coll Cardiol 2003; 41(2):204–10.

51. Barnett CF, Machado RF. Sildenafil in the treatment of pulmonary hypertension. Vasc Health Risk Manag 2006;2(4):411–22.

52. Galie N, Ghofrani HA, Torbicki A, et al. Sildenafil citrate therapy for pulmonary arterial hypertension. N Engl J Med 2005;353(20):2148–57.

53. Galiè N, Brundage BH, Ghofrani HA, et al. Tadalafil therapy for pulmonary arterial hypertension. Circulation 2009;119(22):2894–903.

54. Kumar P, Francis GS, Tang WH. Phosphodiesterase 5 inhibition in heart failure: mechanisms and clinical implications. Nat Rev Cardiol 2009; 6(5):349–55.

55. Goldsmith SR. Type 5 phosphodiesterase inhibition in heart failure: the next step. J Am Coll Cardiol 2007;50(22):2145–7.

56. Alaeddini J, Uber PA, Park MH, et al. Efficacy and safety of sildenafil in the evaluation of pulmonary hypertension in severe heart failure. Am J Cardiol 2004;94(11):1475–7.

57. Lepore JJ, Maroo A, Bigatello LM, et al. Hemodynamic effects of sildenafil in patients with congestive heart failure and pulmonary hypertension: combined administration with inhaled nitric oxide. Chest 2005; 127(5):1647–53.

58. Lewis GD, Lachmann J, Camuso J, et al. Sildenafil improves exercise hemodynamics and oxygen uptake in patients with systolic heart failure. Circulation 2007;115(1):59–66.

59. Guazzi M, Samaja M, Arena R, et al. Long-term use of sildenafil in the therapeutic management of heart failure. J Am Coll Cardiol 2007;50(22): 2136–44.

60. Guazzi M, Vicenzi M, Arena R, et al. PDE5-inhibition with sildenafil improves left ventricular diastolic function, cardiac geometry and clinical status in patients with stable systolic heart failure: results of a 1-year prospective, randomized, placebo-controlled study. Circ Heart Fail 2011;4(1):8–17.

61. Guazzi M, Vicenzi M, Arena R. Phosphodiesterase 5 inhibition with sildenafil reverses exercise oscillatory breathing in chronic heart failure: a long-term cardiopulmonary exercise testing placebo-controlled study. Eur J Heart Fail 2012;14(1):82–90.

62. Guazzi M, Vicenzi M, Arena R, et al. Pulmonary hypertension in heart failure with preserved ejection fraction/clinical perspective. Circulation 2011; 124(2):164–74.

63. Klotz S, Wenzelburger F, Stypmann J, et al. Reversible pulmonary hypertension in heart transplant candidates: to transplant or not to transplant. Ann Thorac Surg 2006;82(5):1770–3.

64. Beyersdorf F, Schlensak C, Berchtold-Herz M, et al. Regression of "fixed" pulmonary vascular resistance in heart transplant candidates after unloading with ventricular assist devices. J Thorac Cardiovasc Surg 2010;140(4):747–9.

65. Sansone F, Rinaldi M. Oral sildenafil: potential role in heart transplantation. Review of the literature and personal experience. J Cardiol 2010;55(3):291–5.

66. Garrity ER, Moore J, Mulligan MS, et al. Heart and lung transplantation in the United States, 1996–2005. Am J Transplant 2007;7:1390–403.

67. Deuse T, Sista R, Weill D, et al. Review of heart-lung transplantation at Stanford. Ann Thorac Surg 2010; 90(1):329–37.

68. Nair PK, Kormos RL, Teuteberg JJ, et al. Pulsatile left ventricular assist device support as a bridge to decision in patients with end-stage heart failure complicated by pulmonary hypertension. J Heart Lung Transplant 2010;29(2):201–8.

69. Zimpfer D, Zrunek P, Sandner S, et al. Post-transplant survival after lowering fixed pulmonary hypertension using left ventricular assist devices. Eur J Cardiothorac Surg 2007;31(4):698–702.

Pulmonary Hypertension in Parenchymal Lung Disease

Rosechelle M. Ruggiero, MD, MSCS[a],
Sonja Bartolome, MD[a],*, Fernando Torres, MD[a,b]

KEYWORDS

- Pulmonary hypertension • Interstitial lung disease • Chronic obstructive pulmonary disease
- Idiopathic pulmonary fibrosis

KEY POINTS

- The prevalence of pulmonary hypertension (PH) in parenchymal lung disease is common.
- The pathophysiology of pulmonary hypertension (PH) in parenchymal lung diseases is partially, if not mostly, related to hypoxic pulmonary vasoconstriction.
- The pathophysiology of PH in chronic obstructive pulmonary disease is poorly described, but likely involves an interaction between hypoxic vasoconstriction, vascular inflammation, and a loss of capillaries in the diseased lung.
- Restrictive lung diseases are characterized by pulmonary parenchymal abnormalities rather than the obstruction of airflow and are often associated with PH through hypoxic pulmonary vasoconstriction and varying degrees of inflammation.
- Systemic disorders can also affect the pulmonary parenchyma and be associated with PH.
- PH treatment is controversial for patients with parenchymal lung disease.

INTRODUCTION

Pulmonary hypertension (PH) is an umbrella term that encompasses all disease states that elevate the pressures in the pulmonary circulation. It is defined as a mean pulmonary artery pressure (mPAP) of greater than 25 mm Hg.[1] The term is nonspecific and includes diseases that increase pressures from the pulmonary venous circulation, such as congestive heart failure; conditions that affect the small pulmonary arteries, such as idiopathic pulmonary arterial hypertension; and conditions characterized by hypoxic vasoconstriction, such as chronic obstructive pulmonary disease

(COPD). These conditions all result in elevation of pulmonary pressures but have distinct pathophysiology, prognoses, and treatment. A classification scheme for PH was introduced at the World Health Organization conference in 1973 to organize these conditions according to cause and treatment.[2] This classification scheme has undergone several revisions in the past—the most recent in 2008 (**Table 1**).[3]

This article focuses on group III PH, namely PH attributable to lung disease and/or hypoxia. Group III PH includes COPD and interstitial lung disease (ILD)—the most common parenchymal lung diseases associated with PH. It also includes

This work was supported by F32 training grant: NIH 5T32HL098040-01.

Financial disclosures: Dr Torres is on the speaker's bureau or has participated in advisory boards for Actelion Pharmaceuticals, Gilead, United Therapeutics, and Pfizer. Dr Bartolome is on the speaker's bureaus or has participated in advisory boards for Actelion Pharmaceuticals, Gilead, and United Therapeutics. Dr Torres and Dr Bartolome participate in clinical research at UT Southwestern, which is funded by Gilead, United Therapeutics, Pfizer, Novartis, Bayer, and GeNO.

[a] Division of Pulmonary and Critical Care Medicine, UT Southwestern Medical Center, 5323 Harry Hines Boulevard, Dallas, TX 75390-8550, USA; [b] Lung Transplant and Pulmonary Hypertension Program, UT Southwestern, 5323 Harry Hines Boulevard, Dallas, TX 75390-8550, USA

* Corresponding author.

E-mail address: Sonja.Bartolome@utsouthwestern.edu

Heart Failure Clin 8 (2012) 461–474
doi:10.1016/j.hfc.2012.04.010
1551-7136/12/$ – see front matter Published by Elsevier Inc.

Table 1	
World Health Organization classification of pulmonary hypertensive diseases	
Group I	Pulmonary arterial hypertension
Group II	PH attributable to left heart disease
Group III	PH owing to lung diseases and/or hypoxia
	COPD
	ILD
	Other pulmonary diseases with mixed restrictive and obstructive patterns
	Sleep-disordered breathing
	Alveolar hypoventilation disorders
	Chronic exposure to high altitude
	Developmental abnormalities
Group IV	Chronic thromboembolic PH
Group V	PH with unclear multifactorial mechanisms

sleep-disordered breathing and hypoventilation from any cause. Also discussed are other parenchymal lung diseases associated with PH, namely sarcoidosis and systemic vasculitides (group V) (see **Table 1**).[3]

The overall prevalence of PH in parenchymal lung disease is difficult to assess. In a national hospital discharge survey, it was demonstrated that use of the *International Classification of Diseases, Ninth Revision* code for PH has increased over the past two decades. In patients with chronic lower respiratory diseases listed as the first diagnosis, PH was listed as secondary diagnoses on hospital discharge with a range from 12.9% to 23.1%.[4]

The pathophysiology of PH in parenchymal lung diseases is partially, if not mostly, related to hypoxic pulmonary vasoconstriction.[5–7] Indeed, studies have shown that long-term oxygen therapy (>16 h/d) slows the progression of PH in patients with parenchymal lung disease.[8] In most these patients, the severity of PH is in the mild-to-moderate range and the clinical course is relatively stable.[9,10] However, there is a subset of patients with parenchymal lung disease who will develop severe PH that is deemed out of proportion to their parenchymal lung disease as measured by pulmonary function testing and/or oxygen saturation. These patients exhibit decreased functional status and a significantly worse prognosis when compared with patients with parenchymal disease alone. It is speculated that this subset may benefit from PH-specific therapy.

A diagnosis of PH should be entertained when a patient's clinical symptoms seem out of proportion to the degree of parenchymal lung disease or when there is a worsening of clinical symptoms that does not correspond to pulmonary function testing or radiographic findings. The diagnosis of PH with underlying lung disease is challenging because the typical screening tests can be unreliable. Patients with PH often exhibit a low 6-minute walk test (6MWT) and DLCO in the pulmonary function lab. However, these abnormalities are also seen with parenchymal lung disease alone. Additionally, transthoracic echocardiography may be unreliable owing to distortion of the acoustic windows by air trapping and/or fibrotic lung parenchyma.[9,11–13] Because of the limited utility of the screening tools available in our armamentarium, a low threshold for right-heart catheterization (RHC) is required to make the diagnosis.

PH treatment is controversial for patients with parenchymal lung disease. There is little evidence for the safety and efficacy of PH-specific treatment in this population. Additionally, the available treatments for PH may worsen ventilation-perfusion mismatch by vasodilating in areas of diseased lung and, therefore, worsen hypoxemia. Because patients with PH and parenchymal lung disease exhibit poorer functional capacity and shorter survival times than those with parenchymal disease alone, PH-specific treatment is attractive. Ongoing clinical trials are attempting to identify the safety, efficacy, and appropriate patient selection for therapy. The following sections review the data describing PH in specific parenchymal diseases.

OBSTRUCTIVE LUNG DISEASE AND PH

Pulmonary vascular constriction is the compensatory response to alveolar hypoxia and, therefore, an elevation in pulmonary vascular resistance is associated with any obstructive lung disease with uncontrolled airflow limitation. Hypoxia-driven vasoconstriction can result in elevated pulmonary pressures in diseases such as uncontrolled asthma, bronchiolitis obliterans, and COPD. The best-described associations are between PH and two entities: (1) COPD and (2) a new syndrome termed combined pulmonary fibrosis and emphysema (CPFE).

COPD

PH is prevalent in the COPD population and, when severe, is a poor prognostic indicator. The true prevalence of PH in COPD is unknown because of the difficulty in obtaining population-based data. Clinical trials are hampered by both the poor positive predictive value of echocardiogram to detect PH in COPD patients and the ethical issues associated with widespread RHC.[13,14] To date, there are three large trials describing the pulmonary pressures of patients with advanced emphysema and one large hospital-based registry of patients with COPD. Scharf and colleagues[10] evaluated the cohort of patients that were screened for the National Emphysema Treatment Trial (NETT). Three of the 17 participating centers performed RHCs as part of their screening protocol, yielding 120 subjects. Of these, the mPAP was 26.3 ± 5.2 mm Hg. Ninety-one percent of this sample had pulmonary artery pressures (PAP) greater than 20 mm Hg, largely accepted as the upper limit of normal. Thus, PH was extremely prevalent in patients with advanced emphysema but was typically in the mild-to-moderate range, with a smaller portion (5%) presenting with severe PH (mPAP >35). Additionally, a significant number of patients had PH accompanied by an elevated pulmonary capillary wedge pressure, indicating that part of this prevalence was due to left-sided heart dysfunction.

Thabut and colleagues[15] performed a retrospective review of 215 patients referred for lung volume reduction surgery (LVRS) or lung transplantation, all with severe COPD. RHC revealed PH in 50% of subjects with an mPAP of 26.9 mm Hg. Again, most these had mild PH. However, 9.8% were classified as moderate PH (mPAP >35 mm Hg) and 3.7% fell into the severe category (mPAP >45 mm Hg) (**Fig. 1**). The study also described a small subgroup of patients (n = 16) with severe elevations in PAP that seemed incongruent with their moderate impairment in spirometry. Finally, Vizza and colleagues[16] reported a retrospective review

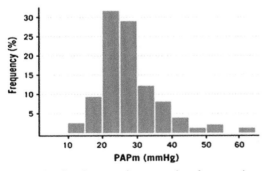

Fig. 1. The distribution of mPAPs taken from a cohort of candidates evaluated for both lung transplantation or LVRS. As indicated, the mPAPs fall in the mild-to-moderate range. (*From* Thabut G, Dauriat G, Stern JB, et al. Pulmonary hemodynamics in advanced COPD candidates for lung volume reduction surgery or lung transplantation. Chest 2005;127(5):1531–6; with permission.)

of patients with parenchymal lung disease referred for transplantation, 156 of whom had COPD. Again, the mPAP was mildly elevated at 25 ± 6 mm Hg.

These studies show an overall prevalence of PH in COPD patients ranging from 50% to 91%. It must be emphasized, however, that these studies were done in patients with advanced disease referred for either LVRS or lung transplantation. Therefore, the data may not be representative of the general population of COPD patients. In that vein, a chart review of 998 patients with COPD who underwent RHC was performed. Taking a random sampling of those patients, they found that approximately 50% had mPAPs above 20 mm Hg.[17] Taken together, the data indicate that in patients with moderate COPD without other co-morbidities, the prevalence of PH is about 50% and, in patients with advanced disease, it is significantly higher. Additionally, PH in the COPD population is generally mild-to-moderate (mPAP 25–40), but there seems to be a small subset of patients who develop severe PH. The aforementioned retrospective review of 998 patients with COPD identified 27 patients with severe PH (mPAP >40 mm Hg). Of those 27 patients, 11 had no other identifiable cause of PH and their degree of obstruction was classified in the mild-to-moderate range. Survival was significantly reduced in this subset of patients (**Fig. 2**).[17]

The pathophysiology of PH in COPD is poorly described but likely involves an interaction between hypoxic vasoconstriction, vascular inflammation, and a loss of capillaries in the diseased lung. Hypoxic pulmonary vasoconstriction, known as the von Euler-Liljestrand mechanism, has been well described throughout the past four decades (**Fig. 3**). Briefly, pulmonary arteries constrict in the presence of localized or diffuse hypoxia. Usually, this occurs in the presence of pneumonia, atelectasis, or lung infarction and is a protective mechanism that minimizes ventilation-perfusion mismatch. However, when this process becomes widespread and/or chronic, it results in a sustained increase in pulmonary vascular resistance. Over time, the pulmonary vasculature not only vasoconstricts, it also remodels.[14,18] Autopsy examination of patients with severe COPD reveals muscularization of the pulmonary arterioles and thickening of the medial and intimal vascular layers of the vessel wall.[19] Additionally, inflammatory cells have been noted in the pulmonary vascular walls of patients with COPD, and levels of proinflammatory cytokines, such as interleukin-6 and chemoattractant protein-1, correlate with mPAP in these patients.[19,20] Finally, patients with COPD exhibit a reduction in the total number of pulmonary vessels on pathology and pulmonary angiography.[14]

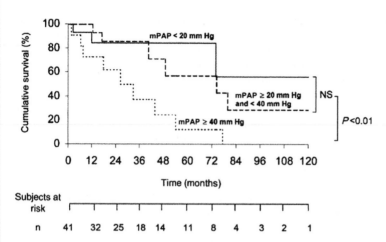

Fig. 2. Survival of patients with COPD and no other detectable cause of PH. The Kaplan-Meier curve of groups according to mPAP levels. mPAP <20 mm, n = 14; mPAP >20, <40, n = 16; mPAP >40, n = 11. (*From* Chaouat A, Bugnet AS, Kadaoui N, et al. Severe pulmonary hypertension and chronic obstructive pulmonary disease. Am J Respir Crit Care Med 2005;172(2):189–94; with permission.)

Symptoms of PH consist of dyspnea, exercise intolerance, and hypoxia and are hard to distinguish from the underlying obstructive airways disease. Thus, suspicion of PH should be piqued when these symptoms seem out of proportion to the degree of obstruction or when there is a worsening of symptoms without an associated decrease in spirometry.

Several investigators have evaluated the natural history of PH in association with COPD. In general, PH in COPD is slowly progressive and patients exhibit relative stability over time. Weitzenblum and colleagues[9] examined 84 patients with COPD who underwent two RHC at least 3 years apart. Initial hemodynamics showed 32 out of 85 patients with an mPAP greater than 20 mm Hg. At follow-up, the range was 27.7 to 31 mm Hg, indicating relative stability in pulmonary hemodynamics with a change of +0.5 to 0.6 mm Hg/y. Additional data on 131 patients with COPD who did not qualify for oxygen therapy were collected over an average of 6 years with two RHCs. At the end of the study period, 25% of the patients had an mPAP over 20 mm Hg, and all elevations were in the mild range.[21]

Although, normally, the overall progression of PH in COPD is slow, the presence of more severe PH is a predictor of early mortality. Oswald-Mammosser

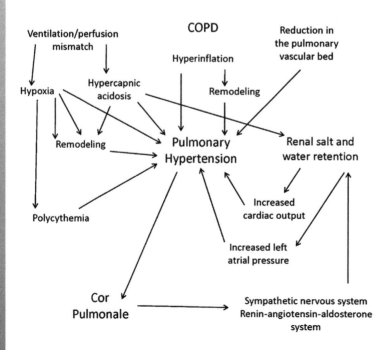

Fig. 3. Confirmed and suspected mechanisms leading to PH in COPD. (*Adapted from* Naeije R, MacNee W. Pulmonary circulation. In: Calverely P, MacNee W, Pride P, et al, editors. Chronic obstructive pulmonary disease. 2nd edition. London: Arnold Health Sciences; 2003. p. 228–42; with permission.)

and colleagues[22] examined the survival of 84 patients with COPD who were being initiated on long-term oxygen therapy. An RHC was performed before the onset of oxygen therapy. Patients with an initial mPAP of 25 mm Hg or less (n = 44) exhibited a 5-year survival of 62.2% versus 36.3% in those with significant elevations in their mPAP.

The treatment of PH related to COPD is focused on treatment of the underlying obstructive lung disease and correction of hypoxemia. Bronchodilators and long-acting inhaled corticosteroids remain the mainstay of pharmacologic treatment of COPD. However, the only two therapies shown to decrease mortality in COPD are smoking cessation and supplemental oxygen; these are paramount in the treatment of COPD both with and without PH.[23–25] Pulmonary rehabilitation programs improve quality of life and the ability to perform activities of daily living for patients with COPD; therefore, they are also recommended.[26]

Fifteen percent of patients with COPD have concomitant obstructive sleep apnea (OSA). In and of itself, OSA leads to PH, likely owing to nocturnal hypoxemia. A formal polysomnogram is recommended for those patients with COPD who exhibit nocturnal desaturation or symptoms of sleep apnea.

COPD patients also are at increased risk for venous thromboembolism and pulmonary emboli compared with the general population, and thromboembolic disease may increase pulmonary pressures. CT angiogram is recommended for evaluation of patients with an otherwise unexplained exacerbation of their pulmonary symptoms.[27,28]

The aforementioned therapies are typically used in mild-to-moderate PH that is commonly seen in COPD. However, as previously noted, there is a subset of patients with out-of-proportion PH that exhibit significant symptoms and worsened survival compared with those with COPD alone. The prevalence of severe PH in these COPD cohorts is similar to that seen in the general population. Because of their increased symptoms and poor outcomes, it is postulated that this group of patients may benefit from PH-specific therapy. Although this theory is attractive, the data supporting PH-specific therapy for patients with group III PH is restricted to small trials and case reports, and larger clinical trials are ongoing.

The phosphodiesterase type 5 (PDE5) inhibitor sildenafil (Revatio, Viagra) has been investigated in small observational trials. The administration of sildenafil to patients with COPD and PH results in acute (1 hour) hemodynamic improvements but not an increase in exercise capacity. This hemodynamic improvement was accompanied with worsened hypoxia, likely due to the drug's inhibition of hypoxic vasoconstriction in diseased areas of lung and, thus, ventilation-perfusion mismatch.[29,30] Additionally, two small cohorts of patients were followed after 3 months of oral sildenafil with conflicting results. One cohort showed statistically significant improvement in hemodynamics and exercise capacity; the other cohort was a negative trial.[31,32] Further work should help elucidate the role, if any, of PDE5 inhibitors in these patients.

Endothelin receptor antagonists (ERAs) are routinely used in the treatment of moderate idiopathic PH. This class of drugs has yet to show benefit in the patient with underlying COPD. In a recent trial, 30 patients with severe COPD (but not PH) were randomized to receive bosentan (Tracleer) or placebo for 12 weeks. There was no change in exercise capacity, PAP, or lung function. Additionally, oxygenation and quality of life decreased.[33] ERAs reportedly improved hemodynamics and functional status of patients with COPD and PH; however, thus far, the data are limited to abstracts and case reports.[34]

Intravenous epoprostenol (Flolan) was evaluated in COPD patients with significant PH (mPAP >30 mm Hg) who were admitted to the hospital with acute respiratory failure requiring mechanical ventilation. Subjects were randomized to receive epoprostenol or placebo. There was an initial decrease in pulmonary vascular resistance in the treatment arm, but this effect was not sustained at 24 hours. A decline in PaO_2 was also demonstrated in the treatment arm.[35]

In contrast to intravenous prostacyclins, which nonselectively vasodilate the pulmonary vessels, inhaled prostacyclins are thought to be distributed preferentially in the healthier areas of the lung. Because of this, it is postulated that this route could minimize the deleterious effect on gas exchange. To investigate this theory, inhaled iloprost (Ventavis) was given to men with both COPD and elevated PAP on ECG. The subjects lung function, ventilatory equivalents, arterial blood gases, and 6MWT distances were determined 30 min after a dose of inhaled iloprost. After treatment, the subjects gas exchange improved and their 6MWT improved by nearly 50 minutes.[36]

Other small studies have examined the use of cicletanine (an experimental agent in the United States that enhances the production of endogenous prostacyclin) and pravastatin (Pravachol) (which has antiinflammatory properties and enhances endothelial nitric oxide production) in the treatment of PH. These have shown initial positive results; however, additional studies are needed before formal recommendations can be made.[37,38]

Although these therapies seems attractive for patients with COPD and PH, the safety and efficacy of PH-specific therapy in these patients is unproven. Given the poor prognosis of severe PH in COPD patients, referral to a PH center for inclusion in a clinical trial should be considered. In patients with progressive respiratory failure due to COPD with or without PH, lung transplantation is curative. Survival after lung transplantation for COPD is 83.9% at 1 year and 66.5% at 3 years.[39]

The Syndrome of CPFE

The syndrome of CPFE was characterized in 2005 and because of its strong association with PH, was added to the PH classification scheme in 2008 (see **Table 1**).[40] This syndrome is characterized by a history of smoking, severe dyspnea, primarily upper lobe emphysema, primarily lower-lobe pulmonary fibrosis, a severely reduced DLCO, and unexpectedly preserved spirometry findings.[41] These patients exhibit a markedly increased prevalence of PH (reported 50%–90%) and exhibit significant mortality rates with a reported 25% 5-year survival.[40,42] Clinical trials with PH-specific agents have not been done; however, referral to a PH Center is prudent because the mortality rate may be driven primarily by the presence of PH.

RESTRICTIVE LUNG DISEASE AND PH

Restrictive lung disease is characterized by pulmonary parenchymal abnormalities rather than by the obstruction of airflow. It is also often associated with PH through hypoxic pulmonary vasoconstriction and varying degrees of inflammation. PH can complicate any restrictive lung disease associated with hypoxia, such as pneumoconiosis, hypersensitivity pneumonitis, nonspecific interstitial pneumonia, or idiopathic pulmonary fibrosis (IPF). Because of the rarity of most of these entities, most of the data have been collected on IPF.

IPF

The reported prevalence of PH in IPF varies widely and may be related to the timing of initial evaluation for PH. The prevalence in most studies ranges from 30% to 80%. These studies suffer the same selection bias as those for COPD and PH, with most patients recruited from lung transplant clinic and, therefore, having advanced disease. Nadrous and colleagues[43] evaluated 136 patients with IPF who underwent echocardiogram screening. In 88 of these patients, an estimate of the right ventricular systolic pressure was obtained. There was evidence of PH (sPAP >35 mm Hg at rest) in 74 patients (84%). In these patients, higher estimated pulmonary artery systolic pressures portended a shortened survival (**Fig. 4**). Although these are compelling data, echocardiogram is not a definitive diagnostic test for PH, particularly in patients with parenchymal lung disease.[11]

In a recent study in which RHC was used for diagnosis, 79 patients with IPF were evaluated and PH was present in 32% of this population. The mPAP correlated positively with mortality and there was a striking difference. One year mortality was 28% in the group with PH and IPF versus 5.5% in the group with IPF alone. Additionally, patients with PH and IPF have worsened oxygenation, exercise

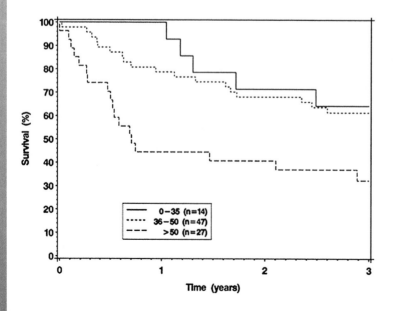

Fig. 4. Kaplan-Meier survival curve of idiopathic pulmonary fibrosis (IPF) patients stratified by their systolic pulmonary artery pressure. (*From* Nadrous HF, Pellikka PA, Krowka MJ, et al. Pulmonary hypertension in patients with idiopathic pulmonary fibrosis. Chest 2005;128(4):2393–9; with permission.)

capacity, and DLCO than those with IPF alone.[44,45] Evaluation of the United Network for Organ Sharing registry indicates that of those patients listed for lung transplant for IPF between 1995 and 2004, 45% had PH. However, as with COPD, most of these were in the mild-to-moderate range, with only 9% exhibiting severe PH (mPAP >40).[46] Long-term follow-up of transplant candidates with IPF illustrates worsening PAP over time. Nathan and colleagues[47] performed a retrospective review of IPF patients who had an RHC at the time of transplant evaluation and then at the time of transplantation. The mPAP of the population at baseline was 22.5 mm Hg and 17 out of 44 (39%) qualified as having PH. At follow-up, the mPAP was 32.7 mm Hg with 38 out of 44 (86%) with PH. The mean interval between PAP measurements was 258 days for the final cohort (range 25–936). This might lead one to think that patients with more severe IPF will develop more PH, but studies have not confirmed this theory. In the aforementioned retrospective review of 118 patients with IPF, the presence of PH did not correlate with the severity of lung function abnormalities. In fact, there was a trend toward increased prevalence of PH in IPF patients with better lung function, indicating that the interaction between PH and IPF is more complex than parenchymal destruction alone.[45] Zisman and colleagues[48] published further evidence of this incongruity in 2007. They performed a cross-sectional study of 65 patients trying to predict the presence of PH in IPF patients by findings on high-resolution CT scanning. Despite an exhaustive analysis, including a fibrosis score, quantification of ground glass infiltrates, total profusion score, honeycombing score, and the diameter of the pulmonary arteries, no CT finding correlated with the presence of PH on RHC. This

is further evidence that the interaction between PH and IPF is more complex than simple progression of parenchymal damage or hypoxia.

The pathophysiology of PH in IPF remains poorly defined. As with COPD, hypoxic vasoconstriction plays a role in the pathology by causing not only vasoconstriction but also vascular remodeling. However, in addition to the typical hypoxic pulmonary vascular changes (muscularization of the small pulmonary arteries, and collagen and elastin deposition in the medial layer) patients with IPF and PH display intimal hyperplasia and fibrosis and reduplication of the internal elastic lamina more typical of other kinds of PH. Additionally, although there is a reduction in the net area of the vascular bed from the parenchymal destruction related to the fibrosis, abnormal pulmonary vessels are observed even in areas of relatively normal lung, perhaps indicating an ongoing vascular inflammation independent of the surrounding parenchymal damage (**Fig. 5**).[49] Similarly to IPAH, an inflammatory environment has been described in the pulmonary vasculature of patients with IPAH and IPF, and elevated levels of endothelin-1, interleukin-6, and transforming growth factor-β have been demonstrated.[50–53]

The treatment of PH in IPF is challenging, again owing to worsening ventilation-perfusion mismatch with the use of pulmonary vasodilators. In COPD, the mainstay of treatment is focused on the obstructive lung disease; IPF, on the other hand, does not have an efficacious specific treatment and is progressive. There have been a few studies evaluating PH-specific therapy in patients with IPF.

Endothelin antagonists are an attractive possibility as endothelin is thought to participate in the fibrotic process. Minai and colleagues[54] performed a retrospective review of 19 patients with ILD who

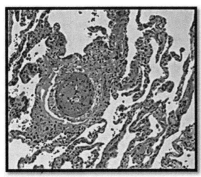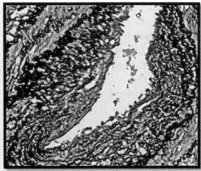

Fig. 5. Marked medial thickening in a distal pulmonary artery surrounded by relatively nonfibrotic lung tissue in an IPF patient (*left*). Medial thickening, intimal thickening, and elastic tissue duplication in a patient with PH and IPF (*right*, elastic von Gieson stain). (*From* Patel NM, Lederer DJ, Borczuk AC, et al. Pulmonary hypertension in idiopathic pulmonary fibrosis. Chest 2007;132:998–1006; with permission.)

were treated with either bosentan or epoprostenol. There was an initial improvement in 6MWD in treated patients, but this was not sustained. A large multicenter trial, the BUILD (Bosentan Use in Interstitial Lung Disease) trial, was reported in 2008. It was a randomized, placebo-controlled trial of bosentan versus placebo for 1 year; 158 patients with IPF, but without known PH, were enrolled. The primary endpoint was improvement in exercise capacity, and the treatment arm did not perform better than placebo.[55] The ARTEMIS and ARTEMIS-PH multicenter trials of ambrisentan (Letairis) (an endothelin-A receptor antagonist) in patients with IPF with and without PH were recently discontinued prematurely because of lack of efficacy.

Sildenafil has been evaluated for this group of patients in several small trials. Acutely, sildenafil treatment did not worsen ventilation-perfusion mismatch in a small cohort of IPF patients.[56] A small open-label study of sildenafil reported a mean improvement in walk distance of 49.0 minutes after 3 months of therapy.[57] Larger trials are currently ongoing.

Inhaled therapy remains an attractive treatment option for PH in parenchymal lung disease because it may minimize ventilation-perfusion mismatch. Thus, inhaled prostacyclins and inhaled nitric oxide (NO) are being investigated in patients with ILD and PH. In a small, single-center study, eight patients with lung fibrosis and PH were given intravenous prostacyclin, inhaled NO, and inhaled iloprost sequentially but in randomized order.[58] As expected, intravenous prostacyclin resulted in a significant drop in arterial pressure and worsened shunt fraction. Aerosolized prostacyclin resulted in a decrease in mPAP from 44.1 ± 4.2 to 31.6 ± 3.1 mm Hg, and pulmonary vascular resistance from 810 ± 226 to 386 ± 69 dyne/s/cm5 ($P<.05$, respectively). There was no significant change in blood pressure, saturation, or shunt fraction. Inhaled NO similarly resulted in selective pulmonary vasodilatation, with pulmonary vascular resistance decreasing from 726 ± 217 to 458 ± 81 dyne/s/cm5. Although promising, longer and larger studies are needed.

IPF is a progressive disease, which responds poorly to current therapy. The concomitant presence of PH reduces a patient's functional capacity and hastens mortality. PH should be suspected in those patients whose dyspnea seems out of proportion to their pulmonary parenchymal disease. Because of their rapidly declining course, these patients should be prioritized into clinical trials and referred for lung transplantation early.[59]

SLEEP-DISORDERED BREATHING AND PH

Class III PH also includes sleep-disordered breathing. OSA is the most common and most widely studied of the sleep disorders.[60]

OSA and PH

OSA is associated with cardiovascular complications, such as hypertension and atrial fibrillation, as well as sudden cardiac death.[60] PH is also associated with OSA, although its presence is less well-documented.[61–63]

Several retrospective studies of severe sleep apnea (apnea hypopnea index >30) have suggested the prevalence of PH is anywhere from 20% to 70%. The prevalence rate decreases to 20% to 40% when patients with confounding diagnoses are removed from the analysis. As with other diseases in group III, PH has been found to be in the mild-to-moderate range (mPAP 25–40) in patients with sleep-disordered breathing.[63–66]

The presence of OSA plus an additional cardiopulmonary disease increases the risk of development of PH. Specific comorbidities that substantially increase the risk of PH in patients with OSA are COPD (the so-called overlap syndrome), obesity, and left-sided heart disease.[65,67–69] Hypertension and obesity increase the likelihood of pulmonary venous hypertension (pulmonary capillary wedge pressure >15 mm Hg), which additionally confounds the diagnosis of PH in this demographic.

The pathophysiology of PH in OSA patients is poorly understood, but again it is postulated to be related to hypoxic events. Intermittent hypoxia (as little as 4 h/d) has a known association with elevated PAP.[70] Other contributing factors unique to OSA include the wide intrathoracic swings in pressure that occur when there are inspiratory efforts made against an occluded glottis and the sympathetic swings with wide heart rate and blood pressure variability that may affect filling pressures in the heart during periods of apnea.[62,71]

As in all other class III PH, the treatment of PH associated with OSA is aimed at treatment of the underlying disease. Proper diagnosis, titration, and adherence to continuous positive airway pressure (CPAP) have been shown to decrease PAP after 6 months of therapy. Positive pressure splints the upper airway open, decreasing apneas, nocturnal hypoxemia, and nocturnal intrathoracic pressure fluctuations.[72–74] In cases in which CPAP is not tolerated or OSA is extremely severe, tracheostomy may be a consideration. Weight loss is an important treatment modality and referral to a nutritionist should be made early; bariatric surgery should also be considered. As of yet, there is no role for pharmaceutical treatment of PH in patients with sleep-disordered breathing.

ALVEOLAR HYPOVENTILATION AND HIGH ALTITUDE AND PH

Alveolar hypoxemia caused by either hypoventilation or chronic exposure to a lower partial pressure of oxygen is associated with PH. This can often be reversed with disorder-specific intervention.

Alveolar Hypoventilation

Alveolar hypoventilation occurs in patients with kyphoscoliosis and other chest wall deformities, neuromuscular diseases, and metabolic diseases causing hypoventilation. It also includes the obesity hypoventilation syndrome (formerly the Pickwickian syndrome).[75] As above, the pathophysiology is hypoxia-induced vasoconstriction and subsequent vascular remodeling. Identifying and treating hypoxemia with oxygen supplementation improves PAP.[76] As with sleep-disordered breathing, there is no data supporting pharmaceutical treatment of PH caused by hypoxemia.

High Altitude

High-altitude PH is a well-documented phenomenon. It remains a concern because 140 million people live at altitudes above 2500 meters.[77] Residents of high altitudes frequently exhibit chronic mountain syndrome, which is characterized by hypoxemia, polycythemia, and PH. The prevalence has been evaluated in the Andes, the Rocky Mountains, and the Himalayas with estimates between 5% and 18%, with PAPs 40 and 45 mm Hg.[78–80] In patients who are symptomatic or who exhibit severely elevated PAPs, the recommendation is to relocate to lower altitudes. Acetazolamide may help pulmonary hemodynamics by increasing the urinary excretion of bicarbonate and improving hypoventilation.[81] Additionally, treatment with sildenafil has been shown to improve hemodynamics and 6MWT at 3 months.[82]

PH WITH UNCLEAR OR MULTIFACTORIAL CAUSES

Systemic disorders can also affect the pulmonary parenchyma and be associated with PH. Because this group of disorders is heterogeneous and complex, they are categorized with group V in the clinical classification of PH. Included in this group are disorders such as pulmonary Langerhans cell histiocytosis, lymphangioleiomyomatosis, neurofibromatosis, vasculitides, and sarcoidosis.

Sarcoidosis

The association between PH and sarcoidosis is well documented and the prevalence has been reported as 1% to 28% depending on the characteristics and severity of the population studied.[83–85] A prevalence greater than 50% was reported in sarcoid patients awaiting lung transplantation.[46,83]

Patients with sarcoidosis and PH are more likely to display a lower total lung capacity, DLCO, and have stage IV disease.[86,87] The natural history of sarcoid-associated PH is poorly studied but small studies indicate that these patients need more help with activities of daily living and have higher oxygen requirements, lower exercise capacity, and higher mortality than those who have sarcoidosis without PH.[83,86,88,89]

The pathophysiology of sarcoidosis is different than in the other parenchymal lung diseases. With COPD and ILD, the degree of fibrosis and hypoxia is thought to play a role; however, PAPs are often higher for any given degree of fibrosis in sarcoidosis versus idiopathic pulmonary fibrosis.[46] Also, sarcoidosis patients awaiting lung transplantation have higher mPAPs (34 mm Hg) compared with their IPF counterparts (26 mm Hg).[90] Sarcoidosis and its characteristic granulomatous inflammation may directly affect the pulmonary arteries, but the systemic affects of sarcoidosis can contribute to additional causes of PH. Sarcoidosis patients are more likely have diastolic dysfunction than patients with other parenchymal lung diseases and this may further raise the PAPs.[46,83,91] Additionally, sarcoidosis can cause mediastinal lymphadenopathy that may mechanically impinge on the pulmonary arteries or involve the pulmonary veins. Sarcoidosis may also cause liver dysfunction and contribute to portopulmonary hypertension. However, it is the direct pulmonary vascular compression and/or involvement of the sarcoid granulomas that is believed to be the major cause of the PH. The granulomas in sarcoidosis are found lining the lymphatics, which surround the bronchovascular bundle in the lungs. Because of this, the granulomatous inflammation impinges on the vascular structures (**Fig. 6**).[92]

In the late 1970s, Rosen and colleagues[93] examined open lung biopsies of 128 patients with diagnosed sarcoidosis. All specimens showed granulomas, as expected, with 69% demonstrating granulomatous angiitis. Venous involvement was seen in 60% of these patients and occlusive narrowing of small pulmonary vessels was also frequently observed. In another series, 40 autopsies of patients with sarcoidosis were examined; vascular granulomas were seen

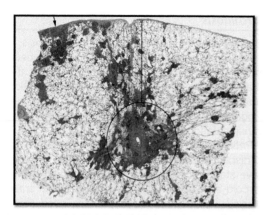

Fig. 6. Sarcoidosis granulomas can be found in several areas of the pulmonary lobule. They are classically found in a lymphatic distribution. The lymphatics are located in the bronchovascular bundle (*circled area*). Granulomas can also compress the pulmonary veins found in the interlobular septae abutting the line drawn above. Finally, granulomas can also bee see in the subpleural area (*arrow*) (Hematoxylin and eosin). (*From* Diaz-Guzman E, Farver C, Parambil J, et al. Pulmonary hypertension caused by sarcoidosis. Clin Chest Med 2008;29(3):549–63, x; with permission.)

in all patients, with the venous involvement greater than the arterial involvement. Medial involvement frequently occurred. In addition, healed granulomatous lesions were seen in pulmonary vessels.[94] This pulmonary venous pathophysiology may cause sarcoidosis-related PH to behave more like pulmonary venoocclusive disease, which has a worse prognosis than other forms of PH and does not respond to PH-specific therapy.[95,96]

The cornerstone of treatment for sarcoidosis is corticosteroids and these are sometimes accompanied by other immunusuppressants. However immunosuppressants do not seem to improve the PH in sarcoidosis to the same degree as they do the parenchymal disease. In one observational study, after 12 months of immunosuppressants, lung parenchymal improvement occurred in 22 out of 24 patients but improvement in hemodynamics was only seen in 12 out of 24.[97]

As in other forms of parenchymal lung disease, therapy with PH-specific medications may worsen hypoxia. Additionally, if a particular patient's pathologic condition is dominated by pulmonary vein involvement, PH-specific therapy may both exacerbate hypoxia and cause pulmonary edema. There have been very few studies with PH-specific therapy in patients with sarcoidosis, all of them small and retrospective. A retrospective chart review of five patients with sarcoidosis and moderate-to-severe PH who received epoprostenol reported an improvement in New York Heart Association functional class at a mean follow-up of 29 months.[98] In another retrospective review of 12 patients with sarcoidosis who were given sildenafil, an improvement in hemodynamics was seen, but this did not manifest in an improved 6MWT distance.[99] A few case reports have reported improvement after initiation of endothelin receptor antagonists.[100,101] Clinical trials are ongoing to identify the efficacy, safety, and appropriate patient selection for PH-specific therapy in this group of patients.

Given the increased mortality in patients with sarcoidosis and significant PH, early lung transplant referral should be considered.[39,83,92]

Vasculitides and PH

Wegener's granulomatosis and other antineutrophil cytoplasmic antibody-associated vasculitides have shown an association with PH in a number of case series.[102] It is likely that vasculitic inflammation in the pulmonary vasculature is the pathophysiologic derangement in these patients. Similar associations have been seen with Takayasu arteritis, which is a large vessel disease, and with Behçet syndrome, which affects blood vessels of all sizes.[103–105] Although large prospective studies have not been performed, treatment of the underlying disease is recommended to treat both the primary vasculitis and improve hemodynamics.

SUMMARY

Pulmonary parenchymal disease is commonly associated with elevations in PAP and resultant cor pulmonale. Generally, these alterations are related to pulmonary hypoxic vasoconstriction. But, there are subsets of these patients who seem to have PH out of proportion to their pulmonary parenchymal disease. PH-specific therapy is an attractive option for these patients. Clinical trials are ongoing to determine the safety, efficacy, and appropriate patient selection for PH-specific treatments in this broad population.

REFERENCES

1. Badesch DB, Champion HC, Sanchez MA, et al. Diagnosis and assessment of pulmonary arterial hypertension. J Am Coll Cardiol 2009;54(Suppl 1): S55–66.
2. Hatano S, Strasser R. Primary pulmonary hypertension. Geneva (Switzerland): World Health Organization; 1975.
3. Simonneau G, Robbins IM, Beghetti M, et al. Updated clinical classification of pulmonary hypertension. J Am Coll Cardiol 2009;54(Suppl 1):S43–54.

4. Hyduk A, Croft JB, Ayala C, et al. Pulmonary hypertension surveillance—United States, 1980–2002. MMWR Surveill Summ 2005;54(5):1–28.

5. Howell K, Ooi H, Preston R, et al. Structural basis of hypoxic pulmonary hypertension: the modifying effect of chronic hypercapnia. Exp Physiol 2004; 89(1):66–72.

6. MacNee W. Pathophysiology of cor pulmonale in chronic obstructive pulmonary disease. Part One. Am J Respir Crit Care Med 1994;150(3):833–52.

7. MacNee W. Pathophysiology of cor pulmonale in chronic obstructive pulmonary disease. Part two. Am J Respir Crit Care Med 1994;150(4):1158–68.

8. Levine BE, Bigelow DB, Hamstra RD, et al. The role of long-term continuous oxygen administration in patients with chronic airway obstruction with hypoxemia. Ann Intern Med 1967;66(4):639–50.

9. Weitzenblum E, Loiseau A, Hirth C, et al. Course of pulmonary hemodynamics in patients with chronic obstructive pulmonary disease. Chest 1979;75(6): 656–62.

10. Scharf SM, Iqbal M, Keller C, et al. Hemodynamic characterization of patients with severe emphysema. Am J Respir Crit Care Med 2002;166(3): 314–22.

11. Nathan SD, Shlobin OA, Barnett SD, et al. Right ventricular systolic pressure by echocardiography as a predictor of pulmonary hypertension in idiopathic pulmonary fibrosis. Respir Med 2008; 102(9):1305–10.

12. Fisher MR, Criner GJ, Fishman AP, et al. Estimating pulmonary artery pressures by echocardiography in patients with emphysema. Eur Respir J 2007; 30(5):914–21.

13. Arcasoy SM, Christie JD, Ferrari VA, et al. Echocardiographic assessment of pulmonary hypertension in patients with advanced lung disease. Am J Respir Crit Care Med 2003;167(5):735–40.

14. Chaouat A, Naeije R, Weitzenblum E. Pulmonary hypertension in COPD. Eur Respir J 2008;32(5):1371–85.

15. Thabut G, Dauriat G, Stern JB, et al. Pulmonary hemodynamics in advanced COPD candidates for lung volume reduction surgery or lung transplantation. Chest 2005;127(5):1531–6.

16. Vizza CD, Lynch JP, Ochoa LL, et al. Right and left ventricular dysfunction in patients with severe pulmonary disease. Chest 1998;113(3):576–83.

17. Chaouat A, Bugnet AS, Kadaoui N, et al. Severe pulmonary hypertension and chronic obstructive pulmonary disease. Am J Respir Crit Care Med 2005;172(2):189–94.

18. Naeije R, MacNee W. Pulmonary circulation. London: Arnol Health Sciences; 2003.

19. Wright JL, Levy RD, Churg A. Pulmonary hypertension in chronic obstructive pulmonary disease: current theories of pathogenesis and their implications for treatment. Thorax 2005;60(7):605–9.

20. Eddahibi S, Chaouat A, Tu L, et al. Interleukin-6 gene polymorphism confers susceptibility to pulmonary hypertension in chronic obstructive pulmonary disease. Proc Am Thorac Soc 2006;3(6):475–6.

21. Kessler R, Faller M, Weitzenblum E, et al. "Natural history" of pulmonary hypertension in a series of 131 patients with chronic obstructive lung disease. Am J Respir Crit Care Med 2001;164(2):219–24.

22. Oswald-Mammosser M, Weitzenblum E, Quoix E, et al. Prognostic factors in COPD patients receiving long-term oxygen therapy. Importance of pulmonary artery pressure. Chest 1995;107(5):1193–8.

23. Continuous or nocturnal oxygen therapy in hypoxemic chronic obstructive lung disease: a clinical trial. Nocturnal Oxygen Therapy Trial Group. Ann Intern Med 1980;93(3):391–8.

24. Weitzenblum E, Sautegeau A, Ehrhart M, et al. Long-term oxygen therapy can reverse the progression of pulmonary hypertension in patients with chronic obstructive pulmonary disease. Am Rev Respir Dis 1985;131(4):493–8.

25. Zielinski J, Tobiasz M, Hawrylkiewicz I, et al. Effects of long-term oxygen therapy on pulmonary hemodynamics in COPD patients: a 6-year prospective study. Chest 1998;113(1):65–70.

26. Ries AL, Bauldoff GS, Carlin BW, et al. Pulmonary rehabilitation: joint ACCP/AACVPR evidence-based clinical practice guidelines. Chest 2007; 131(Suppl 5):4S–42S.

27. Tillie-Leblond I, Marquette CH, Perez T, et al. Pulmonary embolism in patients with unexplained exacerbation of chronic obstructive pulmonary disease: prevalence and risk factors. Ann Intern Med 2006;144(6):390–6.

28. Ambrosetti M, Ageno W, Spanevello A, et al. Prevalence and prevention of venous thromboembolism in patients with acute exacerbations of COPD. Thromb Res 2003;112(4):203–7.

29. Holverda S, Rietema H, Bogaard HJ, et al. Acute effects of sildenafil on exercise pulmonary hemodynamics and capacity in patients with COPD. Pulm Pharmacol Ther 2008;21(3):558–64.

30. Blanco I, Gimeno E, Munoz PA, et al. Hemodynamic and gas exchange effects of sildenafil in patients with chronic obstructive pulmonary disease and pulmonary hypertension. Am J Respir Crit Care Med 2010;181(3):270–8.

31. Alp S, Skrygan M, Schmidt WE, et al. Sildenafil improves hemodynamic parameters in COPD—an investigation of six patients. Pulm Pharmacol Ther 2006;19(6):386–90.

32. Rietema H, Holverda S, Bogaard HJ, et al. Sildenafil treatment in COPD does not affect stroke volume or exercise capacity. Eur Respir J 2008;31(4):759–64.

33. Stolz D, Rasch H, Linka A, et al. A randomised, controlled trial of bosentan in severe COPD. Eur Respir J 2008;32(3):619–28.

34. Valerio G, Bracciale P, Grazia D'Agostino A. Effect of bosentan upon pulmonary hypertension in chronic obstructive pulmonary disease. Ther Adv Respir Dis 2009;3(1):15–21.

35. Archer SL, Mike D, Crow J, et al. A placebo-controlled trial of prostacyclin in acute respiratory failure in COPD. Chest 1996;109(3):750–5.

36. Dernaika TA, Beavin M, Kinasewitz GT. Iloprost improves gas exchange and exercise tolerance in patients with pulmonary hypertension and chronic obstructive pulmonary disease. Respiration 2010; 79(5):377–82.

37. Saadjian A, Philip-Joet F, Paganelli F, et al. Long-term effects of cicletanine on secondary pulmonary hypertension. J Cardiovasc Pharmacol 1998;31(3): 364–71.

38. Lee TM, Chen CC, Shen HN, et al. Effects of pravastatin on functional capacity in patients with chronic obstructive pulmonary disease and pulmonary hypertension. Clin Sci (Lond) 2009;116(6): 497–505.

39. Christie JD, Edwards LB, Kucheryavaya AY, et al. The Registry of the International Society for Heart and Lung Transplantation: twenty-seventh official adult lung and heart-lung transplant report—2010. J Heart Lung Transplant 2010;29(10):1104–18.

40. Cottin V, Nunes H, Brillet PY, et al. Combined pulmonary fibrosis and emphysema: a distinct underrecognised entity. Eur Respir J 2005;26(4): 586–93.

41. Brillet PY, Cottin V, Letoumelin P, et al. Combined apical emphysema and basal fibrosis syndrome (emphysema/fibrosis syndrome): CT imaging features and pulmonary function tests. J Radiol 2009;90(1 Pt 1):43–51 [in French].

42. Mejia M, Carrillo G, Rojas-Serrano J, et al. Idiopathic pulmonary fibrosis and emphysema: decreased survival associated with severe pulmonary arterial hypertension. Chest 2009;136(1):10–5.

43. Nadrous HF, Pellikka PA, Krowka MJ, et al. Pulmonary hypertension in patients with idiopathic pulmonary fibrosis. Chest 2005;128(4):2393–9.

44. Lettieri CJ, Nathan SD, Barnett SD, et al. Prevalence and outcomes of pulmonary arterial hypertension in advanced idiopathic pulmonary fibrosis. Chest 2006;129(3):746–52.

45. Nathan SD, Shlobin OA, Ahmad S, et al. Pulmonary hypertension and pulmonary function testing in idiopathic pulmonary fibrosis. Chest 2007;131(3):657–63.

46. Shorr AF, Wainright JL, Cors CS, et al. Pulmonary hypertension in patients with pulmonary fibrosis awaiting lung transplant. Eur Respir J 2007;30(4): 715–21.

47. Nathan SD, Shlobin OA, Ahmad S, et al. Serial development of pulmonary hypertension in patients with idiopathic pulmonary fibrosis. Respiration 2008;76(3):288–94.

48. Zisman DA, Karlamangla AS, Ross DJ, et al. High-resolution chest CT findings do not predict the presence of pulmonary hypertension in advanced idiopathic pulmonary fibrosis. Chest 2007;132(3): 773–9.

49. Colombat M, Mal H, Groussard O, et al. Pulmonary vascular lesions in end-stage idiopathic pulmonary fibrosis: histopathologic study on lung explant specimens and correlations with pulmonary hemodynamics. Hum Pathol 2007;38(1):60–5.

50. Rubens C, Ewert R, Halank M, et al. Big endothelin-1 and endothelin-1 plasma levels are correlated with the severity of primary pulmonary hypertension. Chest 2001;120(5):1562–9.

51. Yamakami T, Taguchi O, Gabazza EC, et al. Arterial endothelin-1 level in pulmonary emphysema and interstitial lung disease. Relation with pulmonary hypertension during exercise. Eur Respir J 1997; 10(9):2055–60.

52. Lesur OJ, Mancini NM, Humbert JC, et al. Interleukin-6, interferon-gamma, and phospholipid levels in the alveolar lining fluid of human lungs. Profiles in coal worker's pneumoconiosis and idiopathic pulmonary fibrosis. Chest 1994;106(2): 407–13.

53. Saleh D, Furukawa K, Tsao MS, et al. Elevated expression of endothelin-1 and endothelin-converting enzyme-1 in idiopathic pulmonary fibrosis: possible involvement of proinflammatory cytokines. Am J Respir Cell Mol Biol 1997;16(2):187–93.

54. Minai OA, Sahoo D, Chapman JT, et al. Vaso-active therapy can improve 6-min walk distance in patients with pulmonary hypertension and fibrotic interstitial lung disease. Respir Med 2008;102(7): 1015–20.

55. King TE Jr, Behr J, Brown KK, et al. BUILD-1: a randomized placebo-controlled trial of bosentan in idiopathic pulmonary fibrosis. Am J Respir Crit Care Med 2008;177(1):75–81.

56. Ghofrani HA, Wiedemann R, Rose F, et al. Sildenafil for treatment of lung fibrosis and pulmonary hypertension: a randomised controlled trial. Lancet 2002; 360(9337):895–900.

57. Collard HR, Anstrom KJ, Schwarz MI, et al. Sildenafil improves walk distance in idiopathic pulmonary fibrosis. Chest 2007;131(3):897–9.

58. Olschewski H, Ghofrani HA, Walmrath D, et al. Inhaled prostacyclin and iloprost in severe pulmonary hypertension secondary to lung fibrosis. Am J Respir Crit Care Med 1999;160(2):600–7.

59. Kreider M, Kotloff RM. Selection of candidates for lung transplantation. Proc Am Thorac Soc 2009; 6(1):20–7.

60. Young T, Peppard PE, Gottlieb DJ. Epidemiology of obstructive sleep apnea: a population health perspective. Am J Respir Crit Care Med 2002; 165(9):1217–39.

61. Marrone O, Bonsignore MR, Romano S, et al. Slow and fast changes in transmural pulmonary artery pressure in obstructive sleep apnoea. Eur Respir J 1994;7(12):2192–8.

62. Marrone O, Bellia V, Ferrara G, et al. Transmural pressure measurements. Importance in the assessment of pulmonary hypertension in obstructive sleep apneas. Chest 1989;95(2):338–42.

63. Sajkov D, McEvoy RD. Obstructive sleep apnea and pulmonary hypertension. Prog Cardiovasc Dis 2009;51(5):363–70.

64. Sanner BM, Doberauer C, Konermann M, et al. Pulmonary hypertension in patients with obstructive sleep apnea syndrome. Arch Intern Med 1997;157(21):2483–7.

65. Bady E, Achkar A, Pascal S, et al. Pulmonary arterial hypertension in patients with sleep apnoea syndrome. Thorax 2000;55(11):934–9.

66. Sajkov D, Cowie RJ, Thornton AT, et al. Pulmonary hypertension and hypoxemia in obstructive sleep apnea syndrome. Am J Respir Crit Care Med 1994;149(2 Pt 1):416–22.

67. Fletcher EC, Schaaf JW, Miller J, et al. Long-term cardiopulmonary sequelae in patients with sleep apnea and chronic lung disease. Am Rev Respir Dis 1987;135(3):525–33.

68. Laaban JP, Cassuto D, Orvoen-Frija E, et al. Cardiorespiratory consequences of sleep apnoea syndrome in patients with massive obesity. Eur Respir J 1998;11(1):20–7.

69. O'Hearn DJ, Gold AR, Gold MS, et al. Lower extremity edema and pulmonary hypertension in morbidly obese patients with obstructive sleep apnea. Sleep Breath 2009;13(1):25–34.

70. Kay JM, Suyama KL, Keane PM. Effect of intermittent normoxia on muscularization of pulmonary arterioles induced by chronic hypoxia in rats. Am Rev Respir Dis 1981;123(4 Pt 1):454–8.

71. Tilkian AG, Guilleminault C, Schroeder JS, et al. Hemodynamics in sleep-induced apnea. Studies during wakefulness and sleep. Ann Intern Med 1976;85(6):714–9.

72. Sajkov D, Wang T, Saunders NA, et al. Continuous positive airway pressure treatment improves pulmonary hemodynamics in patients with obstructive sleep apnea. Am J Respir Crit Care Med 2002; 165(2):152–8.

73. Arias MA, Garcia-Rio F, Alonso-Fernandez A, et al. Pulmonary hypertension in obstructive sleep apnoea: effects of continuous positive airway pressure: a randomized, controlled cross-over study. Eur Heart J 2006;27(9):1106–13.

74. Alchanatis M, Tourkohoriti G, Kakouros S, et al. Daytime pulmonary hypertension in patients with obstructive sleep apnea: the effect of continuous positive airway pressure on pulmonary hemodynamics. Respiration 2001;68(6):566–72.

75. Kessler R, Chaouat A, Schinkewitch P, et al. The obesity-hypoventilation syndrome revisited: a prospective study of 34 consecutive cases. Chest 2001; 120(2):369–76.

76. Weitzenblum E, Chaouat A, Kessler R, et al. Daytime hypoventilation in obstructive sleep apnoea syndrome. Sleep Med Rev 1999;3(1):79–93.

77. Xu XQ, Jing ZC. High-altitude pulmonary hypertension. Eur Respir Rev 2009;18(111):13–7.

78. Hultgren H. Chronic mountain sickness. San Francisco (CA): Hultgren Publication; 1997.

79. Penaloza D, Arias-Stella J. The heart and pulmonary circulation at high altitudes: healthy highlanders and chronic mountain sickness. Circulation 2007;115(9): 1132–46.

80. Aldashev AA, Sarybaev AS, Sydykov AS, et al. Characterization of high-altitude pulmonary hypertension in the Kyrgyz: association with angiotensin-converting enzyme genotype. Am J Respir Crit Care Med 2002;166(10):1396–402.

81. Rivera-Ch M, Huicho L, Bouchet P, et al. Effect of acetazolamide on ventilatory response in subjects with chronic mountain sickness. Respir Physiol Neurobiol 2008;162(3):184–9.

82. Aldashev AA, Kojonazarov BK, Amatov TA, et al. Phosphodiesterase type 5 and high altitude pulmonary hypertension. Thorax 2005;60(8):683–7.

83. Shorr AF, Helman DL, Davies DB, et al. Pulmonary hypertension in advanced sarcoidosis: epidemiology and clinical characteristics. Eur Respir J 2005;25(5):783–8.

84. Handa T, Nagai S, Miki S, et al. Incidence of pulmonary hypertension and its clinical relevance in patients with sarcoidosis. Chest 2006;129(5):1246–52.

85. Rizzato G, Pezzano A, Sala G, et al. Right heart impairment in sarcoidosis: haemodynamic and echocardiographic study. Eur J Respir Dis 1983; 64(2):121–8.

86. Sulica R, Teirstein AS, Kakarla S, et al. Distinctive clinical, radiographic, and functional characteristics of patients with sarcoidosis-related pulmonary hypertension. Chest 2005;128(3):1483–9.

87. Bourbonnais JM, Samavati L. Clinical predictors of pulmonary hypertension in sarcoidosis. Eur Respir J 2008;32(2):296–302.

88. Shorr AF, Davies DB, Nathan SD. Predicting mortality in patients with sarcoidosis awaiting lung transplantation. Chest 2003;124(3):922–8.

89. Arcasoy SM, Christie JD, Pochettino A, et al. Characteristics and outcomes of patients with sarcoidosis listed for lung transplantation. Chest 2001; 120(3):873–80.

90. Shorr AF, Davies DB, Nathan SD. Outcomes for patients with sarcoidosis awaiting lung transplantation. Chest 2002;122(1):233–8.

91. Fahy GJ, Marwick T, McCreery CJ, et al. Doppler echocardiographic detection of left ventricular

diastolic dysfunction in patients with pulmonary sarcoidosis. Chest 1996;109(1):62–6.

92. Diaz-Guzman E, Farver C, Parambil J, et al. Pulmonary hypertension caused by sarcoidosis. Clin Chest Med 2008;29(3):549–63, x.

93. Rosen Y, Moon S, Huang CT, et al. Granulomatous pulmonary angiitis in sarcoidosis. Arch Pathol Lab Med 1977;101(4):170–4.

94. Takemura T, Matsui Y, Saiki S, et al. Pulmonary vascular involvement in sarcoidosis: a report of 40 autopsy cases. Hum Pathol 1992;23(11):1216–23.

95. Hoffstein V, Ranganathan N, Mullen JB. Sarcoidosis simulating pulmonary veno-occlusive disease. Am Rev Respir Dis 1986;134(4):809–11.

96. Nunes H, Humbert M, Capron F, et al. Pulmonary hypertension associated with sarcoidosis: mechanisms, haemodynamics and prognosis. Thorax 2006;61(1):68–74.

97. Gluskowski J, Hawrylkiewicz I, Zych D, et al. Effects of corticosteroid treatment on pulmonary haemodynamics in patients with sarcoidosis. Eur Respir J 1990;3(4):403–7.

98. Fisher KA, Serlin DM, Wilson KC, et al. Sarcoidosis-associated pulmonary hypertension: outcome with long-term epoprostenol treatment. Chest 2006; 130(5):1481–8.

99. Milman N, Burton CM, Iversen M, et al. Pulmonary hypertension in end-stage pulmonary sarcoidosis: therapeutic effect of sildenafil? J Heart Lung Transplant 2008;27(3):329–34.

100. Foley RJ, Metersky ML. Successful treatment of sarcoidosis-associated pulmonary hypertension with bosentan. Respiration 2008;75(2):211–4.

101. Girgis RE. Pulmonary hypertension associated with sarcoidosis. Adv Pulm Hypertens 2009;8(3):148–53.

102. Launay D, Souza R, Guillevin L, et al. Pulmonary arterial hypertension in ANCA-associated vasculitis. Sarcoidosis Vasc Diffuse Lung Dis 2006; 23(3):223–8.

103. Raz I, Okon E, Chajek-Shaul T. Pulmonary manifestations in Behçet's syndrome. Chest 1989;95(3): 585–9.

104. Grenier P, Bletry O, Cornud F, et al. Pulmonary involvement in Behcet disease. AJR Am J Roentgenol 1981;137(3):565–9.

105. Lande A, Bard R. Takayasu's arteritis: an unrecognized cause of pulmonary hypertension. Angiology 1976;27(2):114–21.

Chronic Thromboembolic Pulmonary Hypertension

Robert J. Moraca, MD[a],*, Manreet Kanwar, MD[b]

KEYWORDS

- Pulmonary hypertension • Chronic thromboembolic pulmonary hypertension
- Pulmonary thromboendarterectomy • Pulmonary endarterectomy

KEY POINTS

- Chronic thromboembolic pulmonary hypertension (CTEPH) is defined as pulmonary hypertension associated with an elevated mean pulmonary artery (PA) pressure (>25 mm Hg) as assessed by right heart catheterization, caused by thromboemboli to the pulmonary arterial system.
- The occurrence of CTEPH in patients surviving an acute pulmonary embolism (PE) is considered rare, with a reported incidence between 0.1% and 0.5%.
- The general criteria to assess operability include: (1) symptoms in New York Heart Association functional class III or IV; (2) a preoperative pulmonary vascular resistance greater than 300 dyne/s/cm^5 and/or a mean PA pressure greater than 40 mm Hg; (3) surgically accessible thrombus (in the main, lobar, or segmental PA), as determined by all appropriate radiographic studies; and (4) no severe comorbidities.
- In the last 2 decade the results of pulmonary endarterectomy surgery in experienced centers has been performed with low operative mortality, 1-year survival rates of greater than 95%, and clinical evidence to suggest a curative result.

INTRODUCTION

Chronic thromboembolic pulmonary hypertension (CTEPH) is a potentially life-threatening condition characterized by obstruction of pulmonary artery (PA) vasculature by acute or recurrent thromboemboli with subsequent organization, leading to progressive pulmonary hypertension (PH) and right heart failure.[1–3] CTEPH is now considered one of the leading causes of severe PH, although the exact prevalence is unknown. Several aspects of the underlying pathogenesis are not fully realized and continue to pose a challenge. Recent literature has suggested that obliteration of central PAs caused by organized thrombi may not be the sole underlying mechanism leading to the progressive PH and right heart failure. While thromboemboli may be the inciting event, the role of pulmonary microvascular arteriopathy is gaining recognition as an important contributor to disease progression.[4–6] Until relatively recently, CTEPH was a diagnosis made primarily at autopsy, but advances made in diagnostic modalities and surgical pulmonary endarterectomy techniques have made this disease treatable and even potentially curable. The European Society of Cardiology in association with the European Respiratory Society published guidelines for the diagnostic and therapeutic approach to patients with CTEPH, which were endorsed by the International Society of Heart

Disclosure: The authors have no funding or financial relationships to disclose.
[a] Department of Thoracic and Cardiovascular Surgery, Gerald McGinnis Cardiovascular Institute, Allegheny General Hospital, 320 East North Avenue, Pittsburgh, PA 15212, USA; [b] Department of Cardiology, Gerald McGinnis Cardiovascular Institute, Allegheny General Hospital, 320 East North Avenue, 16th Floor South Tower, Pittsburgh, PA 15212, USA
* Corresponding author.
E-mail address: rmoraca@wpahs.org

Heart Failure Clin 8 (2012) 475–483
doi:10.1016/j.hfc.2012.04.003
1551-7136/12/$ – see front matter © 2012 Elsevier Inc. All rights reserved.

and Lung Transplant (**Box 1**). However, in the absence of randomized controlled trials there is a lack of standardization, and treatment options have to be individualized.

DEFINITION

CTEPH is defined as PH associated with an elevated mean PA pressure ($\geq$25 mm Hg) as assessed by right heart catheterization, caused by thromboemboli to the pulmonary arterial system. Hemodynamic measurements are consistent with pulmonary capillary wedge pressure $\leq$15 mm Hg,

---

Box 1
Current recommendations for CTEPH

Class I

1. Diagnosis of chronic thromboembolic pulmonary hypertension (CTEPH) is based on the presence of pulmonary hypertension (PH) (mean pulmonary artery pressure $\geq$25 mm Hg, pulmonary capillary wedge pressure $\leq$15 mm Hg, pulmonary venous resistance >2 Wood units) in patients with organized thrombi/emboli in the pulmonary artery (level of evidence: C)

2. Lifelong anticoagulation in patients with CTEPH (level of evidence: C)

3. Surgical pulmonary endarterectomy (PEA) as a choice of treatment in qualifying patients with CTEPH (Level of evidence: C)

Class IIa

1. Once perfusion scanning and/or computed tomographic angiography show signs compatible with CTEPH diagnosis, the patient should be referred to a center with expertise in surgical PEA (level of evidence: C)

2. Selection of patients for surgery should be based on the extent and location of the organized thrombi, degree of PH, and presence of comorbidities (level of evidence: C)

Class IIb

1. Drug therapy specific to pulmonary arterial hypertension may be indicated in selected CTEPH patients who are not surgical candidates or have residual PH after PEA.

Adapted from Galiè N, Hoeper NM, Humbert M, et al. Guidelines for the diagnosis and treatment of pulmonary hypertension. The Task Force for the Diagnosis and Treatment of Pulmonary Hypertension of the European Society of Cardiology (ESC) and the European Respiratory Society (ERS), endorsed by the International Society of Heart and Lung Transplantation (ISHLT). Eur Heart J 2009;30:2493–537; with permission.

---

pulmonary venous resistance (PVR) >2 Wood units, and a normal or reduced cardiac output.[7,8]

EPIDEMIOLOGY

Accurate incidence or prevalence of CTEPH is yet to be determined. The occurrence of CTEPH in patients surviving an acute pulmonary embolism (PE) is considered rare, with a reported incidence of between 0.1% and 0.5%.[9] This figure may underestimate the true frequency of CTEPH, as the disease is often misdiagnosed because of nonspecific symptoms and a variable disease course. More recently, it was reported that the cumulative incidence of symptomatic CTEPH is approximately 1%, 3%, and 4% at 6 months, 1 year, and 2 years in a prospective follow-up study of 223 patients who presented with acute PE.[10] In another prospective study of 78 survivors of acute PE, persistent PH and/or right ventricular dysfunction were present on follow-up echocardiograms in 44% of the patients after 1 year.[11] Defining the true incidence of CTEPH is hindered by the observation that up to two-thirds of these patients have no known history of pulmonary embolism.[12] In fact, CTEPH is often identified during diagnostic workup in patients with unexplained PH with no history suggesting previous venous thrombosis or PE. Further prospective epidemiologic studies are needed to better define the incidence and prevalence of CTEPH.

PATHOGENESIS AND RISK FACTORS

The current model of CTEPH pathogenesis is based on gradual formation of organized thromboemboli after deep venous thrombosis and PE. However, it is unclear why some patients have incomplete resolution of pulmonary emboli and go on to develop CTEPH whereas others do not. Pulmonary thromboembolism or in situ thrombosis may be initiated or aggravated by abnormalities in the clotting cascade, endothelial cells, or platelets, all of which interact in the coagulation process.[12] No abnormality of the coagulation or fibrinolytic pathway or of the pulmonary endothelium has been consistently identified, except for antiphospholipid antibody and elevated levels of factor VIII. Thrombophilia studies have shown that lupus anticoagulant may be found in approximately 10% of such patients, and 20% carry antiphospholipid antibodies, lupus anticoagulant, or both.[13] An observational study found elevated factor VIII levels in 41% of 122 patients with CTEPH compared with 5% of 82 healthy control subjects.[14] There is no difference in the level of persistent PH and severity of right ventricular dysfunction whether PE is due to procoagulant states such as antithrombin III, protein C or protein S deficiency, or Factor II and Factor V Leiden mutations, in comparison with CTEPH in control subjects without these risk factors.[13–16]

Certain conditions appear to be independent risk factors for CTEPH, although the underlying mechanisms linking them are unclear (**Box 2**). These factors include previous splenectomy, infected intravenous lines, ventriculoatrial shunt, thyroid hormone replacement, myeloproliferative disorders, and chronic inflammatory diseases.[17] The hypothesis that chronic inflammatory states may cause a prothrombotic state and impair resolution of thromboemboli is supported by numerous experimental findings.[18,19] Plasma levels of the proinflammatory cytokine macrophage chemoattractant protein 1 are elevated in patients with CTEPH and correlate with the magnitude of PH.[20]

It has been proposed that an acute PE may just be an initiating event, but progression of PH results from progressive pulmonary vascular remodeling, that is, small-vessel disease. Persistent obstruction of pulmonary arteries may result in distal small-vessel arteriopathy caused by high shear stress, leading to elevated PA pressures. The microvascular disease is possibly modified by infection, immune phenomena, chronic inflammatory disorders, and malignancy.[13,17,21] Once vessel obliteration is sufficient to cause increases in the PA pressure, a process of pulmonary vascular remodeling is started that self-perpetuates the progression of PH, even in the absence of further thromboembolic events. The pathologic lesions that develop are characterized by organized thrombi tightly attached to the PA medial layer in the elastic pulmonary arteries, replacing the normal intima. These lesions may completely occlude the lumen or form different grades of stenosis, webs, and bands. The distal pulmonary vasculopathy is characterized by lesions indistinguishable from that of PA hypertension, including plexiform lesions.[22–24] Collateral vessels from the systemic circulation can grow to reperfuse, at least partially, the areas distal to complete obstructions.

CTEPH may also develop in the absence of previous PE. In these cases, the disease is probably initiated by thrombotic or inflammatory lesions in the pulmonary vasculature. Pulmonary microvascular changes manifesting as pulmonary hypertensive arteriopathy likely contribute to disease progression. In fact, in situ thrombosis of pulmonary vessels is a well-recognized complication in patients with severe PH of other etiology. Most experts now believe that in affected patients, minor or major thromboembolic events in combination with infection, inflammation, autoimmunity, or malignancy trigger an intravascular remodeling process that involves the thrombus itself as well as small resistance vessels.

Some patients are more genetically susceptible to develop CTEPH than others, although the genetic variants associated with this increased risk are yet to be determined.[6] Mutations in bone morphogenetic protein receptor type 2 (BMPR-2) have been linked to vascular remodeling and smooth-muscle cell proliferation in other forms of PH, but have not been described in CTEPH.[25,26] However, expression of BMPR-1A, a transmembrane protein required for BMPR-2 signaling, is markedly downregulated in lungs from patients with CTEPH.[25] Angiopoietin-1, a signaling molecule involved in angiogenesis and smooth-muscle cell proliferation, is upregulated in the lungs from CTEPH patients.[27] Angiopoietin-1 shuts off BMPR-1A expression and thereby blocks BMPR-2 signaling even in the absence of germline BMPR-2 mutations. These mechanisms seem to play a role in several forms of PH including, but not restricted to, CTEPH. Further studies are required for a better understanding of the sequence of events that eventually result in pulmonary vascular remodeling.

CLINICAL PRESENTATION

The hemodynamic evolution of CTEPH is not fully understood, and the disease is usually advanced by the time of diagnosis. In the initial period of pulmonary vascular obstruction, the patients are usually minimally symptomatic. However, as the disease progresses, worsening exertional dyspnea, exercise intolerance, syncope, and symptoms of right ventricular failure ensue. Many patients describe a history consistent with an

---

Box 2
Clinical risk factors for development of CTEPH

1. Large thrombus burden/inadequate anticoagulation

2. Chronic inflammatory state (inflammatory bowel disease, malignancy)

3. Splenectomy

4. Infected ventriculoatrial shunt

5. Infected indwelling venous lines/pacemaker leads

6. Myeloproliferative disorders

7. Thyroid hormone replacement therapy

8. Circulating antiphospholipid antibodies

9. Elevated plasma coagulation factor VIII

acute pulmonary embolic event in the past, although a formal diagnosis may have not been made.

Physical findings are often subtle early in the course and may include a left parasternal heave, a prominent pulmonic component of S2, and a systolic murmur of tricuspid regurgitation. More obvious signs of right heart failure (jugular venous distension, edema, and ascites) occur late in the course of the disease. A highly specific but rarely demonstrated clinical finding for CTEPH is bruits over peripheral lung fields, which result from turbulent blood flow through partially occluded pulmonary arteries, heard best during breath-holding.[28]

DIAGNOSIS

Any patient with unexplained PH should be evaluated for the presence of CTEPH. Suspicion should be high when the patient presents with a previous history of venous thromboembolism. Electrocardiography demonstrates right ventricular hypertrophy and strain. A chest radiograph may be normal or show hilar fullness with peripheral pruning or oligemia. Echocardiography usually provides the initial objective evidence of PH. If the survivors of acute PE show echocardiographic evidence of PH or right ventricular dysfunction, follow-up echocardiography should be done 3 to 6 months after discharge to determine whether PH has resolved.[11] In patients with unexplained PH, a ventilation/perfusion (V/Q) lung scan is recommended to exclude CTEPH. A completely normal perfusion study practically excludes the diagnosis of CTEPH.[29–31] The presence of multiple, small, subsegmental defects make idiopathic PA hypertension or another form of small-vessel PH (pulmonary veno-occlusive disease, pulmonary capillary hemangiomatosis, pulmonary vasculitis, or PA sarcoma) more likely, whereas 1 or more mismatched segmental or larger defects generally indicate CTEPH.[32–34] Multiple-row computed tomographic angiography (CTA) is indicated when the V/Q lung scan is indeterminate or reveals perfusions defects. No prospective studies have evaluated the most appropriate diagnostic approach to CTEPH, and both V/Q scanning and CTA have been known to underestimate clot burden. Magnetic resonance (MR) imaging and MR angiography have been used to visualize the pulmonary vasculature and provide detailed information about right ventricular size and function, but are used infrequently.[35]

Once ventilation/perfusion scanning and/or CTA show signs compatible with CTEPH, the patient should be referred to a center with expertise in the medical and surgical management of these

patients.[7,8] Invasive tools including right heart catheterization and traditional, gold-standard pulmonary angiography are usually required to determine the appropriate therapeutic strategy. These tests should be performed at the expert center rather than at the referring hospitals. The use of bilateral pulmonary branch selective injections, serial pictures, and multiple views is recommended. Computed tomographic or angiographic evidence of CTEPH includes pouching, webs, or bands with or without poststenotic dilatation, intimal irregularities, abrupt narrowing, or total occlusion.[36,37] The final diagnosis of CTEPH is based on the presence of precapillary PH (mean PA pressure $\geq$25 mm Hg, pulmonary capillary wedge pressure $\leq$15 mm Hg, and PVR >2 Wood units) in patients with multiple chronic/organized occlusive thrombi/emboli in the pulmonary arteries.[7]

TREATMENT

The decision on how to treat patients with CTEPH should be made at referral centers, based on interdisciplinary discussion among cardiologists, pulmonologists, radiologists, and surgeons. The need to treat patients with PE with residual mild PH, no or minimal clinical impairment, and normal right ventricular function is debatable, as the natural history of these patients has never been studied prospectively. These patients may be followed with regular clinical assessments and echocardiographic monitoring. Unless contraindicated, all patients should receive lifelong anticoagulation therapy, usually with vitamin K antagonists (target international normalized ratio between 2.0 and 3.0). As in other forms of PH, diuretics and oxygen are used as indicated. If the presenting systolic PA pressure at the time of acute PE exceeds 50 mm Hg, the likelihood of these patients developing CTEPH is higher. If these patients are stable, hemodynamic improvement can be anticipated over the next 3 months with anticoagulation. However, if hemodynamic compromise occurs or PH persists after 3 months, a full diagnostic workup for surgical candidacy should be considered.

Given the potential for nonocclusive small-vessel vasculopathy, pharmacologic therapies approved for use in treating idiopathic PA hypertension are being studied in CTEPH. Several uncontrolled clinical studies suggest that prostanoids, endothelin receptor antagonists, and phosphodiesterase type 5 inhibitors may exert hemodynamic and clinical benefits in patients with CTEPH, irrespective of their candidacy for surgery.[38–41] However, most clinical evidence is currently limited to small, uncontrolled trials. The only randomized, placebo-controlled clinical trial that has so far addressed the safety and efficacy of medical treatment was the BENEFIT study, which investigated the effects of bosentan in patients with inoperable CTEPH for a 16-week period.[42] This study revealed a significant drop in PVR in the bosentan group but no change in the 6-minute walking distance (6MWD), functional class, or time to clinical worsening.

Drug therapy specific to PA hypertension may play a role in selected CTEPH patients for the following scenarios. (1) When patients are not considered candidates for PEA because of significant distal disease. (2) In high-risk patients with extremely poor hemodynamics, intravenous epoprostenol may be considered to improve hemodynamics as a therapeutic bridge to PEA.[39] Such individuals include those with functional class IV symptoms, mean PA greater than 50 mm Hg, cardiac index less than 2.0 L/min/m^2, and PVR greater than 1000 dyne/s/cm^5. (3) In patients with persistent PH after PEA (about 10%–15%), and who often have significant residual distal pathology. (4) When surgery is contraindicated because of significant comorbidities.[38]

Given these limited data, further studies are necessary to obtain reliable long-term data on the effects of medical therapies in patients with CTEPH, and these patients should be treated within clinical trials whenever possible. For the present, no medical therapy has been approved for CTEPH in Europe or the United States.

SURGICAL TREATMENT

The only curative option for patients with CTEPH is surgical removal of all thromboembolic material and obstructive lesions within the pulmonary arteries, either by pulmonary endarterectomy (PEA) or bilateral lung transplantation.[7,43] PEA is a well-described procedure pioneered and developed at The University of San Diego, California (UCSD) for the treatment of CTEPH,[44] where the first PEA was performed in 1970. Since then more than 2200 PEA procedures have been performed at UCSD, thereby constituting the world's largest single-center experience.[45] The goals of PEA as outlined by the UCSD group are as follows: (1) hemodynamic: to improve right ventricular function by reducing the PVR and PA pressure; (2) respiratory: to restore perfusion to the large areas of ventilation; and (3) prophylactic: to prevent further deterioration in the right ventricular function and progressive, secondary arteriopathic changes in the pulmonary vasculature. Experienced centers now report a low operative mortality, with 1-year survival rates of greater than 95% and clinical evidence to suggest a curative result.[45–47] The contemporary results of lung transplantation for CTEPH with a 1-year survival of 80% and 5-year survival ranging from 52% to 60%, coupled with the need for lifelong immunosuppression, has limited its role for patients deemed surgically inoperable. Such patients would include those with predominant distal arterial disease, a previous unsuccessful PEA, severe underlying restrictive or obstructive lung disease, and end-stage cardiopulmonary failure.[48,49] Hence, PEA has become the gold standard for treatment of CTEPH, resulting in a significant reduction of PA pressure and improvement in right ventricular function, quality of life, and survival.[7,43,50]

ASSESSMENT OF OPERABILITY

The current lack of specific medical therapy for CTEPH necessitates that all patients should undergo a thorough evaluation by an experienced CTEPH team to identify surgical candidacy. Although there is no widely accepted preoperative CTEPH classification scheme that allows for risk stratification to identify good operative candidates, several different guidelines have been proposed. Clinical guidelines provided by the American College of Chest Physicians provide a basic framework to assess the operability of patients with CTEPH (Box 3).[51] General criteria include: (1) New York Heart Association (NYHA) functional class III or IV symptoms; (2) a preoperative PVR greater than 300 dyne/s/cm^5 and/or a mean PA pressure greater than 40 mm Hg; (3) surgically accessible thrombus (in the main, lobar, or segmental pulmonary arteries) as determined by all appropriate radiographic studies; and (4) no severe comorbidities. Although no exact PVR has been established as a criterion for pulmonary endarterectomy, Dartevelle and colleagues[52] recommended that

---

Box 3
Assessment of operability

1. NYHA functional class III or IV symptoms
2. Preoperative PVR >300 dyne/s/cm^5
3. Mean PA pressure >40 mm Hg
4. Surgically accessible thrombus in the main, lobar, or segmental pulmonary arteries
5. No severe medical comorbidities
6. Predicted reduction of pulmonary resistance of more than 50%
7. Absence of secondary arteriopathy
8. Center experience
9. Patient consent

patients should be selected for PEA only if a reduction of PVR of greater than 50% can be expected. Other groups have expanded criteria to include more diverse factors such as absence of secondary arteriopathy, center experience, and patient consent.[45] In addition, the evaluation should include an analysis of PVR, preoperative diffusion capacity, upstream resistance, and precise assessment of right ventricular function.[7] The most common reasons patients are not considered operative candidates are severe comorbidities, a preponderance of distal PA disease, with PH out of proportion to radiographic disease.

The most widely adopted postoperative classification system for patients with CTEPH that correlates well with operative success and mortality was proposed by Thistlethwaite and colleagues[53] (**Box 4**). These investigators classified CTEPH patients into 4 types based on obstructive lesions categorized at the time of surgery. This classification system identified that the operative mortality in patients with disease of types I to III ranged from 3.9% to 6.3%, while patients with type IV disease suffered from a mortality rate of greater than 16%.[45] Although this classification system is not applicable to screen CTEPH patients preoperatively, it has helped to realize the fact that patients with type IV disease with predominantly distal arteriopathy may not be ideal candidates for PEA. It has also become increasingly clear that the key factor for success is a complete endarterectomy with a significant reduction in PVR to less than 500 dyne/s/cm[5]. The most compelling evidence comes from UCSD experience, demonstrating 30.6% in-hospital mortality if the postoperative PVR is greater than 500 dyne/s/cm[5], compared with 0.9% in-hospital mortality in patients with lower postoperative PVR values.[45]

PROCEDURE

PEA is a well described procedure of complete removal of all obstructive material within the PAs.

It should be noted that the procedure is not an embolectomy with removal of thrombus alone, but rather a meticulous complete endarterectomy of the entire PA tree. Operative details for PEA are well described elsewhere, with the following key elements: approach via median sternotomy, use of deep hypothermic circulatory arrest at a temperature of 18° to 20°C, and a bilateral complete and meticulous PEA of main, lobar, segmental, and subsegmental PA branches.[44] CTEPH results in large systemic-pulmonary collaterals that obscure the anatomic planes in the segmental and subsegmental arteries, requiring the use of deep hypothermic circulatory arrest as an essential tool to maintain a bloodless field. Deep hypothermic circulatory arrest should be limited to 40 to 50 minutes before an increased risk of central neurologic injury. Some groups, including the authors', have used selective bilateral cerebral perfusion at low flows to minimize the risk of cerebral complications, and may extend the circulatory arrest times beyond 40 to 50 minutes thus permitting a safer, more thorough PEA.[54]

COMPLICATIONS

PEA surgery is a complex procedure that requires experienced centers and physicians familiar with the perioperative management of hemodynamics as well as respiratory and fluid balance necessary to achieve a successful outcome. The UCSD group reported results from a single institution on 1500 patients undergoing PEA, with complications including reperfusion pulmonary edema (16.2%), pneumonia (9.5%), reoperation for bleeding (3.5%), cerebrovascular accident (0.4%), and a mortality of 4.7%.[45] An international registry report of 679 patients found that 49.2% of patients had major complications[47] including infection (18.8%), persistent PH (16.7%), neurologic (11.2%) or bleeding (10.2%) complications, pulmonary reperfusion edema (9.6%), pericardial effusion (8.3%), need for extracorporeal membrane oxygenation (3.1%), and in-hospital mortality due to perioperative complications (4.7%). These 2 large series highlight the potential for significant complications and warrant an experienced team able to prevent, recognize, and manage complex perioperative issues such as persistent PH and reperfusion pulmonary edema.

OUTCOMES

Outcome measures typically reported include in-hospital mortality, reduction in PA pressure and PVR, and improvement in NYHA heart failure classification, 6MWD, and long-term survival. Operative mortality rates after PEA range from 4% to

---

Box 4
Postoperative classification of CTEPH
Type I: fresh thrombus within the main and/or lobar pulmonary arteries
Type II: intimal thickening and fibrosis proximal to the segmental arteries
Type III: disease within the distal segmental arteries only
Type IV: distal arterial vasculopathy with no visible thromboembolic material

30% depending on center experience, patient selection, and comorbidities.[45,47,54,55] An international registry report demonstrated that within 1 year after surgery the median PVR had decreased from 698 to 235 dyne/s/cm^5 and the median 6MWD had increased from 362 to 459 m.[47] In 2008, the Cambridge group evaluated 229 patients who survived PEA surgery, reporting on the hemodynamic and functional outcome 1 year after PEA.[54] At 3 months after surgery, there was a significant reduction in mean PA pressure (from 47 to 25 mm Hg, $P<.001$), a significant increase in cardiac index (from 1.9 to 2.5 min/m^2, $P<.001$), and a significant increase in 6MWD (from 269 to 375 m, $P<.001$), which persisted at 1-year follow-up. Survival following discharge from hospital was 92.5% at 5 years and 88.3% at 10 years. In a Dutch study, Saouti and colleagues[56] examined 72 patients after PEA, and reported in-hospital mortality of 6.9% with 3- and 5-year survival rates of 91.2% and 88.7%, respectively. Before surgery patients were in NYHA functional class III and IV, yet almost all patients returned to functional class I or II at 1-year follow-up ($P = .0001$). Also, mean PA pressure decreased from 42 to 22 mm Hg ($P = .0001$), NT-proBNP improved from 1527 to 160 pg/mL ($P = .0001$), and 6MWD increased from 359 to 518 m ($P = .0001$).

Klepteko and colleagues[43] outlined the general predictors of successful outcomes from PEA as (1) prior history of PE and/or deep venous thrombosis, (2) a honeymoon period of months to years between the embolic event and clinical development of CTEPH, (3) appropriate association between anatomic lesions and PH/PVR, and (4) angiographic lesions located in the proximal PA and lobar branches. The predictors of high operative risk include (1) a history of myeloproliferative syndrome, (2) normal bronchial arteries, (3) distal thromboembolic disease, (4) PH out of proportion to angiographic disease, and (5) no history of thromboembolic events implying other etiology for PH.[46] Thus, PEA can be performed in experienced centers with modest in-hospital morbidity and low mortality, with dramatic improvement in hemodynamics, quality of life, and survival.

SUMMARY

CTEPH is a life-threatening condition that imparts a negative impact on hemodynamics, quality of life, and long-term survival. At present there are no approved or efficacious medical therapies. The gold-standard treatment is PEA, which in experienced centers improves long-term survival and quality of life, and reverses the complex spiral of right heart failure and early death.

REFERENCES

1. Dartevelle P, Fadel E, Mussot S, et al. Chronic thromboembolic pulmonary hypertension. Eur Respir J 2004;23:637–48.
2. Fedullo PF, Auger WR, Kerr KM, et al. Chronic thromboembolic pulmonary hypertension. N Engl J Med 2001;345:1465–72.
3. Moser KM, Auger WR, Fedullo PF. Chronic major-vessel thromboembolic pulmonary hypertension. Circulation 1990;81:1735–43.
4. Auger WR, Kerr KM, Kim NH, et al. Chronic thromboembolic pulmonary hypertension. Cardiol Clin 2004; 22:453–66.
5. Galiè N, Kim NH. Pulmonary microvascular disease in CTEPH. Proc Am Thorac Soc 2006;3:571–6.
6. Hoeper MM, Mayer E, Simonneau G, et al. Chronic thromboembolic pulmonary hypertension. Circulation 2006;113:2011–20.
7. Galiè N, Hoeper NM, Humbert M, et al. Guidelines for the diagnosis and treatment of pulmonary hypertension. The Task Force for the Diagnosis and Treatment of Pulmonary Hypertension of the European Society of Cardiology (ESC) and the European Respiratory Society (ERS), endorsed by the International Society of Heart and Lung Transplantation (ISHLT). Eur Heart J 2009;30:2493–537.
8. McLaughlin VV, Archer SL, Badesch DB, et al. ACCF/AHA 2009 expert consensus document on pulmonary hypertension. J Am Coll Cardiol 2009; 53:1573–619.
9. Dalen JE, Alpert JS. Natural history of pulmonary embolism. Prog Cardiovasc Dis 1975;17:259–70.
10. Pengo V, Lensing AW, Prins MH, et al. Incidence of chronic thromboembolic pulmonary hypertension after pulmonary embolism. N Engl J Med 2004;350: 2257–64.
11. Ribeiro A, Lindmarker P, Johnsson H, et al. Pulmonary embolism: one-year follow-up with echocardiography Doppler and five-year survival analysis. Circulation 1999;99:1325–30.
12. Lang IM. Chronic thromboembolic pulmonary hypertension: not so rare after all. N Engl J Med 2004;350:2236–8.
13. Wolf M, Boyer-Neumann C, Parent F, et al. Thrombotic risk factors in pulmonary hypertension. Eur Respir J 2000;15:395–9.
14. Bonderman D, Turecek PL, Jakowitsch J, et al. High prevalence of elevated clotting factor VIII in chronic thromboembolic pulmonary hypertension. Thromb Haemost 2003;90:372–6.
15. Hoeper MM, Sosada M, Fabel H. Plasma coagulation profiles in patients with severe primary pulmonary hypertension. Eur Respir J 1998;12: 1446–9.
16. Lang IM, Klepetko W, Pabinger I. No increased prevalence of the factor V Leiden mutation in chronic

major vessel thromboembolic pulmonary hypertension (CTEPH). Thromb Haemost 1996;76:476–7.

17. Bonderman D, Jakowitsch J, Adlbrecht C, et al. Medical conditions increasing the risk of chronic thromboembolic pulmonary hypertension. Thromb Haemost 2005;93:512–6.

18. Fox EA, Kahn SR. The relationship between inflammation and venous thrombosis: a systematic review of clinical studies. Thromb Haemost 2005;94:362–5.

19. Esmon CT. Coagulation inhibitors in inflammation. Biochem Soc Trans 2005;33:401–5.

20. Kimura H, Okada O, Tanabe N, et al. Plasma monocyte chemoattractant protein-1 and pulmonary vascular resistance in chronic thromboembolic pulmonary hypertension. Am J Respir Crit Care Med 2001;164:319–24.

21. Bonderman D, Jakowitsch J, Redwan B, et al. Role for staphylococci in misguided thrombus resolution of chronic thromboembolic pulmonary hypertension. Arterioscler Thromb Vasc Biol 2008;28:678–84.

22. Moser KM, Bloor CM. Pulmonary vascular lesions occurring in patients with chronic major vessel thromboembolic pulmonary hypertension. Chest 1993;103:685–92.

23. Arbustini E, Morbini P, D'Armini AM, et al. Plaque composition in plexogenic and thromboembolic pulmonary hypertension: the critical role of thrombotic material in pultaceous core formation. Heart 2002;88:177–82.

24. Yi ES, Kim H, Ahn H, et al. Distribution of obstructive intimal lesions and their cellular phenotypes in chronic pulmonary hypertension: a morphometric and immunohistochemical study. Am J Respir Crit Care Med 2000;162:1577–86.

25. Du L, Sullivan CC, Chu D, et al. Signaling molecules in nonfamilial pulmonary hypertension. N Engl J Med 2003;348:500–9.

26. Deng Z, Morse JH, Slager SL, et al. Familial primary pulmonary hypertension (gene PPH1) is caused by mutations in the bone morphogenetic protein receptor-II gene. Am J Hum Genet 2000;67:737–44.

27. Sullivan CC, Du L, Chu D, et al. Induction of pulmonary hypertension by an angiopoietin 1/TIE2/serotonin pathway. Proc Natl Acad Sci 2003;100:12331–6.

28. ZuWallack RL, Liss JP, Lahiri B. Acquired continuous murmur associated with acute pulmonary thromboembolism. Chest 1976;70:557–9.

29. Fishman AJ, Moser KM, Fedullo PF. Perfusion lung scans vs pulmonary angiography in evaluation of suspected primary pulmonary hypertension. Chest 1983;84:679–83.

30. Lisbona R, Kreisman H, Novales-Diaz J, et al. Perfusion lung scanning: differentiation of primary from thromboembolic pulmonary hypertension. Am J Roentgenol 1985;144:27–30.

31. Powe JE, Palevsky HI, McCarthy KE, et al. Pulmonary arterial hypertension: value of perfusion scintigraphy. Radiology 1987;164:727–30.

32. Rush C, Langleben D, Schlesinger RD, et al. Lung scintigraphy in pulmonary capillary hemangiomatosis: a rare disorder causing primary pulmonary hypertension. Clin Nucl Med 1991;16:913–7.

33. Kauczor HU, Schwickert HC, Mayer E, et al. Pulmonary artery sarcoma mimicking chronic thromboembolic disease: computed tomography and magnetic resonance imaging findings. Cardiovasc Intervent Radiol 1994;17:185–9.

34. Kerr KM, Auger WR, Fedullo PF, et al. Large vessel pulmonary arteritis mimicking chronic thromboembolic disease. Am J Respir Crit Care Med 1995;152:367–73.

35. Ley S, Fink C, Zaporozhan J, et al. Value of high spatial and high temporal resolution magnetic resonance angiography for differentiation between idiopathic and thromboembolic pulmonary hypertension: initial results. Eur Radiol 2005;15:2256–63.

36. Auger WR, Fedullo PF, Moser KM, et al. Chronic major-vessel thromboembolic pulmonary artery obstruction: appearance at angiography. Radiology 1992;182:393–8.

37. Nicod P, Peterson K, Levine M, et al. Pulmonary angiography in severe chronic pulmonary hypertension. Ann Intern Med 1987;107:565–8.

38. Bresser P, Pepke-Zaba J, Jais X, et al. Medical therapies for chronic thromboembolic pulmonary hypertension: an evolving treatment paradigm. Proc Am Thorac Soc 2006;3:594–600.

39. Kerr KM, Rubin LJ. Epoprostenol therapy as a bridge to pulmonary thromboendarterectomy for chronic thromboembolic pulmonary hypertension. Chest 2003;123:319–20.

40. Nagaya N, Sasaki N, Ando M, et al. Prostacyclin therapy before pulmonary thromboendarterectomy in patients with chronic thromboembolic pulmonary hypertension. Chest 2003;123:338–43.

41. Hoeper MM, Kramm T, Wilkens H, et al. Bosentan therapy for inoperable chronic thromboembolic pulmonary hypertension. Chest 2005;128:2363–7.

42. Jais X, D'Armini AM, Jansa P, et al. Bosentan for treatment of inoperable chronic thromboembolic pulmonary hypertension: BENEFit (Bosentan Effects in iNopErable Forms of chronic Thromboembolic pulmonary hypertension), a randomized, placebo-controlled trial. J Am Coll Cardiol 2008;52:2127–34.

43. Klepetko W, Mayer E, Sandoval J, et al. Interventional and surgical modalities of treatment for pulmonary arterial hypertension. J Am Coll Cardiol 2004;43(12 Suppl S):73S–80S.

44. Thistlethwaite PA, Kaneko K, Madani MM, et al. Technique and outcomes of pulmonary endarterectomy surgery. Ann Thorac Cardiovasc Surg 2008; 14(5):274–82.

45. Jamieson SW, Kapelanski DP, Sakakibara N, et al. Pulmonary endarterectomy: experience and lessons learned in 1,500 cases. Ann Thorac Surg 2003;76: 1457–62.

46. Mayer E, Klepetko W. Techniques and outcomes of pulmonary endarterectomy for CTEPH. Proc Am Thorac Soc 2006;3:589–93.

47. Mayer E, Jenkins D, Lindner J, et al. Surgical management and outcome of patients with chronic thromboembolic pulmonary hypertension: results from an international prospective registry. J Thorac Cardiovasc Surg 2011;141(3):702–10.

48. Fadel E, Mercier O, Mussot S, et al. Long-term outcome of double-lung and heart-lung transplantation for pulmonary hypertension: a comparative retrospective study of 219 patients. Eur J Cardiothorac Surg 2010;38(3):277–84.

49. Fischler M, Speich R, Dorschner L, et al. Pulmonary hypertension in Switzerland: treatment and clinical course. Swiss Med Wkly 2008;138(25–26):371–8.

50. Piazza G, Goldhaber SZ. Chronic thromboembolic pulmonary hypertension. N Engl J Med 2011;364(4): 351–60.

51. Doyle RL, McCrory D, Channick RN, et al. Surgical treatments/interventions for pulmonary arterial hypertension: ACCP evidence-based clinical practice guidelines. Chest 2004;126(Suppl 1):63S–71S.

52. Dartevelle P, Fadel E, Chapelier A, et al. Pulmonary thromboendarterectomy with video-angioscopy and circulatory arrest: an alternative to cardiopulmonary transplantation and post-embolism pulmonary artery hypertension. Chirurgie 1998;123(1):32–40.

53. Thistlethwaite PA, Mo M, Madani MM, et al. Operative classification of thromboembolic disease determines outcome after pulmonary endarterectomy. J Thorac Cardiovasc Surg 2002;124(6):1203–11.

54. Freed DH, Thomson BM, Tsui SS, et al. Functional and haemodynamic outcome 1 year after pulmonary thromboendarterectomy. Eur J Cardiothorac Surg 2008;34(3):525–9.

55. Kunihara T, Gerdts J, Groesdonk H, et al. Predictors of postoperative outcome after pulmonary endarterectomy from a 14-year experience with 279 patients. Eur J Cardiothorac Surg 2011;40(1): 154–61.

56. Saouti N, Morshuis WJ, Heijmen RH, et al. Long-term outcome after pulmonary endarterectomy for chronic thromboembolic pulmonary hypertension: a single institution experience. Eur J Cardiothorac Surg 2009;35(6):947–52.

Exercise-Induced Pulmonary Hypertension

Eduardo Bossone, MD, PhD[a,b,c,*], Robert Naeije, MD, PhD[d,e]

KEYWORDS

- Pulmonary hypertension • Exercise • Stress echocardiography

KEY POINTS

- There is a need for a better definition of invasively measured limits of normal of pulmonary artery pressure (PAP) changes as a function of increased cardiac output at exercise.
- It appears that both PAP and left atrial pressure increase linearly with cardiac output, but with a take-off pattern possibly appearing at the highest levels of exercise.
- Methodological aspects of exercise stress testing have to be looked after very attentively.
- Exercise hemodynamic studies in patients with pulmonary hypertension allow for an improved understanding of functional state, exercise capacity, and effects of therapeutic interventions.
- Improved knowledge of limits of normal and further validation of noninvasive approaches are urgently needed.

INTRODUCTION

After catheterization of the heart was introduced as a diagnostic tool by Cournand and colleagues[1] in the 1940s, it was realized that many diseases are associated with excess pressures in the pulmonary circulation, and that this can be a cause of dyspnea and fatigue symptoms. The questions asked at that time were about the critical levels of pulmonary artery pressure (PAP) that would be of clinical relevance, and whether differences in mechanisms of increased PAP might matter. Accordingly, Paul Wood defined limits of normal based on catheterizations of the heart in 60 healthy subjects at the Brompton hospital, which showed PAP ranging from 8/2 to 28/14 mm Hg, with values never exceeding 30/15, mean 20 mm Hg.[2] However, he thought that "serious pulmonary hypertension" usually would be associated with much higher pressures. This view was at the basis of pulmonary hypertension being defined by a PAP higher than 25 mm Hg, thus with a safety margin of at least 5 mm Hg above the upper limit of normal,[3,4] still agreed on at the most recent expert consensus conference held in Dana Point, California in 2008.[5] Wood and his contemporaries further reasoned on hemodynamic measurements using the Poiseuille-Hagen notion of resistance as a ratio between a driving pressure and flow, extrapolated to the pulmonary circulation as pulmonary vascular resistance (PVR), defined as the ratio between mean PAP and left atrial pressure (LAP) divided by cardiac output (Q).

$$PVR = (PAP - LAP)/Q$$

The simple use of the PVR equation, rewritten as

$$PAP = PVR \times Q + LAP$$

The authors have nothing to disclose.

[a] Division of Cardiology, Cava de'Tirreni-Amalfi Coast Hospital, Salerno, Italy; [b] Department of Cardiology and Cardiac Surgery, University Hospital "Scuola Medica Salernitana", Salerno, Italy; [c] Department of Cardiology and Cardiac Surgery, IRCCS Policlinico San Donato, Milan, Italy; [d] Department of Physiology, Faculty of Medicine, Erasme Academic Hospital, Université Libre de Bruxelles, 808 Lennik Road, B-1070 Brussels, Belgium; [e] Department of Cardiology, Erasme Academic Hospital, Université Libre de Bruxelles, 808 Lennik Road, B-1070 Brussels, Belgium
* Corresponding author. Via Principe Amedeo, 36, 83023 Lauro (AV), Italy.
E-mail address: ebossone@hotmail.com

Heart Failure Clin 8 (2012) 485–495
doi:10.1016/j.hfc.2012.04.007
1551-7136/12/$ – see front matter © 2012 Elsevier Inc. All rights reserved.

was at the basis of a hemodynamic classification of pulmonary hypertension defined as being due to an increased cardiac output, an increased LAP or increased resistance, and identification of associated causal conditions.[2] As it was already known that cardiac output increases linearly with increased oxygen uptake (Vo$_2$) or workload, at was also realized that PAP could remain within limits of normal at rest, but briskly increase with exercise in the presence of increased resistance such as in chronic obstructive lung disease, or increased left atrial pressure resulting from left heart failure or mitral stenosis.[6]

The early hemodynamic exercise studies in normal subjects had reported that LAP remained within normal limits and that mean PAP did not increase much, and actually never rose above 30 mm Hg.[3] Accordingly, exercise-induced pulmonary hypertension was defined by a mean PAP higher than 30 mm Hg.[3,4] However, the participants of the expert consensus conference at Dana Point considered that this cutoff value was not sufficiently supported by the data reported in the literature, and therefore decided to omit exercise testing from any diagnosis of pulmonary hypertension.[5]

THE LIMITS OF NORMAL OF THE PULMONARY CIRCULATION AT EXERCISE

The first catheterizations of the right heart in normal humans at exercise were reported in the late 1940s. The results showed either a small increase, no change, or sometimes a decrease in mean PAP as cardiac output was increased with moderate levels of exercise.[7,8] In 1950, Cournand and colleagues[9] observed a sharp increase in mean PAP when cardiac output was increased to 3.5 times the resting value. A similar sharp increase in mean PAP at flows above 350% of normal was reported a few years later in isolated perfused lungs.[10] However, subsequent studies repeatedly reported a linear increase in mean PAP as a function of flow in isolated perfused lungs, as well as in intact human beings studied using the unilateral balloon occlusion technique (to double the flow in the contralateral lung) and/or exercise. In his review of pulmonary hemodynamics at exercise published in 1969, Fowler[11] concluded that mean PAP-flow relationships are generally best described by a linear approximation until the highest physiologically possible flows, and that previously reported take-off patterns, or disproportionate increase in PAP at the highest flows, were probably explained by a deterioration of the experimental preparation in isolated perfused lung studies, and either methodological problems or diastolic dysfunction with an increase in LAP in intact human studies.

In 1989, Reeves and colleagues[12] reviewed the published data on invasive pulmonary hemodynamic measurements at exercise normal subjects. These investigators collected 196 measurements in the supine posture in 91 subjects (63 men, 28 women) analyzed by oxygen uptake in steps of 50 or 1000 mL/min as workload was increased, reported in 6 previous studies. For each step of oxygen uptake, there were no differences between men and women, so that the data were pooled in the analysis. Also retrieved was a total of 104 measurements in 24 subjects (23 men, 1 woman) in the upright posture and submitted to an exercise test with progressively increased workload, reported in 4 previous studies, and unpublished data provided by Wagner and Moon. This analysis established that supine exercise is associated with no change or a slight decrease in PVR, in keeping with the notion that the normal pulmonary circulation is maximally dilated and relaxed at rest. In the upright position, the initial PVR was found to be higher, which is explained by an initial derecruitment caused by a lower cardiac output (via decreased venous return). An initially higher PVR accounts for more marked and hyperbolic decrease of PVR at exercise reported in upright subjects. However, the upright and supine PVR-workload relationships converge at low levels of exercise, indicating that mean PAP-Q relationships are identical in fully recruited supine or erect lungs.

Reeves and colleagues[12] were able to find measurements at rest and at least 2 levels of exercise in 63 subjects (including 21 women), so that they could calculate linear regressions relating mean PAP to Q in each of them. On average, each liter per minute of increase in cardiac output was accompanied by an increase of 1 mm Hg in mean PAP in young adult men and women. Aging to 60 to 80 years was found to be associated with a more than doubling of the slope of mean PAP-Q relationships, such that:

Mean PAP-Q ≈ 1 mm Hg/min/L in young adults

Mean PAP-Q ≈ 2.5 mm Hg/min/L in old adults

However, there was a large individual variation, with standard deviations in the order of the means, which introduces a difficulty for the estimation of the limits of normal. The best method for a definition of limits of normal would be to adjust multipoint PAP-Q relationships for individual variability, as reported later in limited-size noninvasive studies in young adult volunteers.[13] In this study on 25 healthy subjects aged 35 years, the slope of mean PAP-Q was 1.37 ± 0.65 (mean ± SD) mm Hg/min/L, suggesting a normal range from

0 to 2.7 mm Hg/min/L. This result is not satisfactory because the size of the study was insufficient, the normal age range was not covered, and there is always doubt about the accuracy and precision of noninvasive measurements. There is a need for a better definition of invasively measured limits of normal of PAP changes as a function of increased cardiac output at exercise.

Much of the normal slope of PAP-Q may be accounted for by an exercise-induced LAP. Until the 1980s, the opinion prevailed that LAP does not change at exercise, despite evidence for the contrary.[3] However, Bevegaard and colleagues[14] had already reported increased wedged PAP (PAW) of up to 25 mm Hg in exercising athletes, while Granath and colleagues[15,16] had observed PAW above 30 mm Hg in exercising elderly subjects. This increase in PAW with exercise has been repeatedly confirmed, and found to be strongly correlated to right atrial pressure (RAP), even though RAP rises less than PAW.[17–19] In their analysis of the pulmonary vascular pressure-flow relationships from at least 3 points during exercise, Reeves and colleagues[12] found a linear increase in PAW with Q, with a high correlation between these measurements during either supine or upright exercise, and slopes very close to 1, suggesting a 1-for-1 mm Hg upstream transmission of LAP to PAP.

$$PAP - PAW \approx 1 \text{ mm Hg/mm Hg}$$

There has been discussion as to whether these observations are valid in the presence of higher intrathoracic pressure swings at exercise, in particular with doubt about the reliability of the estimations of LAP from PAW. However, positive and negative intrathoracic pressures at high levels of ventilation probably cancel each other out, and LAP is probably correctly estimated by a PAW in zone III lungs at high levels of cardiac output. Previous studies have reported a good agreement between PAW and invasively measured LAP over a wide range of pressures at exercise.[20] Intrathoracic pressures as a cause of spuriously increased PAW would not explain the proportional increase in RAP.[17]

As for the cause of increased PAW or LAP at exercise, this is likely explained by the left ventricle using the Starling mechanism matching of its flow output to peripheral demand.[17] Left ventricular diastolic compliance decreases with increasing diastolic volume, which reaches a maximum at mild to moderate levels of exercise.[21] This relationship is explained by intrinsic mechanical properties of the left ventricle, with contribution of competition for space with the right ventricle within the relatively nondistensible pericardium and possible activation of the sympathetic nervous

system. Elite endurance athletes present with parallel increases of LAP and RAP that occur at higher levels of exercise than in less well trained or sedentary subjects,[18] suggesting that pericardial constraint is acting in the elite athletes at very high levels of exercise but not in the latter group. This theory is supported by studies on athletic animals showing that when the pericardium is removed, peak end-diastolic volume, stroke volume and maximal oxygen uptake are increased.[22]

Given the hyperbolic relationship between diastolic ventricular pressure and volumes, it is curious that available data rather suggest a linear relationship between PAW and cardiac output during exercise.[12] A possible explanation for this apparent paradox is in the limited number of individual PAW-Q and PAP-Q coordinates reported in studies that examine the shape of the relationships, so that the relationships might have been be spuriously linearized (**Fig. 1**).

This issue was addressed by Stickland and colleagues[18] in an invasive study in healthy athletes. Neither PAW nor RAP increased to above normal before oxygen uptake values of approximately 30 mL/kg/min, corresponding to cardiac outputs in the range of 20 L/min. Above this level of exercise, both PAW and RAP increased rapidly in the less fit subjects, but was very much delayed in the fittest subjects, in whom as expected stroke volume continued to increase (**Fig. 2**).

Whereas Stickland and colleagues[22] favored the hypothesis that elite athletes present with a lesser

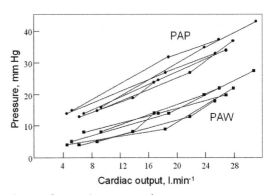

Fig. 1. Three-point mean pulmonary artery pressure (PAP) and wedged PAP (PAW) to estimate left atrial pressure, as a function of cardiac output in 6 triathletes at exercise. These highly trained athletes achieved high levels of exercise and cardiac output, which were associated with increases in PAP to above 30 mm Hg and PAW to above 20 mm Hg. (*From* Naeije R, Mélot C, Niset G, et al. Mechanisms of improved arterial oxygenation after peripheral chemoreceptor stimulation during hypoxic exercise. J Appl Physiol 1993;74:1666–71; with permission.)

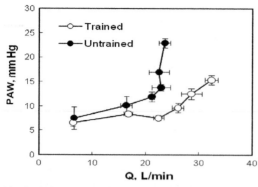

Fig. 2. Pulmonary wedge pressure (PAW) as a function of cardiac output (mean ± SD) in exercising athletes, either highly trained and fit (*empty symbols*) or less trained and fit (*full symbols*). The increase in PAW occurs at higher levels of exercise and cardiac output in the fittest athletes. (*From* Stickland MK, Welsh RC, Petersen SR, et al. Does fitness level modulate the cardiovascular hemodynamic response to exercise? J Appl Physiol 2006;100:1895–901; with permission.)

increase in PAP because of a higher left ventricular compliance, La Gerche and colleagues[23] recently added the notion of the individual variability in exercise-induced decrease in PVR, with the largest decreases possibly detected noninvasively at echocardiography by the shunting of agitated contrast. In the case of both higher left ventricular compliance and exercise-induced decrease in PVR, the right ventricle would be submitted to lesser loading conditions at high cardiac outputs because of lower PAP and would accordingly become less dilated, resulting in decreased LAP because of less ventricular competition for space within the nondistensible pericardium.

Argiento and colleagues[13] calculated LAP from transmitral mitral Doppler and mitral annulus tissue Doppler ratio of E and E′ waves in normal exercising individuals, and could not find a significant change over a range of cardiac outputs from 10 to 26 L/min, mean 18 L/min. Although the measurement has been validated at exercise,[24] the investigators wondered whether this negative result might have been artifactual, or related to the fact that most subjects did not exercise at levels high enough to be associated with a significant increase in LAP.

In summary, based on available exercise measurements in normal subjects, it appears that both PAP and LAP increase linearly with cardiac output, but with a take-off pattern possibly appearing at the highest levels of exercise. Both the slope of pulmonary vascular pressure-flow relationships and eventual take-off would be dependent on the state of the pulmonary circulation and its intrinsic ability to dilate at exercise, and left ventricular diastolic compliance.

EXERCISE STRESS TESTS FOR THE DETECTION OF EARLY OR LATENT PULMONARY HYPERTENSION

The identification of early pulmonary vascular disease has for obvious reasons relied on noninvasive assessments using Doppler echocardiography (**Table 1**).[25–37] Grünig and colleagues[27] implemented systolic PAP calculated from the maximum velocity of tricuspid regurgitation (TR) to detect abnormal pulmonary vascular responses to exercise in 9 subjects with a history of previous high-altitude pulmonary edema (HAPE), known to be associated with excessive increases in PAP when challenged with hypoxic breathing or exercise. Only the subjects with a previous HAPE, and none of the controls, presented with a systolic PAP higher than 40 mm Hg at exercise. The same group coordinated a multicenter European study investigating the TR-derived systolic PAP responses to exercise in relatives of patients with idiopathic pulmonary arterial hypertension (PAH) in comparison with controls. The study included 291 relatives of 114 idiopathic PAH patients. Thirty-two percent of the relatives compared with 10% of the controls presented with a maximum velocity of TR higher than 3.1 m/s corresponding to a systolic PAP higher than 40 mm Hg.[28]

Kovacs and colleagues[36] combined this approach with exercise testing in 52 patients with connective tissue diseases, predominantly systemic sclerosis. The investigators hypothesized that a combination of increased systolic PAP at exercise and a decreased peak Vo_2 would predict PAH. Peak Vo_2 was lower than the 75% predicted in 10 of the patients. Systolic PAP reached values higher than 40 mm Hg in 26 of the patients. Systolic PAP was measured by right heart catheterization in 28 of the patients, 25 of whom had a systolic PAP higher than 40 mm Hg at exercise. The results were in good agreement with TR-derived systolic PAP. In 8 of the invasively studied patients, systolic PAP increased at exercise in relation to increased PAW increased to higher than 20 mm Hg, indicating a left ventricular diastolic dysfunction that had not been looked for at echocardiography.

Although the exercise stress test based solely on systolic PAP and workload measurements may be of some interest in screening programs, the approach is incompletely satisfactory because PAP is a flow-dependent variable, and the cardiac output achieved at a given workload varies from one subject to another.[13] Furthermore, the maximum velocity of TR is markedly dependent on stroke volume, so that a systolic PAP higher than 40 mm Hg is easily achieved by exercising athletes[38] in whom this cutoff value is very close to the upper limit of

Table 1
Pulmonary pressure response to exercise Doppler echocardiography in patients at high risk for pulmonary arterial hypertension

Authors,[Ref.] Year	Associated Disease (No. of Patients; Gender)	Age (Years) Height (cm)/ Weight (kg)	Exercise Protocol	RAP Estimate (mm Hg)	Baseline PAP (mm Hg)	Peak PAP (mm Hg)
Himelman et al,[25] 1989	COPD (n = 36; 21 male)	32–80 —	Supine bicycle (10 or 25 W/2 min)	From IVC	46 ± 20 22 ± 4 (ctrl)	83 ± 30 31 ± 7
Oelberg et al,[26] 1998	Asymptomatic ASD (n = 10; 6 male)	52.9 ± 11.2 167 ± 7/82 ± 20	Upright bicycle (10 W/2 min)	From IVC	31 ± 8 17 ± 8 (ctrl)	51 ± 10 19 ± 8
Grünig et al,[27] 2000	HAPE-S (n = 9 male)	45 ± 8 182 ± 8/82 ± 9	Supine bicycle (25 W/2 min)	Fixed value (5 mm Hg)	28 ± 4 27 ± 4 (ctrl)	55 ± 11 36 ± 3
Grünig et al,[28] 2000	Relatives of iPAH cases (n = 52)	—	Supine bicycle (25 W/2 min)	Fixed value	24 ± 4 (n.r.) 23 ± 3 (a.r.)	37 ± 3 (n.r.) 56 ± 11(a.r.)
Collins et al,[29] 2005	Scleroderma (n = 51; 49 female)	53.9 ± 12.0 —	Treadmill METs 5.9 ± 1.9	Fixed value (10 mm Hg)	24 ± 8	38 ± 12
Alkotob et al,[30] 2006	Scleroderma (n = 65; 56 female)	51 ± 12 —	Treadmill METs 1–13.4	Fixed value (5 mm Hg)	25 ± 8	39 ± 8
Kiencke et al,[31] 2008	HAPE-S (n = 10)	33 ± 2 —	Supine bicycle —	—	19 ± 4 17 ± 3 (ctrl)	23 ± 6 11 ± 5
Steen et al,[32] 2008	Scleroderma (n = 54; 51 female)	—	Treadmill 85% predicted max HR	Fixed value (10 mm Hg)	34.5 ± 11.5	51.4
Grünig et al,[33] 2009	Relatives of iPAH cases (n = 291; 43% female)	37 ± 16 169 ± 9/69 ± 15	Supine bicycle (25 W/2 min)	From IVC	20.7 ± 5.4 20.4 ± 5.3 (ctrl)	39.5 ± 5.6 35.5 ± 5.4
Reichenberger et al,[34] 2009	Scleroderma (n = 33; 31 female)	54 ± 11 —	Supine bicycle (30 W/2 min)	From IVC	23 ± 8	40 ± 11
Möller et al,[35] 2010	ASD and VSD (n = 44; 25 female)	17.5 ± 3.3 167 ± 8.8/59 ± 11	Supine bicycle (25 W/2 min)	From IVC	20.7 ± 5,3 21.8 ± 3.6 (ctrl)	37 (24–76) 39 (17–63)
Kovacs et al,[36] 2010	Connective tissue disease (n = 52; 42 female)	54 ± 11 167 ± 8/69 ± 12	Supine bicycle (25 W/2 min)	From IVC	27 ± 5a 23 ± 3b 23 ± 3c	55 ± 10a 29 ± 8b 30 ± 7c
D'Alto et al,[37] 2011	Systemic sclerosis (n = 172; 155 female)	51.8 ± 21.5 163 ± 9/66 ± 14	Supine bicycle (25 W/2 min)	From IVC	26.2 ± 5.3 20.6 ± 3.7 (ctrl)	36.9 ± 8.7 25.9 ± 3.3

Abbreviations: ASD, atrial septal defect; a.r., abnormal response to exercise; COPD, chronic obstructive pulmonary disease; ctrl, controls; HAPE-S, high-altitude pulmonary edema susceptible; HR, heart rate; iPAH, idiopathic pulmonary arterial hypertension; IVC, inferior vena cava inspiratory collapse; METs, metabolic equivalents; n.r., normal response to exercise; PAP, systolic pulmonary artery pressure; RAP, right atrial pressure; VSD, ventricular septal defect; —, data not available.

a Ex PAPs >40 mm Hg.
b Ex PAPs <40 mm Hg, peak Vo₂ <75%.
c Ex PAPs <40 mm Hg, peak Vo₂ >75%.

normal at rest.[39] Systolic PAP increases with aging and body weight, in relation to decreased left ventricular diastolic compliance and an associated increase in LAP.[40]

Huez and colleagues[41] screened patients with systemic sclerosis at risk of developing PAH with exercise stress tests involving echocardiographic systolic PAP but also cardiac output measurements. The patients achieved the same maximal systolic PAP compared with controls, but at lower cardiac output and workload, so that their PAP-Q relationships presented with abnormally high slopes. Even though the patients also presented with shortened acceleration times of pulmonary flow at rest, in keeping with a suspicion of early pulmonary vasculopathy, the investigators did not report on estimates of LAP at exercise. As there also were altered indices of diastolic function of both ventricles, a contribution of abnormal exercise-induced increase in LAP could not be excluded. Further research has shown the feasibility of the measurement of all the components of the PVR equation by echocardiography until high levels of exercise.[13]

Tolle and colleagues[42] reported on invasive hemodynamic studies in 78 patients referred for a workup of unexplained dyspnea, and who presented with a normal PAP at rest, along with a PVR of 161 ± 60 dyne/s/cm[5], but a mean PAP increased to 37 ± 6 mm Hg at exercise. In these subjects with exercise-induced pulmonary hypertension, defined by a mean PAP below 20 mm Hg at rest increasing to above 30 mm Hg at exercise, aerobic exercise capacity defined by a Vo_2max was significantly decreased, to $67\% \pm 16\%$ predicted, compared with 16 controls with a mean PAP of less than 30 mm Hg at exercise who presented with a Vo_2max of $92\% \pm 14\%$ predicted. In 15 patients with a diagnosis of PAH, Vo_2max was $48\% \pm 11\%$ predicted. A curious feature of this study was the shape of PAP-Vo_2 relationships, expressed as log-log plots, which showed a take-off pattern in normal subjects and a plateau pattern in the patients with exercise-induced pulmonary hypertension (**Fig. 3**). These patterns are probably artifactual in relation to the use of Vo_2 instead of cardiac output and log-log transforms,[13] even though a take-off pattern may indeed occur in normal subjects.[9,18] However, the strength of the study was in the demonstration of exercise-induced pulmonary hypertension as a clinical entity.

In another invasive study on 29 patients with systemic sclerosis and pulmonary hemodynamics at the upper limit of normal, mean PAP increased linearly with cardiac output up to values higher than 30 mm Hg, with a slope very much predicted by baseline PVR.[43] In this study, both resting and

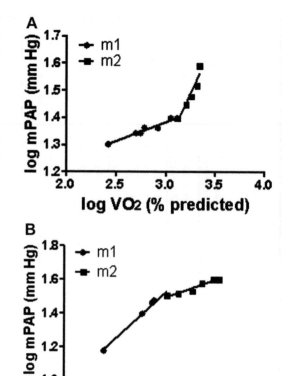

Fig. 3. Log-log plots of mean pulmonary artery pressure (mPAP) as a function of oxygen uptake (Vo_2) in a healthy control (*A*) and in a patient with exercise-induced pulmonary hypertension (*B*). The normal subject presents with a take-off pattern, and the patient with a plateau pattern. (*From* Tolle JJ, Waxman AB, Van Horn TL, et al. Exercise induced pulmonary arterial hypertension. Circulation 2008;118:2183–9; with permission.)

exercise PVR were negatively correlated with exercise capacity, further comforting the clinical relevance of exercise-induced pulmonary hypertension.

As always, methodological aspects of exercise stress testing have to be looked at very attentively. Exercise to increase cardiac output has to be dynamic. Resistive exercise is associated with increased systemic vascular resistance and eventually intrathoracic pressure changes, with unpredictable effects on the pulmonary circulation.[44] Another important issue is the timing of the measurements. The postexercise return to normal of PAP and cardiac output is rapid, with values almost back to baseline after only a few minutes of rest.[13] Finally, good-quality echocardiographic explorations are better performed on adapted exercise tables, as illustrated in **Fig. 4**, allowing for lateral rotation to ease signal sampling and a maximum of internal controls to improve the reliability of the results.

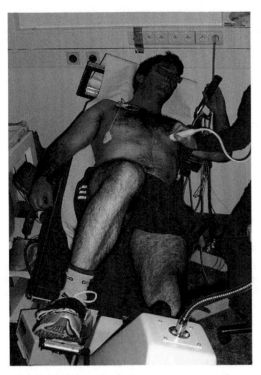
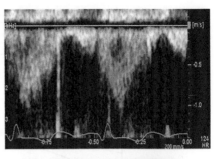
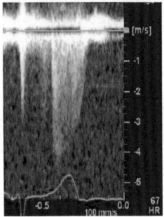

Fig. 4. Noninvasive echocardiographic exercise stress test of the pulmonary circulation. The subject is installed on a specifically designed exercise table. Source aortic flow and tricuspid regurgitant signals are also shown.

EXERCISE STRESS TESTS IN PATIENTS WITH ESTABLISHED PULMONARY HYPERTENSION

Pulmonary vascular pressure-flow relationships have been reported in patients with a variety of lung and cardiac diseases, with flow increased by unilateral balloon occlusion and/or exercise, sometimes with inotropic drug interventions.[45–49] A summary of the mean PAP-Q relationships reported in these studies is shown in **Figs. 5** and **6**. It is interesting that the slope of mean PAP-Q was almost always less than predicted by the PVR equation, suggesting preserved exercise-induced decrease in pulmonary vascular tone.

Janicki and colleagues[47] investigated the pressure-flow responses of the pulmonary circulation in patients with left heart failure without and with pulmonary hypertension (defined by a mean PAP higher than 19 mm Hg), and in patients with various pulmonary vascular diseases. The investigators were able to record 3 to 11 mean PAP-Q coordinates while patients were exercising, with workload increased every 2 minutes up to submaximal or maximal levels. The mean PAP-Q relationships were best described by a linear approximation, and found to be shifted upward with increased slope in proportion to the level of resting mean PAP. In patients with no pulmonary hypertension, the slope of mean PAP-Q was

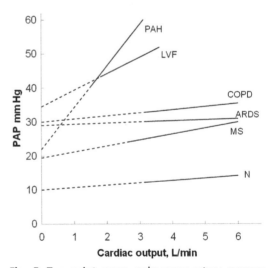

Fig. 5. Two-point mean pulmonary artery pressure (PAP) cardiac output (Q) plots in normal subjects (N), or patients with mitral stenosis (MS), acute respiratory distress syndrome (ARDS), chronic obstructive pulmonary disease (COPD), left ventricular failure (LVF), and pulmonary arterial hypertension (PAH). All PAP-Q plots are shifted upward to higher pressure with an increased extrapolated pressure intercept (*dashed lines*). Left atrial pressure was equal to the extrapolated pressure intercept in LVF. (*Data from* Refs.[44–48,51])

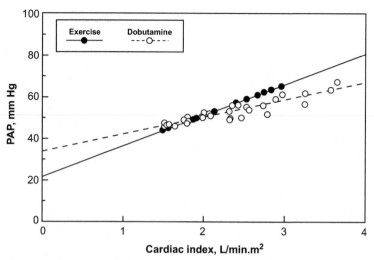

Fig. 6. Poon-adjusted plots of mean pulmonary artery pressure (PAP) as a function cardiac output (Q) in patients with idiopathic pulmonary arterial pressure, with Q increased at exercise or by an infusion of low-dose dobutamine. The slope of PAP-Q was higher with exercise. (*From* Janicki JS, Weber KT, Likoff MJ, et al. The pressure-flow response of the pulmonary circulation in patients with heart failure and pulmonary vascular disease. Circulation 1985;72:1270–8; with permission.)

3 mm Hg/min/L. In patients with pulmonary hypertension secondary to heart failure the slope increased to 5.1 mm Hg/min/L, reaching 7.2 mm Hg/min/L^{-1} in patients with PAH. The changes in extrapolated pressure intercept of mean PAP-Q with exercise were variable, often with values below the resting PAW and even negative in a few patients. This situation is physically impossible in any model of the pulmonary circulation, and has to be explained by exercise-induced pulmonary vasoconstriction and/or increased LAP pressures at the highest levels of exercise.

Kafi and colleagues[48] compared the effects of exercise and an infusion of a low dose of dobutamine assumed to be without effect on pulmonary vascular tone in patients with idiopathic PAH. Slopes and extrapolated pressure intercepts of mean PAP-Q plots were respectively higher and lower with exercise (see **Fig. 5**), which was explained by exercise-induced vasoconstriction related to decreased pH and mixed venous blood Po_2, and also perhaps activation of the sympathetic nervous system.

Castelain and colleagues[50] investigated the effects of intravenous epoprostenol in patients with idiopathic PAH. Six weeks of treatment increased exercise capacity as assessed by a 6-minute walk distance, but resting PVR was unchanged. Hemodynamic measurements at exercise showed a decreased slope of mean PAP-Q relationships, explaining improved exercise capacity by a decreased right ventricular afterload. The average slope of mean PAP-Q decreased from 12 to 7 mm Hg/L/min/m², which was highly significant.

Exercise in patients with pulmonary hypertension is associated with an increase in LAP. In the study by Janicki and colleagues,[47] PAW increased by 14 to 16 mm Hg in patients with heart failure, and by 10 mm Hg in patients with pulmonary vascular diseases. In heart failure, mean PAP closely followed PAW, whereas mean PAP and PAW were less tightly correlated in pulmonary vascular disease. The investigators rightly noted that PAW also increases at exercise in normal subjects, with reported increments up to 5 mm Hg in young adults, but to 10 to 15 mm Hg in elderly normal men, so that the limits of normal of PAP-Q relationships are not exactly known. The fact remains that tight relationships between mean PAP and PAW are characteristic of left heart failure. In cardiac transplantation patients with severe left heart failure, pulmonary hypertension, and very high PAW, the postoperative decrease in PAW was followed by a proportional decrease in mean PAP.[51]

In summary, exercise hemodynamic studies in patients with pulmonary hypertension allow for an improved understanding of functional state, exercise capacity, and effects of therapeutic interventions. Exercise stress tests provide less information about pulmonary vascular function, as the slope and probably also the shape of mean PAP-Q relationships is affected by exercise-induced pulmonary vasoconstriction and changes in LAP. Studies of pulmonary vascular pressure-flow characteristics for different types of pulmonary hypertension would ideally rely on interventions that cause purely passive increases of flow. Whether this might be achieved by low-dose dobutamine requires further confirmation.

SUMMARY

Exercise stress tests of the pulmonary circulation show promise for the detection of early or latent pulmonary vascular disease, and may help us understand the clinical evolution and effects of treatments in patients with established disease. Improved knowledge of limits of normal and further validation of noninvasive approaches are urgently needed. Exercise stresses the pulmonary circulation through increases in cardiac output and LAP. Invasive studies in healthy volunteers have shown that the average slope of PAP-flow relationships is 1 mm Hg/L/min in young adults, increasing to 2.5 mm Hg/L/min after 5 to 6 decades of life. LAP also increases with exercise, with an average upstream transmission to PAP in a manner close to 1-for-1 mm Hg. Measurements can be either invasive or noninvasive using echocardiography, even though the latter approach is still in need of more validation. Exercise has to be dynamic, avoiding the increase in systemic vascular resistance and changes in intrathoracic pressure that occur with resistive exercise, and which might lead to unpredictable effects on the pulmonary circulation. Postexercise measurements are unreliable because of the rapid return of pulmonary vascular pressures and flows to baseline resting state. Recent studies have shown that exercise-induced increase in PAP to a mean higher than 30 mm Hg is associated with dyspnea-fatigue symptomatology, validating the notion of exercise-induced pulmonary hypertension. Exercise in established pulmonary hypertension has no diagnostic relevance, but may help in the understanding of changes in functional state and the effects of therapies.

ACKNOWLEDGMENTS

The authors thank Francesco Ferrara, MD for his work as a research fellow.

REFERENCES

1. Cournand A, Bloomfield RA, Lauson HD. Double lumen catheter for intravenous and intracardiac blood sampling and pressure recording. Proc Soc Exp Biol Med 1945;60:73–5.

2. Wood P. Pulmonary hypertension with special reference to the vasoconstrictive factor. Br Heart J 1958;20:557–70.

3. Fishman AP. Pulmonary circulation. In: Handbook of physiology. The respiratory system. Circulation and non-respiratory functions, sect 3, vol. 1. Bethesda (MD):

American Physiological Society; 1985. p. 93–166. Chapter 3.

4. Rich S, Dantzker DR, Ayres SM, et al. Primary pulmonary hypertension. A national prospective study. Ann Intern Med 1987;107:216–23.

5. Simonneau G, Robbins IM, Beghetti M, et al. Updated clinical classification of pulmonary hypertension. J Am Coll Cardiol 2009;54(Suppl 1): 43S–54S.

6. Naeije R. In defense of exercise stress tests for the diagnosis of pulmonary hypertension. Heart 2011; 97:94–5.

7. Hickman JB, Cargill WH. Effect of exercise on cardiac output and pulmonary artery pressure in normal persons and in patients with cardiovascular disease and pulmonary emphysema. J Clin Invest 1948;27:10–23.

8. Riley RL, Himmelstein A, Motley HL, et al. Studies of the pulmonary circulation at rest and during exercise in normal individuals and in patients with chronic pulmonary disease. Am J Physiol 1948; 152:372–82.

9. Cournand A, Riley RL, Himmelstein A, et al. Pulmonary circulation and alveolar ventilation-perfusion relationships after pneumonectomy. J Thorac Surg 1950;19:80–116.

10. Lategola MT. Pressure-flow relationships in the dog lung during acute subtotal vascular occlusion. Am J Physiol 1958;192:613–9.

11. Fowler NO. The normal pulmonary arterial pressure-flow relationships during exercise. Am J Med 1969; 47:1–6.

12. Reeves JT, Dempsey JA, Grover RF. Pulmonary circulation during exercise. In: Weir EK, Reeves JT, editors. Pulmonary vascular physiology and physiopathology. New York: Marcel Dekker; 1989. p. 107–33. Chapter 4.

13. Argiento P, Chesler N, Mulè M, et al. Exercise stress echocardiography for the study of the pulmonary circulation. Eur Respir J 2010;35:1273–8.

14. Bevegaard S, Holmgren A, Jonsson B. Circulatory studies in well trained athletes at rest and during heavy exercise, with special reference to stroke volume and the influence of body position. Acta Physiol Scand 1963;57:26–50.

15. Granath A, Jonsson B, Strandell T. Circulation in healthy old men, studied by right heart catheterization at rest and during exercise in supine and sitting position. Acta Med Scand 1964;176: 425–46.

16. Granath A, Strandell T. Relationships between cardiac output, stroke volume, and intracardiac pressures at rest and during exercise in supine position and some anthropometric data in healthy old men. Acta Med Scand 1964;176:447–66.

17. Reeves JT, Groves BM, Cymerman A, et al. Operation Everest II: cardiac filling pressures during

cycle exercise at sea level. Respir Physiol 1990; 80:147–54.

18. Stickland MK, Welsh RC, Petersen SR, et al. Does fitness level modulate the cardiovascular hemodynamic response to exercise? J Appl Physiol 2006; 100:1895–901.

19. Naeije R, Mélot C, Niset G, et al. Improved arterial oxygenation by a pharmacological increase in chemosensitivity during hypoxic exercise in normal subjects. J Appl Physiol 1993;74:1666–71.

20. Thadani U, Parker JO. Hemodynamics at rest and during supine and sitting exercise in normal subjects. Am J Cardiol 1978;41:52–9.

21. Sullivan MJ, Cobb FR, Higginbotham MB. Stroke volume increases by similar mechanisms during upright exercise in men and women. Am J Cardiol 1991;67:1405–12.

22. Stray-Gunderson J, Musch TI, Haidot GC, et al. The effects of pericardiectomy on maximal oxygen consumption and maximal cardiac output in untrained dogs. Circ Res 1986;58:523–30.

23. La Gerche A, MacIsaac AL, Burns AT, et al. Pulmonary transit of agitated contrast is associated with enhanced pulmonary vascular reserve and right ventricular function at exercise. J Appl Physiol 2010;109:1307–17.

24. Talreja DR, Nishimura RA, Oh JK. Estimation of left ventricular filling pressure with exercise by Doppler echocardiography in patients with normal systolic function: a simultaneous echocardiographic-cardiac catheterization study. J Am Soc Echocardiogr 2007; 20:477–9.

25. Himelman RB, Stulbarg M, Kircher B, et al. Noninvasive evaluation of pulmonary artery pressure during exercise by saline-enhanced Doppler echocardiography in chronic pulmonary disease. Circulation 1989;79:863–71.

26. Oelberg D, Mascotte F, Kreisman H, et al. Evaluation of right ventricular systolic atrial pressure during incremental exercise by Doppler echocardiography in adults with septal defect. Chest 1998;113:1459–65.

27. Grünig E, Mereles D, Hildebrandt W, et al. Stress Doppler echocardiography for identification of susceptibility to high altitude pulmonary edema. J Am Coll Cardiol 2000;35:980–7.

28. Grünig E, Janssen B, Mereles D, et al. Abnormal pulmonary artery pressure response in asymptomatic carriers of primary pulmonary hypertension. Circulation 2000;102:1145–50.

29. Collins N, Bastian B, Quiqueree L, et al. Abnormal pulmonary vascular responses in patients registered with a systemic autoimmunity database: pulmonary hypertension assessment and screening evaluation using stress echocardiography (PHASE-I). Eur J Echocardiogr 2006;7:439–46.

30. Alkotob ML, Soltani P, Sheatt MA, et al. Reduced exercise capacity and stress-induced pulmonary hypertension in patients with scleroderma. Chest 2006;130:176–81.

31. Kiencke S, Bernheim A, Maggiorini M, et al. Exercise-induced pulmonary artery hypertension: a rare finding? J Am Coll Cardiol 2008;51:513–4.

32. Steen V, Chou M, Shanmugam V, et al. Exercise-induced pulmonary arterial hypertension in patients with systemic sclerosis. Chest 2008;134:146–51.

33. Grünig E, Weissmann S, Ehlken N, et al. Stress Doppler echocardiography in relatives of patients with idiopathic and familial pulmonary arterial hypertension: results of a multicenter European analysis of pulmonary artery pressure response to exercise and hypoxia. Circulation 2009;119:1747–57.

34. Reichenberger F, Voswinckel R, Schulz R, et al. Noninvasive detection of early pulmonary vascular dysfunction in scleroderma. Respir Med 2009;103: 1713–8.

35. Möller T, Brun H, Fredriksen PM, et al. Right ventricular systolic pressure response during exercise in adolescents born with atrial or ventricular septal defect. Am J Cardiol 2010;105:1610–6.

36. Kovacs G, Maier R, Aberer E, et al. Assessment of pulmonary arterial pressure during exercise in collagen vascular disease: echocardiography versus right heart catheterisation. Chest 2010;138(2): 270–8.

37. D'Alto M, Ghio S, D'Andrea A, et al. Inappropriate exercise-induced increase in pulmonary artery pressure in patients with systemic sclerosis. Heart 2011; 97:112–7.

38. Bossone E, Rubenfire M, Bach DS, et al. Range of tricuspid regurgitation velocity at rest and during exercise in normal adult men: implications for the diagnosis of pulmonary hypertension. J Am Coll Cardiol 1999;33:1662–6.

39. D'Andrea A, Naeije R, D'Alto M, et al. Range of pulmonary artery systolic pressure among highly trained athletes. Chest 2011;139:788–94.

40. McQuillan BM, Picard MH, Leavitt M, et al. Clinical correlates and reference intervals for pulmonary artery systolic pressure among echocardiographically normal subjects. Circulation 2001;104:2797–802.

41. Huez S, Roufosse F, Vachièry JL, et al. Isolated right ventricular dysfunction in systemic sclerosis: latent pulmonary hypertension? Eur Respir J 2007;30:928–36.

42. Tolle JJ, Waxman AB, Van Horn TL, et al. Exercise-induced pulmonary arterial hypertension. Circulation 2008;118:2183–9.

43. Kovacs G, Maier R, Aberer E, et al. Borderline pulmonary arterial pressure is associated with decreased exercise capacity in scleroderma. Am J Respir Crit Care Med 2009;181:881–6.

44. MacDougall JD, McKelvie RS, Moroz DE, et al. Factors affecting blood pressure during heavy weight lifting and static contractions. J Appl Physiol 1992;73:1590–7.

45. Even P, Duroux P, Ruff F, et al. The pressure/flow relationship of the pulmonary circulation in normal man and in chronic obstructive pulmonary diseases. Effects of muscular exercise. Scand J Respir Dis 1971;77(Suppl):72–6.

46. Harris P, Segel N, Bishop JM. The relation between pressure and flow in the pulmonary circulation of normal subjects and in patients with chronic bronchitis and mitral stenosis. Cardiovasc Res 1968;2: 73–84.

47. Janicki JS, Weber KT, Likoff MJ, et al. The pressure-flow response of the pulmonary circulation in patients with heart failure and pulmonary vascular disease. Circulation 1985;72:1270–8.

48. Kafi SA, Mélot C, Vachiéry JL, et al. Partitioning of pulmonary vascular resistance in primary pulmonary hypertension. J Am Coll Cardiol 1998;31:1372–6.

49. Zapol WM, Snider MT. Pulmonary hypertension in severe acute respiratory failure. N Engl J Med 1977;296:476–80.

50. Castelain V, Chemla D, Humbert M, et al. Pulmonary artery pressure-flow relations after prostacyclin in primary pulmonary hypertension. Am J Respir Crit Care Med 2002;165:338–40.

51. Naeije R, Lipski A, Abramowicz M, et al. Nature of pulmonary hypertension in congestive heart failure. Effects of cardiac transplantation. Am J Respir Crit Care Med 1994;147:881–7.

Index

Note: Page numbers of article titles are in **boldface** type.

doi:10.1016/S1551-7136(12)00047-5
1551-7136/12/$ – see front matter © 2012 Elsevier Inc. All rights reserved.

heartfailure.theclinics.com

Index

Printed and bound by CPI Group (UK) Ltd, Croydon, CR0 4YY

03/10/2024

01040355-0002

Moving?

Make sure your subscription moves with you!

To notify us of your new address, find your **Clinics Account Number** (located on your mailing label above your name), and contact customer service at:

Email: journalscustomerservice-usa@elsevier.com

800-654-2452 (subscribers in the U.S. & Canada)
314-447-8871 (subscribers outside of the U.S. & Canada)

Fax number: 314-447-8029

Elsevier Health Sciences Division
Subscription Customer Service
3251 Riverport Lane
Maryland Heights, MO 63043

*To ensure uninterrupted delivery of your subscription, please notify us at least 4 weeks in advance of move.

ELSEVIER

Moving?

Make sure your subscription
moves with you!